Mental Health
of Refugees and
Asylum Seekers

Mental Health of Refugees and Asylum Seekers

Edited by

Dinesh Bhugra

Tom Craig

Kamaldeep Bhui

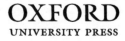

OXFORD
UNIVERSITY PRESS

Great Clarendon Street, Oxford OX2 6DP

Oxford University Press is a department of the University of Oxford.
It furthers the University's objective of excellence in research, scholarship,
and education by publishing worldwide in

Oxford New York

Auckland Cape Town Dar es Salaam Hong Kong Karachi
Kuala Lumpur Madrid Melbourne Mexico City Nairobi
New Delhi Shanghai Taipei Toronto

With offices in

Argentina Austria Brazil Chile Czech Republic France Greece
Guatemala Hungary Italy Japan Poland Portugal Singapore
South Korea Switzerland Thailand Turkey Ukraine Vietnam

Oxford is a registered trade mark of Oxford University Press
in the UK and in certain other countries

Published in the United States
by Oxford University Press Inc., New York

British Library Cataloguing in Publication Data

Data available

Library of Congress Cataloging in Publication Data

Data available

Typeset in Minion by Glyph International, Bangalore, India
Printed in Great Britain
on acid-free paper by
The MPG Books Group, Bodmin and King's Lynn

ISBN 978–0–19–955722–6

10 9 8 7 6 5 4 3 2 1

Preface

Dinesh Bhugra, Tom Craig,
and Kamaldeep Bhui

Refugees and asylum seekers have been described for millennia in human history. Pestilence, war, famine, and flood have long caused human beings to migrate across large distances, and each of these movements has brought with it a set of challenges. It is inevitable that loss of such magnitude will cause psychiatric problems in vulnerable individuals. Loss of home, family, friends, and social support will add stress to an individual's functioning. These changes will produce a range of problems, with additional problems faced by individuals across the age range, which need to be addressed. Political will often controls resources and it is indeed a challenge for clinicians to look after their vulnerable patients under these circumstances, but look after them they must. The act of migration itself is stressful. Cultural factors dictate how emotional distress is expressed and how help is sought, and these, tinged with cultural bereavement, raise significant issues in the planning and delivery of psychiatric services.

The aim of this book is to bring together various facets relating to the management of psychiatric problems in refugees and asylum seekers. It is not a how-to manual, but provides signposts on theoretical and practical factors, which may enable a clinician to provide high-quality services that refugees and asylum seekers will feel comfortable using. We have focused on clinical matters and on using clinical skills to alleviate distress, and not specifically on legal issues, as these vary from country to country.

We have been fortunate in bringing together a group of authors who are experts in the field and who were also committed and conscientious in delivering their manuscripts on time and allowing us to edit these freely. We truly appreciate their help.

We are grateful to Martin Baum at OUP for his sustained and gentle but unobtrusive support, and commitment to the project. Staff at OUP have been wonderful. Our sincere thanks are also due to Andrea Livingstone; without her organizational skills and hard work this volume would not have developed from the chrysalis of our minds to the butterfly it has become.

Contents

Contributors

Dinesh Bhugra
Health Service and Population
Research Department,
Institute of Psychiatry,
King's College London,
London, UK

Kamaldeep Bhui
Wolfson Institute of Preventive
Medicine,
Barts and the London School of
Medicine and Dentistry,
Queen Mary University of London,
UK

Freda Cheung
Department of Psychiatry,
Harbor-UCLA Medical Center,
Torrance, CA, USA

Jim Crabb
Behavioural Psychotherapy Service,
Larbert, Scotland

Tom Craig
Health Service and Population
Research Department,
Institute of Psychiatry,
King's College London,
London, UK

Sean Cross
Specialist Registrar in Liaison
Psychiatry,
St Thomas' Hospital, London;
Volunteer Doctor,
Medical Foundation for the Care of
Victims of Torture,
London, UK

Tonya Fancher
Department of Internal Medicine
and Asian American Center on
Disparities Research, University of
California at Davis,
Davis, CA, USA

Alexander Friedmann
Psychiatric University Clinic
Vienna, Austria

Nick Grey
Centre for Anxiety Disorders and
Trauma,
South London and Maudsley NHS
Foundation Trust,
and Institute of Psychiatry,
Kings College London,
London, UK

Susham Gupta
Consultant Psychiatrist,
East London NHS Foundation Trust,
Assertive Outreach Team–City and
Hackney
London, UK

Helen Herrman
Orygen Youth Health
Research Centre,
Centre for Youth Mental Health,
University of Melbourne,
Melbourne, Australia

David Holzer
Rehalitation Centre for
Neurology and Orthopedy,
Bad Pirawarth,
Austria

Julia Huemer
Department of Child and
Adolescent Psychiatry,
Medical University Vienna,
Austria

Rachel Jenkins
Health Service and Population
Research Department,
Institute of Psychiatry,
King's College London,
London, UK

A.T. Jotheeswaran
Wellcome Trust Research Fellow,
Institute of Community Health,
Voluntary Health Services,
Chennai, India

Ida Kaplan
Victorian Foundation for Survivors
of Torture,
Melbourne, Australia

J. David Kinzie
Oregon Health and Science
University, Department of
Psychiatry,
Portland, USA

J. Mark Kinzie
Oregon Health and Science
University, Department of
Psychiatry,
Portland, USA

Alan K. Koike
Health Sciences Clinical Professor,
University of California,
Davis, School of Medicine,
Department of Psychiatry and
Behavioral Sciences,
Sacramento, CA, USA

Damon Lab
Traumatic Stress Service,
South London and Maudsley NHS
Foundation Trust,
London, UK

Russell F. Lim
Health Sciences Associate
Clinical Professor, University of
California,
Davis, School of Medicine,
Department of Psychiatry and
Behavioral Sciences,
Sacramento,
CA, USA

Keh-Ming Lin
Center for the Advanced Study of
Behavioral Sciences at Stanford,
CA, USA;
and National Health Research
Institutes (NHRI),
Taiwan

Gill Mezey
Division of Mental Health,
St George's University of London,
London, UK

Salaad Mohamud
Wolfson Institute of
Preventive Medicine,
Barts and The London School of
Medicine and Dentistry,
Queen Mary University of London,
UK

Susan Rees
Psychiatry Research and Teaching
Unit, School of Psychiatry,
University of New South Wales,
Australia

Pedro Ruiz
Professor and Executive Vice Chair,
Department of Psychiatry and
Behavioral Sciences,
University of Miami Miller
School of Medicine, Miami,
Florida, USA

Derrick Silove
Centre for Population Mental
Health Research,
Psychiatry Research and
Teaching Unit,
School of Psychiatry,
University of New South Wales,
Sydney, Australia

Daya Somasundaram
Associate Clinical Professor,
University of Adelaide,
Adelaide, Australia

Thomas Stompe
Psychiatric University Clinic,
Vienna, Austria

Josef Szwarc
Victorian Foundation for Survivors
of Torture,
Melbourne, Australia

Ajoy Thachil
Division of Mental Health,
St George's University of London,
London, UK

Lakshmi Vijayakumar
SNEHA and Voluntary Health
Services,
Kotturpuram, Chennai, India

Panos Vostanis
Department of Child Adolescent
Psychiatry,
University of Leicester,
Leicester, UK

Nasir Warfa
Wolfson Institute of Preventive
Medicine, Barts and the London
School of Medicine and Dentistry,
Queen Mary University of London,
London, UK

Wojtek Wojcik
Department of Psychological
Medicine,
Institute of Psychiatry,
King's College London,
London, UK

Kerry Young
Wolfson Institute of Preventive
Medicine,
Barts and the London School of
Medicine and Dentistry,
Queen Mary University of London
London, UK

Chapter 1

Refugees and asylum seekers: conceptual issues

Pedro Ruiz and Dinesh Bhugra

Introduction

Refugees and asylum seekers are individuals who are seeking to settle elsewhere other than their country of origin largely due to persecution due to their political, religious beliefs, or sexual orientation. The definitions are often complicated and dictated by the legal system of the new country. In this chapter we propose to set the scene. Never before has culture, race, and ethnicity been so relevant and important in the mental health field and/or in psychiatric practice, as it is at the present time; additionally, this new conceptualization of psychiatric care is not only quite relevant in industrialized nations such as the United States, England, Germany, and many other similar developed countries, but all over the world as well. In this context, it is important that 'culture', 'race', and 'ethnicity' be defined with respect to mental health and mental illness is concerned (Gonzales, Griffith, and Ruiz, 2001).

Culture: defined as a set of meanings, behavioural norms, and values used by members of a given society as they construct their view of the world. These unique values include language, non-verbal expression of thoughts and emotions, social relationship, religious beliefs, and financial philosophies.

Ethnicity: defined as a subjective sense of belonging to a group of persons who share a common origin and who share similar social beliefs and practices; ethnicity is also an essential component of the sense of identity of every person.

Race: defined as a psychosocial concept under which humans have chosen to group themselves; and is also based primarily on general physiognomy.

Central to the clinical understanding of psychiatric patients from a cultural, racial, and ethnic point of view is the clear conceptualization of 'identity'. In this context, the 'cultural formulation' described in the Diagnostic and Statistical Manual of Mental Health Disorders, 4th Edition (DSM-IV) fully addresses the concept of identity (American Psychiatric Association, 2004). In this regard, the patient's ethnic, racial, and cultural backgrounds must be fully taken into consideration when assessing, diagnosing, and treating psychiatric patients, or any patients for that matter. In this context, the 'cultural' identity of the patient, with attention also given to the cultural, racial, and ethnic backgrounds of the patient, is very important. Additionally, in the case of migrants, refugees, or asylum seekers, the degree of their involvement with both their culture of origin and the culture of the host society or 'majority culture' must be taken into consideration. Moreover, the cultural explanation of the patient's illness, including idioms of distress, ways of manifesting the symptoms and signs of their illnesses, especially somatic manifestations, and/or culture-bound syndromes (Canino *et al.*, 1992; Foulks, 2002), also requires attention and consideration. Cultural factors that relate to the psychosocial environment and the levels of functioning also require exploration and, additionally, the cultural elements of the relationships between the patient and the psychiatric practitioner, as well as the overall cultural assessment of the diagnosis and treatment requires full consideration.

The role of migration within the context of globalization

World War II led to the realization of the complexity and magnitude of mental illnesses and psychiatric disorders, and also helped to better understand the role of culture, race, and ethnicity in this context, given the plurality and multiethnic backgrounds of many of the soldiers involved in this worldwide military conflict (Ruiz, 1995). During the last 15–20 years, however, an extensive globalization process has taken place in all regions of the world. This process has led to millions of persons migrating from their original countries to other places in the world. Of course, behind this globalization process is the desire, on the part of the migrants, to improve their socio-economic conditions prevalent in their countries of origin. Together with such hope and aspiration for an improvement in their socio-economic conditions, they also bring with them their heritages, languages, religions, and traditions; that is, their culture, as well as their racial and ethnic characteristics and/or manifestations.

In many occasions, these migrants are either refugees and/or asylum seekers as a result of the many military and political conflicts faced in many parts of the world nowadays. These migratory processes, whether they are legal or illegal, or due to political and/or military reasons, all convey positive as well as negative implications to both the migrants and the host society. Intrinsic in this migratory process is the 'stress' that it produces to both the majority culture represented by the host society and the minority culture symbolized by the migrant groups. This migratory-produced stress is known as 'acculturative stress', and the process itself is known as the 'acculturation process' (Ruiz, 2004).

In this context, the migrant groups tend to a) 'integrate' within the majority culture; b) 'assimilate' into the majority culture; c) 'reject' the majority culture; or d) 'marginalize' themselves within the host society or majority culture. There are a series of variables that may impact positively or negatively the acculturation process, as represented by integration, assimilation, rejection, or marginalization. They are as follows:

Sociodemographic variables: age, sex, marital status, educational levels, race, ethnicity, religion, climate, geographical locations (rural versus urban), foreign versus local born status, and economic conditions.

Societal variables: pluralistic nature of the majority culture or host society, tolerant nature of the host or majority culture, and racist nature of the host society or majority culture.

Migrant group variables: touristic nature of the migration process, temporary workers, sojourners, immigrants, asylum seekers, and refugees.

Sociological and psychological variables: coping and adaptational styles of the migrants, as well as previous psychosocial conflicts or experiences among the migrants (e.g. childhood traumas, maternal deprivation, homesickness, separation problems, self-identity difficulties, group cohesiveness, degree of powerlessness, generational differences, attitudes/prejudices, level of rigidity, etc).

Behavioural variables: accidents, alcohol/drugs use and abuse, crime, homicide, and suicide.

These variables, as well as the final mode of resolution of the acculturation process, will determine the final degree of positive or negative outcomes when resolving the impact of the acculturative stress.

European trends

The types of outcomes commonly observed among migrants, refugees, or asylum seekers are quite often seen in the European Union as a result of the globalization and migratory process which is lately occurring in many countries of the European Union; for instance, the top asylum countries in the European Union during the period 2000–2004 were the following (Ruiz, 2004):

Countries	Asylum Seekers
Great Britain	300,000
Germany	240,000
France	175,000
Netherlands	95,000
Austria	90,000
Sweden	70,000

Similarly, the legal immigration within the European Union countries in the year 2002 (Ruiz, 2004) was as follows:

Countries	Immigrants
Italy	181,300
Great Britain	140,000
Germany	105,000
France	55,000
Netherlands	53,000
Sweden	24,000
Greece	23,900
Spain	20,800
Ireland	20,000
Austria	17,300
Belgium	12,100
Portugal	11,000
Denmark	10,100
Luxembourg	3,600
Finland	2,400

It is also of interest to note how many countries around the world negatively or positively judge the ethnic/racial groups that immigrate to their countries (Ruiz, 2004). They are as follows:

	agree	disagree
United States	22%	74%
Great Britain	33%	64%
France	32%	66%
Germany	31%	65%
Russia	26%	72%
Turkey	34%	61%

Obviously, these types of statistics clearly demonstrate the ambivalent feelings that still exist in many countries of the world between the majority culture symbolized by the host society and the minority culture represented by the migrant groups. It is also obvious that these feelings also have a major impact on the mental health status and mental illness prevalence in both the majority and the minority cultures. It is, therefore, of major importance for mental health professionals to study, assess, and address these impacts whether they are positives or negatives.

The case of the United States' current immigration trends

The population of the United States has changed a great deal in the last 4–5 decades. As a result of these changes, the US population is no longer a homogenous culture; on the contrary, it has rapidly become a multiethnic and multicultural society (Ruiz, 2005). The description and study of this population leads to a very good understanding and perspective of some of the most relevant therapeutic skills and therapeutic expectations. Actually, the immigration that has taken place in the United States during the last several decades, the acculturation process derived from this immigration, and finally, the coping and adaptational outcomes can all be ideal models for the understanding of the immigration process that is taking place all over the world as a result of the current trends in the globalization tendencies currently observed in all regions of the globe (Ruiz et al., 1995; Ruiz, 1997a; Ruiz, 1998).

In accordance to the year 2000 census (US Census Bureau, 2000) the total population of the United States was approximately 281 million persons; of this number, approximately 12.5% were Hispanics, 12.1% African Americans, 3.7% Asian Americans and 0.7% Native Americans. What is striking in these numbers was that the growth of the Hispanic population during the period 1900 to 2000 was 58%, for the Asian population the growth was 50%, for the Native Americans it was 17%, and for the African Americans it was 16%; for the Caucasian (white) population the growth was only 3%. Certain demographic characteristics are of major importance from a mental health and mental illness point of view; for instance, in accordance to the US Bureau of the Census, 46.7% of the African Americans families were headed by African American females; likewise, 39.4% of the Puerto Rican families from mainland United States were headed by Puerto Rican females. Central and South American female headed families formed 26.8%; in this regard, 20.2% were female headed Mexican families, 16.9% were female headed Cuban American families, 13.2% were female headed Asian families, and 14.2% were female headed Caucasian families. Needless to say, the higher the percentage of female headed families in these ethnic groups, the higher was the potential for prevalence of anxiety, depression, drug and alcohol addiction, drug-related criminality, prostitution, HIV/AIDS infection and other sexually related infections, and suicide (Ruiz, 2005).

Intrinsic to this ethnic minority demographic characteristics are also the disparities that currently exist in the health and mental health care systems not only of the ethnic and racial groups, but also of gender, age cycle, geographical locations, and many other human-related characteristics (Komarony et al., 1996;

Ruiz and Alarcon, 1996; Alegria *et al.*, 2008; Regier *et al.*, 2008). A review of the health and mental health care practices in the United States in recent years depicts clearly the outcome of these major disparities in the health care delivery system of this country; for instance, 33% of the Mexican Americans, 25% of the Cuban Americans, and 20% of the mainland Puerto Ricans residing in the United States do not have medical insurance coverage (Trevino *et al.*, 1991). As a result of this lack of medical insurance coverage, 40% of the Mexican Americans, 40% of the Cuban Americans, and 33% of the mainland Puerto Ricans who reside in the United States do not have any annual medical or psychiatric visits or contacts (Ruiz, 1993). This situation certainly impacts negatively on the therapeutic expectations of this ethnic minority population group. A similar situation prevails in other ethnic minority population groups who live in the United States; especially, the African American population (McCord and Freeman, 1990). Along the lines of health and mental health care disparities, something similar is observed in the United States with respect to socio-economic levels in the population; that is, the higher the socio-economic level of the United States population, the higher the quality of the medical and psychiatric care will be, as well as the mortality of whites in comparison to the mortality of the African Americans (Gift *et al.*, 1986; Rogers, 1992). The last US Census also depicts these types of health care system disparities quite well (US Census Bureau, 2000). The sociodemographic data of this census demonstrate that 15% of the total population in the United States does not have any type of health/mental health insurance coverage; however, the lack of health/mental health insurance coverage for the ethnic minority groups residing in the United States was 32.2%; additionally, the Medicaid programme, which is directed to cover the poor population of the United States medically and psychiatrically, only covered 39.9% of this population. The breakdown of this coverage is 43.7% among Hispanic Americans, 41.7% among Asian Americans, 28.1% among African Americans, and 28% among Caucasians (whites). Working status does not change this negative outcome much; 16.8% of the full-time working class in the United States do not have medical or psychiatric insurance coverage; likewise, 24.1% of the part-time working class in the United States does not have this coverage either; finally, 26.2% of the unemployed class lacks this type of coverage too. Solutions to these very negative trends insofar as the health and mental health insurance coverage in the United States require an urgent solution if one were to expect a higher applicability of therapeutic skills, as well as a higher therapeutic expectation in the health and mental health care of the United States population, and the population for the whole world for that matter; especially, for the ethnic minority groups (Ruiz and Garza Trevino, 1995; Ruiz, 1997b; Ruiz, 2002; Ruiz, 2007).

Conclusions

The psychological and psychiatric needs of refugees and asylum seekers are often stretched to the limits and their physical health may also be jeopardized. It is crucial that psychiatrists and mental health professionals do not get involved in questioning, torture, or physical pain. Specific cultural interventions are discussed later in this volume.

References

Alegria, M., Chatterji, P., Wells, K., *et al.* (2008). Disparity in depression treatment among racial and ethnic minority populations in the United States. *Psychiatric Services* **59**: 1264–1272.

American Psychiatric Association (2004). Diagnostic and statistical manual of mental disorders, 4th edition, Washington DC: American Psychiatric Publishing.

Canino, I.A., Rubio-Stipec, M., Canino, G., and Escobar, J.I. (1992). Functional somatic symptoms: A cross-ethnic comparison. *American Journal of Orthopsychiatry* **62**: 605–612.

Foulks, E.F. (2002). Cultural issues. In M. Hersem and W. Sledge (Eds.) *Encyclopedia of Psychotherapy*, Volume I, pp. 603–613, San Diego: Academic Press.

Gift, T.E., Strauss, J.D., Ritzler, B.A., *et al.* (1986). Social class and psychiatric outcome. *American Journal of Psychiatry* **143**: 222–225.

Gonzales, C.A., Griffith, E.E.H., and Ruiz, P. (2001). Cross-cultural issues in psychiatric treatment. In G.O. Gabbard (Ed.), *Treatment of Psychiatric Disorders*, Third Edition, Volume I, pp. 47–67, Washington DC: American Psychiatric Publishing.

Komarony, M., Grumbach, K., Drake, M. *et al.* (1996). The role of Black and Hispanic physicians in providing health care for underserved populations. *New England Journal of Medicine* **334**: 1305–1310.

McCord, C. and Freeman, H.P. (1990). Excess mortality in Harlem. *New England Journal of Medicine* **322**: 173–177.

Regier, D.A., Bufka, L.F., Whitaker, T. *et al.* (2008). Parity and the use of out-of-network mental health benefits in the FEHB program. *Health Affairs* **27**: w70–w83.

Rogers, R.G. (1992). Living and dying in the USA: Sociodemographic determinants of death among Blacks and Whites. *Demography* **29**: 287–303.

Ruiz, P. (1993). Access to health care for uninsured Hispanics: Policy recommendations. *Hospitals and Community Psychiatry* **44**: 958–962.

Ruiz, P. (1995). Cross-cultural psychiatry – foreword. In J.M. Oldham and M.B. Riba (Eds.) *Review of Psychiatry* 14, pp. 467–476,Washington DC: American Psychiatric Press.

Ruiz, P. (1997a). Issues in the psychiatric care of Hispanics. *Psychiatric Services* **48**(4): 539–540.

Ruiz, P. (1997b). Pobreza y atencion médica: problemas y perspectivas. *Revista Médica Dominicana* **58**(2): 36–39.

Ruiz, P. (1998). The role of culture in psychiatric care. *American Journal of Psychiatry* **155**: 1763–1765.

Ruiz, P. (2002). Consideraciones socioeconomicas en Psiquiatria. *Revista Neuro-Psiquiatrica* **65**: 22–31.

Ruiz, P. (2004). Psychopathology and migration. In Psiquiatria 2004. III symposium Almirall, Libro de Resumenes, pp. 47–60.

Ruiz, P. (2005). La psiquiatria en las minorias etnicas: el ejemplo de las Estados Unidos. In J. Vallejo Ruiloba and C. Leal Cercos (Eds.) *Tratado de Psiquiatria*, Volumen II, pp. 2273–2280, Barcelona: Ars Medica.

Ruiz, P. (2007). Presidential address: Addressing patient needs: Access, parity and humane care. *American Journal of Psychiatry* **164**: 1507–1509.

Ruiz, P. and Alarcon, R.D. (1996). How culture and poverty exclude people from care. *American Journal of Forensic Psychiatry* **17**: 61–73.

Ruiz, P. and Garza Trevino, E.S. (1995). El paciente Hispano y el sistema de Salud Medica y psiquiatria: Problemas y perspectivas. *Revista de Psiquiatria* **2**: 5–12.

Ruiz, P., Venegas Samuels, K. and Alarcon, R.D. (1995). The economics of pain: Mental health care costs among minorities. *Psychiatric Clinics of North America* **18**: 659–679.

Trevino, F.M., Moyer, E., Burciaga Valdes, R., and Stroup-Benham, C.A. (1991): Health insurance coverage and utilization of health services by Mexican Americans, Mainland Puerto Ricans, and Cuban Americans. *Journal of the American Medical Association (JAMA)* **265**(2): 233–237.

US Census Bureau (2000).

Chapter 2

Mental distress and psychological interventions in refugee populations

Tom Craig

Assessing mental health

High rates of emotional distress and mental disorder have been reported by many studies of migrant populations fleeing conflict or other crises. Two chapters (3 and 4) deal with the pre- and post-migration factors that are associated with mental distress and ill health in these populations. In this chapter we provide a brief resumé of the evidence of elevated rates of disorder and of the effectiveness of psychological interventions in migrants from cultures very different from those in which these therapies were first developed.

Until 2005, most of the evidence for elevated rates of disorder came from a plethora of small-scale investigations using non-standardized assessment methods applied to highly selected groups such as those attending out-patient clinics. Not surprisingly, there were hugely differing estimates of the prevalence of common mental disorder. Estimates for post-traumatic stress disorder (PTSD), for example, range between 3 and 86% (Fazel, Wheeler, and Danesh, 2005). Subsequently there have been a number of meta-analyses that have attempted to synthesize the data from the more robust investigations. In the first of these, Porter and Haslam (2005) aimed to provide an estimate of the extent to which broad mental health was less satisfactory in refugees and internally displaced people than in stable comparable populations and to identify the moderators of this psychopathology. Studies were included where there were standardized measures of psychopathology among refugee samples and which included at least one non-refugee comparison group. A total of 56 reports meeting these criteria were identified providing 59 comparisons between 22,221 refugees and 45,073 non-refugees. On a summary estimate of the difference in psychopathology between the two populations, an overall mean effect size was 0.41 (SD 0.02, range, −1.36 to 2.91 [SE 0.01]) indicating fairly conclusively that refugees had poorer mental health than comparable non-refugee populations. Furthermore, worse mental health was reported for refugees living in institutional accommodation (i.e. hostels, temporary residences), those whose occupational opportunity was restricted (i.e. no right to work, or restricted access to employment), those who had been repatriated to a country from which they had previously fled and refugees from countries where there were ongoing conflicts. Greater psychopathology was also associated with older age, higher education, and better pre-displacement social status. The findings also indirectly confirmed that the mental health of refugees is likely to be determined as much by the circumstances after migration as by traumatic experiences preceding it—a fact that is crucial in considering how best to provide care to these populations.

Although demonstrating a significant excess of mental distress and psychopathology, this analysis does not tell us much about which, if any, specific diagnostic conditions were involved. Fazel, Wheeler, and Danesh (2005) assembled data from studies that used clinical research interviews to assess psychosis, major depression, generalized anxiety disorder and PTSD among refugees and asylum seekers in high-income Western countries. The decision to include only interview-based mental health assessments still included a fairly heterogeneous range of assessment methods, including both highly structured interviews administered by lay investigators as well as semi-structured interviews conducted by researchers with a clinical background. The two approaches are known to produce different estimates of 'caseness' when applied in parallel to the same population (Dean, Surtees, and Sashidharan, 1985; Regier, Kaelber, Rae, et al., 1998; Eaton, Neufeld, Chen, et al., 2000) and it is not surprising that even these more sophisticated studies still produce very variable estimates. A total of 20 studies were identified, and provided data on 6,743 adults. The prevalence of PTSD was estimated at 9% (99% CI 8–11%) based on data from 17 studies and 5,499 adults; that for major depression 5% (4–6%) based on 14 studies and 3,616 adults and for generalized anxiety 4% (3–6%) based on just 5 studies and 1,423 adults. There were only 2 studies with a total of 226 adults that reported rates of 2% (99% CI 1–6%) for psychosis. For those studies that examined more than one diagnosis, co-morbidity was common with 71% of people suffering from major depression also having PTSD.

These prevalence estimates are considerably lower than many frequently cited reports, and the confidence intervals for rates for major depression in particular would include the figure reported by several large epidemiological studies of the general population in North America and Europe. Nevertheless, for common mental disorders and PTSD in particular, it appears that the prevalence of diagnosable common mental disorders is indeed elevated over that in the domiciled population. That this is also likely for psychotic disorders is strongly supported by research studies since Ödegaard reported high rates of severe mental illness among Norwegian migrants to the United States (Ödegaard, 1932). Perhaps the most persuasive evidence comes from studies into the incidence of psychosis in people of African and Caribbean origin who migrated to the UK in the 1950s. Studies over the last 30 years have consistently reported rates 2 to 14 times greater in these populations than in White British (e.g. Fearon, Kirkbride, Morgan, *et al.*, 2006). Cantor-Graae and Selten (2005) reported a meta-analysis of worldwide studies of schizophrenia and migration. They included 18 studies that reported incident rates for residents of a particular geographical area, and which included a correction for age differences between the different ethnic groups. All except one study had been carried out in Europe (the majority in Britain). The most common ethnic groups were people of African-Caribbean origin, people of South Asian origin, and smaller numbers of migrants to the Netherlands from Surinam, Morocco and Turkey, and of European migrants to Australia. The meta-analysis of these studies reported an average weighted relative risk of 2.7 (95% CI 2.3–3.2) among first-generation migrants compared to the indigenous population and 4.5 (95% CI 1.5–13.1) for the second generation—a striking finding suggesting quite powerfully that whatever factors are driving the increased incidence, these also affect the children (and indeed grandchildren) of migrants. Furthermore, epidemiological studies carried out in the Caribbean countries of origin of the migrant groups find rates comparable to the White British rate in the UK (Hickling and Rodgers-Johnson, 1995; Bhugra, Hilwig, Hosein, *et al.*, 1996) suggesting that the increase has something to do with exposure subsequent to migration. The meta-analysis also showed that migrants from developing countries were at higher risk than were migrants from developed countries and that migrants from countries where the majority population were 'black' were at greater risk than those from countries where the majority were white (RR 4.8, 95% CI 3.7–6.2).

All these studies, whether of common mental disorders or of psychosis, have estimated rates based on clinical assessments and diagnostic measures developed in a Western biomedical psychiatric system. Refugee status and migration in particular is a complex variable that encompasses a very wide range of experiences (the earlier studies of psychosis were mainly on economic migrants whereas those done more recently include all categories including asylum seekers) and the meta-analyses (and many of the original studies) bring together in one analysis people from many different ethnic and cultural backgrounds. To take the example of psychosis, the African–Caribbean migrants in the European studies came originally from a scattering of islands with substantially different ethnic mixes, language, and culture and are often lumped together in these studies with other 'black' migrants from African countries. There are also problems related to how the participants are recruited to the various studies, which may be particularly problematic for common mental disorders where significant numbers of affected individuals do not contact services. Few studies have employed robust methods to access relevant populations in non-conventional settings. One that attempted this for a Somali migrant population in London, England, recruited participants through probabilistic sampling from a range of non-health-care settings such as the Mosque, Somali cafés and Western Union offices on the high street but even with these approaches ascertainment bias was clearly a problem, particularly for the Somali women (Bhui, Craig, Mohamud, *et al.*, 2006).

The imposition of Western diagnostic systems and the methods for establishing the presence of these disorders in cross-cultural settings has been widely criticized for decades. The problem is particularly challenging for common mental disorders, which overlap with non-pathological distress and where the local idioms of distress have no direct equivalence in the Western-designed measurement tool. In the Somali study mentioned earlier, pathological affective symptoms proved very difficult to convey. For example, the nearest translation for the concept of depression also means headache and migraine, whereas two Somali terms that were eventually used were also general approximations to the concept, one of which was a relatively recent addition to the language and derived from a medical term (see Bhui, Craig, Mohamud, *et al.*, 2006 for further details).

Although there are sometimes no equivalent terms in the local language for Western-derived psychiatric symptoms, there are also numerous examples of expressions of distress that have no simple translation in the other direction but that are core to understanding mental distress in that society. So for example, symptoms of PTSD may be far less meaningful to a sufferer of war-related trauma than some other culturally more salient concept. Miller, Kulkarni, and Kushner (2006) give the example of the Afghan concept of *gigar khun*—a post-traumatic and often persistent state of sadness and withdrawal that is regarded as being far more salient than the intrusive imagery of PTSD, which although recognized, was regarded as transitory and of less significance. Furthermore, even where the constituent symptoms of a Western diagnosis can be identified, Kleinman's categorical fallacy (Kleinman, 1977) tells us that we cannot assume that the diagnosis assembled from these symptoms has the same meaning that it has to natives of, say, North America.

However, despite these caveats, it seems beyond doubt that migration is associated with an increase in mental distress that meets Western-derived 'caseness' criteria and would also be recognized as abnormal and deserving of the attention of healers in the migrant's home society. One example is reported in a study of the prevalence of culture-bound syndromes and their treatment in a study of Guetemalan Myan refugees in UNHCR camps in Mexico (Smith, Sabin, Berlin, *et al.*, 2009). In this study, 179 adults living in 183 households were interviewed about his or her health and 95 answered a child-health questionnaire for their children. Questions concerned the presence of several (but not all) local ethnomedical (i.e. culture-bound) expressions of disorder and treatment-seeking behaviour. Ethnomedical syndromes were common, with 59% of the adults and 48% of the children having experienced *susto* (fright) and 34% of the adults having experienced *ataques de nervios* (nervous attacks) in the week prior to the interview. There was considerable overlap between these conditions and Western concepts of PTSD or major depression. The majority of participants used both Western health care as well as indigenous remedies including medicinal plants and cleansings or other rituals.

Management issues

In their critique of the Western epidemiological approach to the ascertainment of psychopathological responses to trauma, Miller, Kulkarni, and Kushner (2006) point out that relatively little of the available research contains information that is helpful to guide the creation of culturally appropriate interventions and services. They argue that what is needed, in addition to epidemiology, is good-quality information on the ways psychological distress is expressed in the specific cultural context of the refugee, what experiences and stressors are considered most important, what are the traditional ways of coping with distress, and whether there are interventions that have been shown to be helpful in similar situations that might be adapted or copied. To this one might add good-quality outcome studies testing specific interventions in well-described migrant populations.

For any therapy to proceed, an understanding of local idioms of distress within the person's cultural background is essential as is an awareness of the stigma associated with particular traumatic experiences and with mental illness. This information must also take account of the importance of religion and spirituality for the individual and be aware of religious and other socially determined taboos and how these may shape the consultation or contribute to the reluctance a refugee might have of disclosing sensitive personal information. Helping to solve practical problems and to achieve outcomes such as getting a job, sorting out childcare and housing difficulties is likely to be of much greater benefit initially than a focus on emotional responses to trauma

(Summerfield, 2001; Miller, Kulkarni, and Kushner, 2006). Sometimes the most acceptable approach will seem quite contrary to what we in the West might consider as a first choice. For example, Hubbard and Pearson (2004) in a study of Sierra Leoneans in refugee camps in Guinea noted that communal discussion towards resolving social problems was common practice, and found that a group-based approach was preferred over individual counselling as the vehicle for therapy.

Many refugees will have experienced or witnessed violence and abuse. Clinical experience suggests that some forms of this abuse, including torture and sexual violence, is particularly toxic in terms of their propensity to cause lasting distress and mental ill health and that multiple traumas can have a cumulative dose effect on mental health (Mollica, McInnes, Poole, et al., 1998). Rape and other sexual violation may leave no long-term physical sign, yet be profoundly shaming.

Although not doubting the importance of understanding the nature and extent of pre-migration trauma and violence, it is important not to overlook stressors in the current environment that may be more immediately relevant to the individual. Repressive violence and forced migration affect whole families, the consequence of which can persist for years. Children may have to take on caring roles prematurely; family trust may break down and domestic violence may become a way of coping with personal conflict. Many of those whose families have suffered abuse describe guilt at having failed to avert violence to loved ones. These are taboo subjects in most cultures, and it is hardly surprising that many are very reluctant to talk about their experiences. Counselling and the notion of disclosing personal experiences to a relative stranger is an alien experience for many refugees. The last point also needs to be kept in mind where an interpreter is involved. In the worst case, he/she may be a member of a tribe or political party that is opposed to the refugee patient though the more common risk is knowledge of the patient's family or wider circle of acquaintances and fears that confidential matters will leak out. Domestic violence may be particularly difficult to discuss through an interpreter, let alone where the sufferer is accompanied to the clinic by the perpetrator. That said, there are very good guidelines available on the use of interpreter services in the delivery of psychosocial assessment and therapy (Tribe and Morrissey, 2003) and evidence that therapy delivered in this way can be effective. For example, a recent study explored the use of interpreters in therapy comparing three groups of patients receiving CBT—refugees who required an interpreter, those who did not, and English-speaking non-refugee comparison group. All three groups attended a similar number of sessions and all three improved with treatment. Those needing an interpreter fared no worse than those who did not (d'Ardenne, Ruaro, Cestari, *et al.*, 2007).

For the most part, everyday therapy provided to refugees in Western health-care settings is that offered to the indigenous population with only minimal consideration given to whether the therapy model or means of delivery needs specific adaptation. There are, however, a handful of good-quality studies where such adaptations have been taken into account and which demonstrate some limited efficacy. One such adaptation that is worth detailed considera-tion concerned the provision of community-based group interpersonal psy-chotherapy (IPT) to people suffering from depression in rural Uganda (Bolton, Bass, Neugebauer, *et al.*, 2003; Bass, Neugebauer, Clougherty, *et al.*, 2006). In this study, participants suffering from at least one of the two local depression-like syndromes (*Yo'kwekyawa* or *Okwekubazida*) were interviewed using adap-tation of the depression section of the Hopkins Symptom Checklist (Derogatis, *et al.*, 1974) together with a gender-specific questionnaire that assessed func-tional impairment. The resulting data were used to generate a diagnosis of major depression and participants meeting this criterion were eligible to take part in the study. Randomization was at village level, with 116 participants in 15 villages receiving the intervention and 132 in 15 villages assigned to 'treat-ment as usual'. The intervention was carried out in single-gender groups of up to eight participants that met for 90 minutes over 16 weeks. Each group was led by a Ugandan who had no previous mental health or counselling experience other than training in the intervention. Group members were encouraged to provide encouragement and support to one another. At the end of the inter-vention, there was a mean reduction in depression symptoms of 17.47 points compared to a mean of 3.76 in the control group. Functional impairment also improved significantly more in those in the treatment arm. At the end of the intervention, 6.5% of the intervention but 54.7% of the controls continued to meet criteria for major depression. At a six month follow-up, intervention group participants had depression scores of 14.0 (95% CI 12.2–15.8) points lower than those in the control arm. The rate of those meeting criteria for major depression at 6 months was significantly lower for the treatment arm (11.7%) than the control arm (54.4%). It is possible that the longer-term effects were mediated by continuing informal group meetings that continued in an ad hoc manner after the end of the specific time-limited therapy.

A subsequent investigation, also in Uganda and by members of the same research team, compared the efficacy of the group-based IPT intervention to that of a creative play (CP) comparison treatment and a no-treatment waiting list (WL) control in 14–17-year-old Acholi refugees living in two camps in northern Uganda. In a preparatory survey, seven mental health and psychosocial problems were identified that were considered important by young people, caregivers, and key local individuals. Three of these problems were 'depression-like', one 'anxiety-like', one a combination of socially unacceptable behaviours, one PTSD with psychotic symptoms, and one a legitimate fear of future attacks from the Lords Resistance Army. As in the non-refugee study described earlier, questionnaires were developed to assess both symptomatic and functional impairments. Young people were eligible for inclusion if they were considered to have at least one of the 'depression-like' local syndromes and scored more than 32 points on the depression scale, greater than 0 on the functional impairment scale, and had been symptomatic for at least one month. A total of 314 adolescents were randomized to one of the three treatment conditions (105 to IPT, 105 to CP and 104 to WL). The IPT and CP interventions comprised 16 weekly sessions of approximately two hours each. The IPT followed manualized guidelines similar to those used in the earlier Uganda study. The CP intervention was originally developed by War Child Holland on the principle that resilience to stress is increased through participation in creative activities such as music, art, sports, and debates. All three groups showed reductions in depression scores between baseline and end of therapy. The adjusted difference in mean within-subject decline in symptoms between the IPT and WL control groups was 9.79 points (95% CI 1.66 to 17.93, P = 0.02) whereas that for the difference between CP and WL was small and not significant (−2.51 [95% CI 11.4–6.39, p = 0.58]). However, further sub-analyses by gender showed that the significant change for those receiving IPT was confined to girls. The IPT group also showed a small (2-point) reduction in anxiety scores compared to the WL control but had no significant impact on conduct problems. All three groups showed improvements in function scores (Bolton, Bass, Betancourt, et al., 2007).

A quite different approach to the intensive individual therapy of the Ugandan studies has been reported in a study of survivors of the civil war in Mozambique (Igreja, Kleijn, Schreuder, et al., 2004). This used a testimony intervention in which participants described in detail one major traumatic experience, their role in the event, the perceptions and feeling at the time of the event and in recounting it, and feelings about the future. The potential healing effects of testimony are attributed to the psychological alleviation that comes from sharing a trauma story with others. Participants who met criteria for PTSD 'caseness' were randomly allocated to intervention (n = 66) or a no-intervention control group (n = 71). Both groups showed significant reductions in symptoms between baseline and follow-up. There was a small but non-significant benefit in women. The authors point out the difficulty of carrying out a controlled trial in the community setting where there was inevitably a great deal of interaction between the intervention and non-intervention control participants. The intervention itself may have been insufficient, involving only a single session for most participants.

Individualized psychological interventions based on cognitive behaviour therapy (CBT) techniques have also been evaluated. Neuner, Schauer, Klaschik, *et al.*, (2004) report an randomized controlled trial (RCT) carried out with Rwandan and Somali refugees in the Nakivale refugee camp in southern Uganda. A total of 9 refugees were trained in 'trauma counselling' (TC), comprising general counselling skills and a manualized narrative exposure therapy (NET). The NET approach was developed by the authors as a short-term intervention based on cognitive behavioural exposure therapy. Unlike the narrative therapy used in the Mozambique intervention mentioned earlier, NET requires the participant to construct a narration of his whole life up to the present, while focusing also on the traumatic event. The autobiography is recorded by the counsellor and expanded or corrected at each session. During discussion of traumatic experiences the counsellor encourages the reliving of emotional and behavioural reactions to the trauma and the discussion of the traumatic event is only discontinued on habituation of the emotional reactions. The approach had previously been shown to be acceptable and effective when implemented by professional Western therapists in a smaller study with Sudanese refugees.

The study compared the results of implementing this manualized NET approach with TC—in which the counsellors were encouraged to take elements of the NET approach and combine these with other techniques from general counselling including non-directive active listening, problem solving, and discussing coping skills. The TC was less directive and more responsive to the expressed needs of the individual during the therapy session, relating current difficulties to past traumatic problems. Outcomes at the end of treatment and at six month follow-up for both treatment groups were compared with a waiting list 'no treatment' control group. A total of 277 participants were allocated to one of the three groups (NET $n = 111$, TC $n = 111$, MG $n = 55$). Dropout from therapy was greater for the TC group (20%) than the NET group (4%). The outcomes of both the active treatment groups were clinically and statistically superior to the no-treatment control but did not differ from each other. For example, at follow-up, 70% of the NET group and 65% of the TC group but only 37% of the no-treatment controls no longer fulfilled PTSD diagnostic criteria.

These are among the very few studies that have attempted to take a clinical intervention into general community settings. More typical are interventions designed to be delivered to actively help seeking populations. For example, Hinton, Chhean, Pich, *et al.* (2005) have described a culturally adapted cognitive behaviour therapy for Cambodian refugees with treatment resistant PTSD and panic attacks (treatment resistance was defined as still experiencing symptoms despite an adequate trial of a selective serotonin reuptake [SSRI] antidepressant and supportive counselling). Forty patients were randomized to either immediate treatment or a delayed treatment waiting list. The treatment, referred to as 'Sensation Reprocessing Therapy (SRT)', comprised 12 weekly sessions with content based on CBT principles including elements of psychoeducation, muscle relaxation, visualization, cognitive restructuring, and interoceptive exposure to anxiety related sensations, particularly those concerning tension of the neck muscles (a fear of catastrophic rupture of the arteries of the neck with multiple autonomic arousal symptoms was common in this group of patients). There was a clinically and statistically significant improvement for patients in the intervention group compared to those in the waiting list comparison. Improvements were seen across all outcome measures including the clinician-administered PTSD scale score, and symptom checklist 90-R subscales. Improvement was rapid and sustained, so that after the first course of CBT 60% ($n = 12$), the active treatment group no longer met diagnostic criteria for PTSD whereas all the waiting list patients did. It is not possible from this study to know whether the cultural modifications to CBT were all necessary or indeed whether the package as a whole is superior to 'standard' CBT.

One final intervention deserves mention. It is well established that many refugees suffering from mental health problems do not seek advice or help for these and under-utilize mental health services. Weine, Kulauzovic, Klebic, *et al.* (2008) in Chicago, USA, report a multi-family group intervention for refugees from Bosnia-Herzegovina aimed at increasing appropriate health service utilization in refugees suffering from PTSD and other common mental disorders. Previous work had established low health service utilization despite high levels of need in this population, which had not improved despite the provision of no-cost, culturally appropriate clinical services provided by several local agencies in the city. Participants were recruited through community-based organizations. As a first step, research staff screened potential participants for symptoms of PTSD and those meeting research diagnostic criteria were invited to take part in the subsequent treatment trial. A total of 197 adults with PTSD and their families were recruited to the study and randomized to either the intervention ($n = 110$) or no-treatment control condition ($n = 87$). The 'Coffee and Family Education and Support' (CAFES) intervention was delivered over 9 sessions over 16 weeks with approximately 7 families per group. The primary subject and all family members over the age of 17 living in his/her household were invited to attend the sessions. Each session included a fifteen minute didactic presentation followed by a one hour group discussion and covered a diverse range of topics including mental health problems, school problems, mental health services, and family beliefs. Each session was led by lay facilitators, who were Bosnian refugees themselves and had experience of doing group work (e.g. nurses, teachers, and organizers). These facilitators were trained to deliver the intervention and received weekly supervision from the senior research staff with monthly videotapes of CAFES sessions. Outcomes were assessed at baseline, end of treatment, at 6, 12, and 18 months. The results showed that CAFES was effective in increasing access to appropriate mental health services and that two factors, the presence of depression and increased family comfort with discussing trauma, mediated this intervention effect.

This last study calls attention to the importance of considering where to base mental health services for refugees. Although specialist therapies may be developed and tested within specialist mental health settings, experts agree that treatment needs to be delivered in primary health-care settings where the majority of sufferers will attend.

Conclusions

The past three decades has seen an explosion in interest in the mental health of refugees and internally displaced people. Much of this interest has been in documenting rates of disorder as defined by Western biomedical diagnostic systems and in applying therapies similarly developed by Western medicine and psychology. However, for more effective treatment, clearer understanding of the overlap of these Western diagnoses with the idioms of distress popular in particular refugee groups, and a clearer understanding of local treatment-seeking behaviours is critical for developing more effective health care for these populations. Health-care providers need to know more about how distress is experienced and expressed in particular cultural contexts, what problems are considered most important and also be aware of the wider impact of pre-migration trauma on the families and wider support networks of the people referred for help. Although there are promising results from a number of recent studies to suggest that with adaptations, the psychological therapies developed in the West can also be of value in other settings, we also need more carefully constructed clinical trials to establish what interventions work best with what populations.

References

Bass, J., Neugebauer, R., Clougherty, K., *et al.* (2006). Group interpersonal psychotherapy for depression in rural Uganda: 6-Month outcomes. Randomised controlled trial. *British Journal of Psychiatry* **188**: 567–573.

Bhui, K., Craig, T., Mohamud, S., *et al.* (2006). Mental disorders among Somali refugees: Developing culturally appropriate measures and assessing sociocultural risk factors. *Social Psychiatry and Psychiatric Epidemiology* **41**: 400–408.

Bolton, P., Bass, J., Betancourt, T., *et al.* (2007). Interventions for depression symptoms amongst adolescent survivors of war and displacement in Northern Uganda: A randomized controlled trial. *Journal of American Medical Association* **298**: 519–527.

Bolton, P., Bass, J., Neugebauer, R., *et al.* (2003). Group interpersonal psychotherapy for depression in rural Uganda: A randomized controlled trial. *Journal of American Medical Association* **289**: 3117–3124.

Bhugra, D., Hilwig, M., Hosein, B., *et al.* (1996). First contact incidence rates of schizophrenia in Trinidad and one year follow-up. *British Journal of Psychiatry* **169**: 587–592.

Cantor-Graae, E., and Selten, J.P. (2005). Schizophrenia and migration: A meta-analysis and review. *American Journal of Psychiatry* **162**: 12–24.

d' Ardenne, P., Ruaro, L., Cestari, L., *et al.* (2007). Does interpreter-mediated CBT with traumatized refugee people work? A comparison of patient outcomes in East London. *Behavioural and Cognitive Psychotherapy* **35**: 293–301.

Dean, C., Surtees, P.G., and Sashidharan, S.P. (1985). Comparison of research diagnostic systems in an Edinburgh community sample. *British Journal of Psychiatry* **142**: 247–256.

Derogatis, L.R., Lipman, R.S., Rickels, K., Uhlenhuth, E.H., and Covi, L. (1974). The Hopsins Symptom Checklist (HSCL): A self-report symptom inventory. *Behavioural Science* **19**: 1–5.

Eaton, W.W., Neufeld, K., Chen, L., *et al.* (2000). A comparison of self-report and clinical diagnostic interviews for depression: diagnostic interview schedule and schedules for clinical assessment in neuropsychiatry in the Baltimore Epidemiologic Catchment Area Follow-Up. *Archives of General Psychiatry* **57**: 217–222.

Fazel, M., Wheeler, J., and Danesh, J. (2005). Prevalence of serious mental disorders in 7000 refugees resettled in western countries: A systematic review. *Lancet* **365**: 1309–1314.

Fearon, P., Kirkbride, J.K., Morgan, C., *et al.* (2006). Incidence of schizophrenia and other psychoses in ethnic minority groups: Results from the MRC AESOP study. *Psychological Medicine* **36**: 1541–1550.

Hickling, F.W. and Rodgers-Johnson, P. (1995). The incidence of first-contact schizophrenia in Jamaica. *British Journal of Psychiatry* **167**: 193–196.

Hinton, D.E., Chhean, D., Pich, V., *et al.* (2005). A randomized controlled trial of cognitive-behaviour therapy for Cambodian refugees with treatment-resistant PTSD and panic attacks: A cross-over design. *Journal of Traumatic Stress* **18**: 617–629.

Hubbard, J. and Pearson, N. (2004). Sierra Leonean refugees in Guinea: addressing the mental health effects of massive community violence. In K.E. Miller and L.M. Rasco (Eds.), *The Mental Health of Refugees: Ecological Approaches to Healing and Adaptation,* pp. 95–132, Mahwah, NJ: Erlbaum.

Igreja, V., Kleijn, W.C., Schreuder, B.J.N., *et al.* (2004). Testimony method to ameliorate post-traumatic stress symptoms. *British Journal of Psychiatry* **184**: 251–257.

Kleinman, A. (1977). Depression, somatization and the new cross-cultural psychiatry. *Social Science and Medicine* **11**: 3–10.

Miller, K.E., Kulkarni, M., and Kushner, H. (2006). Beyond trauma-focused psychiatric epidemiology: Bridging research and practice with war-affected populations. *American Journal of Orthopsychiatry* **76**: 409–442.

Mollica, R.F., McInnes, K., Poole, C., *et al.* (1998). Dose effect relationship of trauma to symptoms of depression and post traumatic stress disorder among Cambodian survivors of mass violence. *British Journal of Psychiatry* **173**: 482–488.

Neuner, F., Schauer, M., Klaschik, C., *et al.* (2004). A comparison of narrative exposure therapy, supportive counselling and psychoeducation for treating posttraumatic stress disorder in an African refugee settlement. *Journal of Consulting and Clinical Psychology* **72**: 579–587.

Ödegaard, Ö. (1932). Emigration and insanity. *Acta Psychiatrica et Neurologica Scandinavica*, **7**: 1–206.

Porter, M. and Haslam, N. (2005). Predisplacement and postdisplacement factors associated with mental health of refugees and internally displaced persons: A meta-analysis. *Journal of American Medical Association* **294**: 602–611.

Regier, D.A., Kaelber, C.T., Rae, D.S., *et al.* (1998). Limitations of diagnostic criteria and assessment instruments for mental disorders: Implications for research and policy. *Archives of General Psychiatry* **55**: 109–115.

Smith, B.D., Sabin, M., Berlin, E.A., *et al.* (2009). Ethnomedical syndromes and treatment-seeking behaviour among Mayan refugees in Chiapas, Mexico. *Culture, Medicine and Psychiatry* **33**: 366–381.

Summerfield, D. (2001). Asylum seekers, refugees and mental health services in the UK. *Psychiatric Bulletin* **25**: 161–163.

Tribe, R. and Morrissey, J. (2003). The refugee context and the role of interpreters. In R. Tribe and H. Raval (Eds.), *Working with Intepreters in Mental Health*. London: Brunner-Routledge.

Weine, S., Kulauzovic, Y., Klebic, A., *et al.* (2008). Evaluating a multiple-family group access intervention for refugees with PTSD. *Journal of Marital and Family Therapy* **34**: 149–164.

Chapter 3

Pre-migration and mental health of refugees

Thomas Stompe, David Holzer, and Alexander Friedmann

Introduction

In 2008, more than 200,000,000 people voluntarily or involuntarily left their countries of origin to take the chance for a better future for themselves and their relatives. Therefore the term migrant is not based on constant biological, cultural, religious, or other characteristics, but on the biographical event of migration (for whatever reason) and the resulting peculiarities of life circumstances. Migration is a dynamic, long-lasting process with impact over years after physical relocation. This process is inevitably stressful, often leading to mental illness.

For a better understanding of migration, it is important to distinguish between pre-migration, migration, and post-migration. Migration may be temporary or permanent. Migration can have a variety of motives, but in general we should separate voluntary migrants like labour migrants, students, diplomats, charity workers, etc. from involuntary migrants like asylum seekers and refugees. Whereas an asylum seeker is a person who has applied for asylum in another country and whose asylum application is still under consideration, a refugee has a granted refugee status by the new country. Migration can open new chances, but more often it is a negative stressful life event associated with a high prevalence of different mental illnesses like schizophrenia (Ödegaard, 1932; Cochrane and Bal, 1987; Harrison *et al.*, 1997; Hutchinson and Haasen, 2004; Cantor-Graae and Selten, 2005; Fearon *et al.*, 2006; Cooper *et al.*, 2008), mood disorders (Bhugra, 2003; Fazel *et al.*, 2005; Swinnen and Selten, 2007) and especially post-traumatic stress disorder (PTSD) (Fazel *et al.*, 2005).

This chapter describes the potential effects of the pre-migration stage on mental health.

Factors related to mental illness

Several biological, environmental, and sociocultural factors are interacting during development of every human being, forming an individual who is more or less vulnerable or resilient against severe stressors.

Biological background

The stage of pre-migration begins before the birth of the later migrant and ends with the process of migration. Every human being has a genetic equipment promoting resilience and vulnerability towards extreme stressful situations (de Jong, 2007). Cavalli-Sforza *et al.* (1994) and other researchers in population genetics had collected an amount of data on genetic population units during the last 30 years showing the variability of the distribution of complex gene patterns in different ethnic and racial groups. Cluster analyses of a database of 76,676 gene frequencies from 6633 samples with different geographical locations resulted in a final sample of 42 populations (Cavalli-Sforza *et al.*, 1994). Other biological factors associated with the geographical origin, which may influence the individual vulnerability are poor prenatal and perinatal care especially in developing countries, malnutrition, and infections like malaria, parasites, or diarrhoeal diseases, which may negatively influence the cognitive development (Mung'Ala-Odera *et al.*, 2004; Bangirana *et al.*, 2006) and therefore the capacity to cope with stressful situations.

Ethnicity and culture

Despite the fact that ethnic groups and cultures are not natural species, every human being is part of a self-organizing process of co-evolution between the individual development and the historical situation of a society.

According to the classic definition of Max Weber (1972), published 1922 in his book *Wirtschaft und Gesellschaft* (*Economics and Society*), an ethnic group is characterized by a common culture, mediated by a collective memory, a commonness of life style, shared traditions, values, religion or language, as well as allegiance, independent of biological origin. Therefore ethnicity is a social category, which classifies humans according to cultural differences. In epidemiology ethnicity describes a group to which a person belongs by self-attribution or attribution by others. In Anglo-American studies ethnicity often is applied similar to race. Originally, race was an exclusively biological–genetic defined category, classified according to phenotypical attributes like colour of the skin or structure of the hair. Later, this definition was enlarged by the inclusion of cultural and social attributes.

Culture is a term with a long history. In 1952 Alfred Kroeber and Clyde Kluckhohn published a list of 164 definitions of culture. In the twentieth century, culture emerged as a central concept to anthropology, encompassing all human forms of expression that are not purely results of human genetics. Specifically, the term culture in American anthropology had two meanings: (1) the evolved human capacity to classify and represent experiences with symbols, and to act imaginatively and creatively; and (2) the distinct ways in which people living in different parts of the world classify and represent their experiences and actions. Culture area is a geographic region and time sequence characterized by substantially uniform environment and culture.

Members of certain society share a bulk of cultural memories (Assmann, 1988). Cultural memory preserves the store of knowledge from which a group derives an awareness of its unity and peculiarity. The objective manifestations of cultural memory are defined through identification in a positive ('We are this') or in a negative ('That's our opposite') sense. Cultural memory reconstructs the distinct history of a community within its contemporary frame of reference. The objectivation of communicated meaning and collectively shared knowledge is a prerequisite of its transmission into the culturally institutionalized heritage of a society. The normative self-image of the group includes a system of values and differentiations in importance, which structures the cultural supply of knowledge and symbols. Individuals internalize cultural schemes or paradigms by means of socialization and education as well as through mass media. These schemes consist of a loosely organized set of socially shared practices, norms, and values, basically influencing the development of the personality (Triandis and Suh, 2002). They play a constitutive role in the evolution of the self-concept (Markus and Kitayama, 1991) and of the self-regulation (Tweed and Lehmann, 2002). Differences in this culture-based self-construal may also have an impact in the vulnerability or resilience of migrants: Path analyses have revealed that an independent self-construal was positively related to direct coping strategies, which predicted reduced levels of stress (Cross, 1995). These effects of self-construal and coping are moderated by culture (Tweed *et al.*, 2004). Illness beliefs and idioms of distress, which have crucial influence on the presentation of symptom of the later migrant, are also part of the self-evident cultural knowledge of a certain society.

Labour migrants as well as refugees show a variable prevalence and phenomenology of mental illness dependent on their cultural and ethnical origins. Several studies indicated an increased risk for schizophrenia and schizophrenia-like psychoses especially among African Caribbean immigrants (Harrison *et al.*, 1997; Sharpley *et al.*, 2001). A study from the Netherlands found an increased risk for schizophrenia in subjects born in Morocco, Surinam, and Dutch Antilles, but not in subjects from Turkey or Western countries (Selten *et al.*, 2001). These results point to the importance of the culture-specific development in the pre-migration stage as well as social post-migration factors for the incidence of schizophrenia in migrant groups.

Socio-economic factors

The majority of migrants stem from countries with severe socio-economic problems. Epidemiological studies in many developing countries have attributed the high rates of several mental disorders to factors such as discrimination, unemployment, and living in a period of rapid social change (Rumble *et al.*, 1996). Illiteracy and poor education too are consistent risk factors for mental disorders. Poverty in general is likely to be associated with malnutrition, lack of access to clean water, inadequate housing, accidents, and other risk factors associated with poor physical and mental health (Patel and Kleinman, 2003). Family disruption caused by parental illness and death affect the quality of attachment and the development of the personality and are therefore suited to contribute to the outbreak of mental disorders under the pressure of migration.

Traumatic life events

Principally refugees present a unique risk profile due to their exposure to violence in their homelands. Research on traumatized refugees started after World War II with studies of the Jewish survivors of the Holocaust. These studies documented the severe effects of massive trauma like anxiety, depression, paranoia, and personality change (Benshein and Die, 1960; Klein, 1974). A recent survey with young immigrants in California found a high level of exposure to pre- as well as post-migration violence (Jaycox *et al.*, 2002). Thirty-two percent of these immigrants reported clinical levels of PTSD symptoms. These levels of exposure and symptoms are comparable with those found in migrant groups from Kosovo (Turner *et al.*, 2003; Roth *et al.*, 2006), Bosnia (Mollica *et al.*, 2001; Sundquist *et al.*, 2005), Tamils (Silove *et al.*, 1997, 2002, 2007; Steel *et al.*, 2002), Afghanistan (Kalafi *et al.*, 2002), Korea (Lee *et al.*, 2001), Vietnam (Steel *et al.*, 2004), Cambodia (Cheung, 1994; Rousseau *et al.*, 2003), Burma (Allden *et al.*, 1996), Bhutan (Mills *et al.*, 2008), Middle East (Lindencrona *et al.*, 2008), Ethiopia (Finklestein and Solomon, 2009), Somalia (Bhui *et al.*, 2003), Senegal (Tang and Fox, 2001), Sierra Leone (Fox and Tang, 2000), West Nile (Neuner *et al.*, 2004), or Mexico (Heileman *et al.*, 2005) (Table 3.1).

An overview of these studies shows remarkable differences of the risk for depression, anxiety disorder, and PTSD in refugees. This might depend

Table 3.1 Selected studies on prevalence rates for depression, anxiety disorder, or post-traumatic stress disorder in refugees

Authors (year)	Host country	Country of origin	Prevalence rates in %
Allden et al. (2007)	Thailand	Burma	Depression: 16% Anxiety: 17%
Bhui et al. (2003)	UK	Somalia	Depression and/or anxiety: 24%
Fox, Tang (2000)	Gambia	Sierra Leone	Depression: 49% Anxiety: 80% PTSD: 86%
Kalafi et al. (2002)	Iran	Afghanistan	Depression and/or anxiety: 35%
Lee et al. (2001)	China	Korea	Depression: 81% Anxiety: 90% PTSD: 18%
Marshall et al. (2005)	USA	Cambodia	Depression: 51% PTSD: 62%
Mollica et al. (1993)	Thailand	Cambodia	Depression: 55% PTSD: 15%
Mollica et al. (1999)	Croatia	Bosnia	Depression: 39% PTSD: 26%
Roth et al. (2006)	Sweden	Kosovo	PTSD: 36%
Sabin et al. (2003)	Mexico	Guatemala	Depression: 39% Anxiety: 54% PTSD: 13%
Schweitzer et al. (2006)	Australia	Sudan	Depression: 13% PTSD: 13%
Steel et al. (2002)	Australia	Vietnam	Depression: 3% Anxiety: 5% PTSD: 4%
Sundquist et al. (2005)	Sweden	Bosnia	PTSD: 28%
Tang, Fox (2001)	Gambia	Senegal	Depression: 59% Anxiety: 47% PTSD: 10%
Turner et al. (2003)	UK	Kosovo	Depression: 62% Anxiety: 57% PTSD: 68%

not only on methodological issues, but also on the differences in the burden with traumatic experiences and culture specific strategies to cope with extreme stress. According to de Jong (2007) the collective dimension of culture represents schemes that give meaning to processes of suffering, healing, and reconciliation after severe traumatic experiences. A further factor that might be associated with an increased risk for depression, anxiety disorders, and PTSD seems to be the cultural distance between the country of origin and the host country.

Empirical part

To explore the impact of some of these pre-migration factors on the development of different mental disorders, we evaluated the data of the outpatient facility of the Department for Psychiatry of the Medical University of Vienna. The data were consecutively collected between 1995 and 2007. All patients had been investigated by one of the authors. They were classified according to ICD-10 and DSM-IV. SCID-1 and CroCuDoc, an instrument for the acquisition of sociocultural data and of data related to traumatic experiences and migration, were administered, if necessary, with the support of professional interpreters.

The composition of the sample

The sample finally comprised 1,771 subjects (856 male, 915 female; age: 35.6 ± 10.5 yrs; age with migration: 24.8 ± 10.8 yrs) from 93 countries. These countries from all five continents were pooled into eight geo-cultural regions of origin. Ninety three migrants of the 2nd generation represented an additional part of the sample (Fig. 3.1).

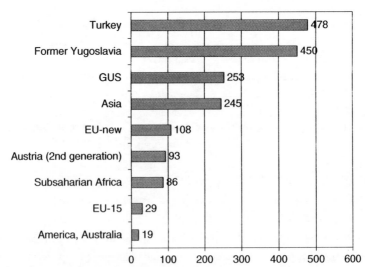

Fig. 3.1 Region of origin of migrants treated in the transcultural psychiatric outpatient facility, Vienna, between 1995 and 2007 (N = 1,771).

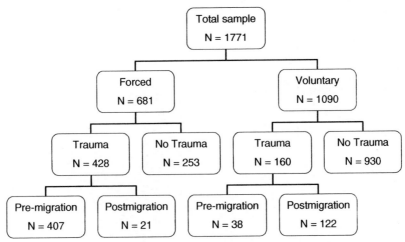

Fig. 3.2 Trauma and migration motives.

Most patients came from Turkey (N = 488), followed by migrants from former Yugoslavia and the states of the former USSR (GUS), most of them from civil war regions like Chechnya. This is not consistent with the Austrian resident population where Turkish are only the third biggest ethnic group behind migrants from former Yugoslavia and Germany. Two hundred and forty-five patients came from Asia, 86 from Sub-Saharan Africa, 137 from the EU, 29 of them from one of the EU-15 states and only 19 came from America or Australia (Fig. 3.2). We distinguished 681 (38.5%) forced and 1090 (61.5%) voluntary migrants, most of them labour migrants (N = 812). The others were students, family members of labour migrants, and tourists.

We further distinguished migrants with and without traumatic experiences. As expected, forced migrants were more often exposed to traumatic situations than voluntary migrants (N = 428), most of them in the pre-migration stage (N = 407). But 160 (14.7%) subjects of the voluntary migrant group reported traumatic experiences too, 122 of them of the stage of post-migration, only 38 of the tome before migration.

Motives of migration, region of origin, and diagnoses

Schizophrenia was statistically significantly overrepresented in voluntary migrants and neurotic disorders in forced migrants. Neurotic disorders were classified in 617 (34.8%) patients; 1154 (65.2%) of the cases fulfilled the criteria of a mood disorder, 214 (12.1%) of a primary or comorbid personality disorder, 169 (9.5%) of schizophrenia, 89 (5%) of a substance abuse disorder (first or comorbid diagnosis), 57 (3.2%) of an organic mental disorder, 55 (3.1%) and only 9 (0.5%) of a mental retardation (Table 3.2).

Table 3.2 Diagnoses (1st + 2nd + 3rd diagnoses) and migration motives with migrants (N = 1.771; multiple diagnoses are possible)

	F0 (n = 57)	F1 (n = 89)	F2 (n = 169)	F3 (n = 306)	F4 (n = 1154)	F5 (n = 55)	F6 (n = 214)	F7 (n = 9)
Forced migration (n = 681)	3.7%	4.7%	7.2%	15.6%	76.2%	2.9%	12.9%	0.3%
Voluntary migration (n = 1.090)	2.9%	5.2%	11.0%	18.3%	58.3%	3.2%	10.7%	0.6%
p	0.408	0.656	0.008	0.138	0.000	0.780	0.178	0.452

ICD-10: F.00–F09 = Organic, including symptomatic, mental disorders; F10–F19 = Mental and behavioural disorders due to psychoactive substance use; F20–29 = Schizophrenia, schizotypal and delusional disorders; F30–39 = Mood (affective) disorders; F40–49 = Neurotic, stress-related, and somatoform disorders; F50–69 = Behavioural syndromes associated with physiological disturbances and physical factors; F60–69 = Disorders of adult personality and behaviour; F70–79 = Mental retardation.

Chi-Square Test.

To further explore the impact of culture on the development of distinct mental diseases, we divided the forced and the voluntary migrant groups according to the region of origin (Table 3.3). With the exception of migrants from the new EU countries, the rates of organic mental disorder were more or less equally distributed. Forced migrants from the new EU states (former Eastern Bloc countries) showed a typical mental health profile with high prevalence of organic mental disorders, substance abuse disorders, and personality disorders.

Voluntary migrants from countries with a large Muslim population had a lower prevalence of substance abuse disorders than patients from countries with a Christian majority (GUS states, EU 15, Africa, and America). With the exception of Turkish migrants, all voluntary migrants had an increased risk for schizophrenia compared with forced migrants. Voluntary migrants from former Yugoslavia, former USSR, and Asia showed higher rates of affective disorders compared to forced migrants from these regions, as well as with voluntary migrants from other regions of origin.

The highest prevalence of neurotic disorders was found in forced migrants from Asia and Sub-Saharan Africa. As mentioned earlier, independent of the migrant status migrants from the new EU countries, the former Eastern bloc states, showed the highest rates of personality disorders. As behavioural syndromes associated with physiological disturbances and mental retardation were so infrequent, we didn't expect to find distinct cultural differences.

Pre-migration traumas

Four hundred and forty-five patients (407 forced, 38 voluntary migrants) reported traumatic stress in their native countries. Of them, 63.4% experienced two or more of situations like war or torture; 11.3% had been traumatized by having observed violence against others; 10% were victims by the police, military, or paramilitary and organized criminality; 5.5% were victims of rape; 2.3% of family violence (Fig. 3.3).

Traumatic stress in the pre-migration stage was associated with higher rates of neurotic disorders and with lower rates of schizophrenia, affective disorders, and behavioural symptoms associated with physiological disturbances (Fig. 3.4).

As expected, traumatized migrants showed a high prevalence rate for stress-related disorders (Fig. 3.5); 32.3% fulfilled the diagnosis of an adjustment disorder; 30.7% of PTSD; and 9.3% of an enduring personality change (Fig. 3.5).

Table 3.3 Migration motives, region of origin, and diagnoses (1st + 2nd + 3rd diagnoses); multiple diagnoses are possible (N = 1.771)

Forced	F0	F1	F2	F3	F4	F5	F6	F7
Turkey	2.0%	2.0%	10.2%	16.3%	73.5%	2.0%	12.2%	–
Ex-Yugos.	1.9%	3.8%	3.2%	13.2%	75.3%	2.5%	7.6%	1.3%
GUS	4.1%	3.2%	3.2%	13.2%	75.3%	2.7%	8.7%	–
Asia	1.3%	6.3%	9.4%	12.6%	80.5%	2.0%	11.9%	–
EU – new	21.1%	10.5%	13.2%	31.6%	47.4%	3.1%	26.3%	–
Africa	3.7%	5.6%	3.7%	23.4%	85.2%	3.7%	9.3%	–
p	0.000	0.032	0.112	0.063	0.001	0.990	0.008	0.476

Voluntary	F0	F1	F2	F3	F4	F5	F6	F7
Turkey	1.8%	2.3%	7.3%	15.7%	61.0%	2.1%	11.8%	–
Ex-Yugos.	3.8%	5.5%	10.3%	22.9%	64.0%	4.1%	14.3%	–
GUS	2.9%	11.8%	8.8%	26.5%	61.8%	5.9%	12.0%	0.7%
Asia	3.5%	4.7%	15.1%	22.1%	60.5%	7.0%	12.1%	0.5%
EU – new	5.7%	4.3%	21.4%	15.7%	54.3%	1.4%	20.9%	–
2nd generation	3.3%	11.0%	13.2%	11.0%	39.6%	2.2%	8.8%	1.1%
Africa	3.1%	15.6%	21.9%	12.5%	46.9%	9.4%	20.1%	2.3%
EU-15	1.7%	10.3%	17.2%	24.1%	37.9%	–	–	–
America	5.9%	11.8%	17.6%	23.5%	41.2%	–	12.5%	–
p	0.662	0.001	0.005	0.089	0.000	0.089	0.356	0.698

ICD-10: F.00–F09 = Organic, including symptomatic, mental disorders; F10–F19 = Mental and behavioural disorders due to psychoactive substance use; F20–29 = Schizophrenia, schizotypal and delusional disorders; F30–39 = Mood [affective] disorders; F40–49 = Neurotic, stress-related, and somatoform disorders; F50–69 = Behavioural syndromes associated with physiological disturbances and physical factors; F60–69 = Disorders of adult personality and behaviour; F70–79 = Mental retardation.

Chi-Square Test.

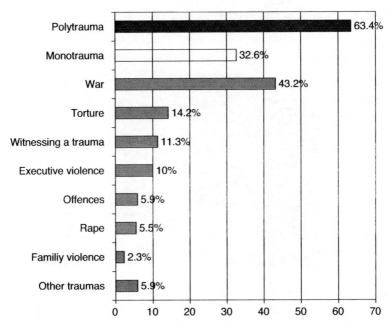

Fig. 3.3 Type of pre-migration trauma (N = 445).

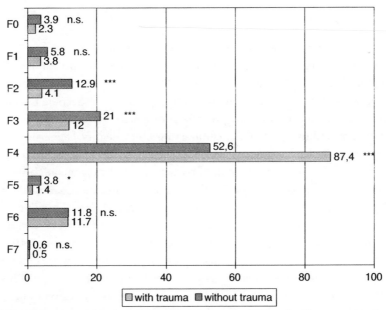

Fig. 3.4 Diagnoses of patients without traumas (n = 978) and with a pre-migration trauma (n = 423).

ICD-10: F.00–F09 = Organic, including symptomatic, mental disorders; F10–F19 = Mental and behavioural disorders due to psychoactive substance use; F20–29 = Schizophrenia, schizotypal and delusional disorders; F30–39 = Mood [affective] disorders; F40–49 = Neurotic, stress-related, and somatoform disorders; F50–69 = Behavioural syndromes associated with physiological disturbances and physical factors; F60–69 = Disorders of adult personality and behaviour; F70–79 = Mental retardation.

Chi-Square Test; * p <0.05; ** p <0.01; *** p < 0.001.

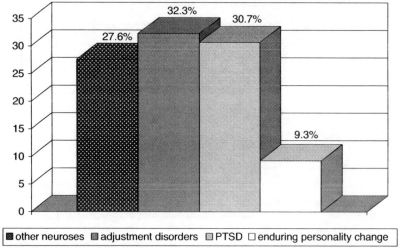

Fig. 3.5 Stress-related disorders and other neurotic and somatoform disorders in patients with reported pre-migration traumas.

Conclusions

The process of migration is not a homogenous phase in human life. Post-migration factors like positive or negative life events in the host country, the cultural distance, or bereavement issues related to the loss of relationship, of social support, and of social and professional prestige may become relevant. The factors associated with the pre-migration phase are difficult to narrow down, because most of them (like cultural values and identity, personality, and cognitive skills) are important to cope with the new situation in the host country too. The first and perhaps most important step is the distinction between voluntary and forced migrants. But also within these two groups, migrants of different origin have different vulnerabilities for distinct mental health problems. One of the most important results is the fact that the high prevalence of schizophrenia in migrants described in literature (e.g. Selten *et al.*, 2001) is mainly caused by voluntary migrants. In contrast, migrants with stressful pre-migration experiences exhibit higher rates of neurotic disorders, especially of stress-related disorders like PTSD. Our data show that the region of origin also plays a decisive role. Additional research is necessary for a better understanding of the impact of factors like cultural identity and personality, illness concepts, and culture-specific coping style for the vulnerability or resilience of migrants.

References

Allden, K., Poole, C., Chantavanich, S., Ohmar, K., Aung, N.N., and Mollica, R.F. (1996). Burmese political dissidents in Thailand: Trauma and survival among young adults in exile. *American Journal of Public Health* **86**: 1561–1569.

Assmann, J.(1988). Kollektives Gedächtnis und kulturelle Identität. In J. Assmann (Ed), *Hölscher T. Kultur und Gedächtnis.* pp. 9–19, Frankfurt am Main: Suhrkamp.

Bangirana, P., Idro, R., John, C.C., and Boivin, M.J. (2006). Rehabilitation for cognitive impairments after cerebral malaria in African children: Strategies and limitations. *Tropical Medicine and International Health* **11**: 1341–1349.

Benshein, H. and Die, K.Z. (1960). Neurose der rassischen Verfolgten: Ein eintrag zur psychopathologie der neurosen. *Der Nervenarzt* **31**: 462–469.

Bhugra, D. (2003). Migration and depression. *Acta Psychiatrica Scandinavia Supplementum* **418**: 67–72.

Bhui, K., Abdi, A., Abdi, M., *et al.* (2003). Traumatic events, migration characteristics and psychiatric symptoms among Somali refugees—preliminary communication. *Social Psychiatry and Psychiatric Epidemiology* **38**: 35–43.

Cantor-Graae, E. and Selten, J. (2005). Schizophrenia and migration: A meta-analysis and review. *American Journal of Psychiatry* **162**: 12–24.

Cavalli-Sforza, L.L., Menozzi, P., and Piazza, A. (1994). *The History and Geography of Human Genes.* Princeton University Press.

Cheung, P. (1994). Posttraumatic stress disorder among Cambodian refugees in New Zealand. *International Journal of Social Psychiatry* **40**: 17–26.

Cochrane, R. and Bal, S. Migration and schizophrenia: An examination of five hypotheses. *Social Psychiatry* **22**: 181–191.

Cooper, C., Morgan, C., Byrne, M., *et al.* (2008). Perceptions of disadvantage, ethnicity and psychosis. *British Journal of Psychiatry* **192**: 185–190.

Cross, S.E. (1995). Self-construals, coping, and stress in cross-cultural adaptation. *Journal of Cross-Cultural Psychology* **26**(6): 673–697.

de Jong, J. (2007). Traumascape: an ecological-cultural-historical model for extreme stress. In D. Bhugra and K. Bhui (Eds.), *Textbook of Cultural Psychiatry* pp. 347–363, Cambridge: Cambridge University Press.

Fazel, M., Wheeler, J., and Danesh, J. (2005). Prevalence of serious mental disorder in 7000 refugees resettled in western countries: A systematic review. *Lancet* **36**: 1309–1314.

Fearon, P., Kirkbride, J.B., Morgan, C., *et al.* (2006). Incidence of schizophrenia and other psychoses in ethnic minority groups: Results from the MRC AESOP study. *Psychological Medicine* **36**: 1541–1550.

Finklestein, M. and Solomon, Z. (2009). Cumulative trauma, PTSD and dissociation among Ethiopian refugees in Israel. *Journal of Trauma Dissociation* **10**: 38–56.

Fox, S.H. and Tang S.S. (2000). The Sierra Leonean refugee experience: Traumatic events and psychiatric sequelae. *Journal of Nervous and Mental Disorders* **188**: 490–495.

Harrison, G., Glazebrook, C., Brewin, J., *et al.* (1997). Increased incidence of psychotic disorders in migrants from the Caribbean to the United Kingdom. *Psychological Medicine* **27**: 799–806.

Heilemann, M.V., Kury, F.S., and Lee, K.A. (2005). Trauma and posttraumatic stress disorder symptoms among low income women of Mexican descent in the United States. *Journal of Nervous and Mental Disorders* **193**: 665–672.

Hutchinson, G. and Haasen, C. (2004). Migration and schizophrenia. *Social Psychiatry and Psychiatric Epidemiology* **39**: 350–357.

Jaycox, L.H., Stein, B.D., Kataoka, S.H., *et al.* (2002). Violence exposure, posttraumatic stress disorder, and depressive symptoms among recent immigrant schoolchildren. *Journal of American Academy of Child Adolescence Psychiatry* **41**: 1104–1110.

Kalafi, Y., Hagh-Shenas, H., and Ostovar, A. (2002). Mental health among Afghan refugees settled in Shiraz, Iran. *Psychological Reports* **90**: 262–266.

Klein, H. (1974). Delayed effects and after-effects of severe traumatization. *Israel Annals of Psychiatry* **12**: 293–303.

Kroeber, A.L. and Kluckhohn, C. (1952). *Culture: A Critical Review of Concepts and Definitions.* New York: Vintage Books.

Lee, Y., Lee, M.K., Chun, K.H., and Yoon, S.J. (2001). Trauma experience of North Korean refugees in China. *American Journal of Preventive Medicine* **20**: 225–229.

Lindencrona, F., Ekblad, S., and Hauff, E. (2008). Mental health of recently resettled refugees from the Middle East in Sweden: The impact of pre-resettlement trauma, resettlement stress and capacity to handle stress. *Social Psychiatry and Psychiatric Epidemiology* **43**: 121–131.

Markus, H.R. and Kitayama, S. (1991). Culture and self: Implications for cognition, emotion, and motivation. *Psychological Review* **98**: 224–253.

Marshall, G.N., Schell, T.L., Elliott, M.N., Berthold, S.M., and Chun, C.A. (2005). Mental health of Cambodian refugees 2 decades after resettlement in the United States. *Journal of American Medical Association* **294**(5): 571–579.

Mills, E., Singh, S., Roach, B., and Chong S. (2008). Prevalence of mental disorders and torture among Bhutanese refugees in Nepal: A systemic review and its policy implications. *Medicine, Conflict, and Survival* **24**: 5–15.

Mollica, R.F., Donelan, K., Tor, S., *et al.* (1993). The effect of trauma and confinement on functional health and mental health status of Cambodians living in Thailand–Cambodia border camps. *Journal of American Medical Association* **270**: 581–586.

Mollica, R.F., Sarajlic, N., Chernoff, M., Lavelle, J., Vukovic, I.S., and Massagli, M.P. (2001). Longitudinal study of psychiatric symptoms, disability, mortality, and emigration among Bosnian refugees. *Journal of American Medical Association* **286**: 546–554.

Mung'Ala-Odera, V., Snow, R.W., and Newton, C.R. (2004). The burden of the neurocognitive impairment associated with plasmodium falciparum malaria in Sub-Saharan Africa. *American Journal of Tropical Medicine and Hygiene* **71**(2 Suppl): 64–70.

Neuner, F., Schauer, M., Karunakara, U., Klaschik, C., Robert, C., and Elbert, T. (2004). Psychological trauma and evidence for enhanced vulnerability for posttraumatic stress disorder through previous trauma among West Nile refugees. *Biomedical Central Psychiatry* **4**: 34.

Ödegaard, Ö. (1932). Emigration and insanity: A study of mental disease among the Norwegian-born population of Minnesota. *Acta Psychiatrica et Neurologica Scandinavica* **4**: 1–206.

Patel, V. and Kleinman, A. (2003). Poverty and common mental disorders in developing countries. *Bull World Health Organization* **81**: 609–615.

Roth, G., Ekblad, S., and Agren, H. (2006). A longitudinal study of PTSD in a sample of adult mass-evacuated Kosovars, some of whom returned to their home country. *European Psychiatry* **21**(3): 152–159.

Rousseau, C., Drapeau, A., and Rahimi, S. (2003). The complexity of trauma response: A 4-year follow-up of adolescent Cambodian refugees. *Child Abuse and Negligence* **27**: 1277–1290.

Rumble, S., Swartz, L., Parry, C., and Zwarenstein, M. (1996). Prevalence of psychiatric morbidity in the adult population of a rural South African village. *Psychological Medicine* **26**: 997–1007.

Sabin, M., Lopes Cardozo, B., Nackerud, L., Kaiser, R., and Varese, L. (2003). Factors associated with poor mental health among Guatemalan refugees living in Mexico 20 years after civil conflict. *Journal of American Medical Association* **290**: 635–642.

Schweitzer, R., Melville, F., Steel, Z., and Lacherez, P. (2006). Trauma, post-migration living difficulties, and social support as predictors of psychological adjustment in resettled Sudanese refugees. *Australia and New Zealand Journal of Psychiatry* **40**: 179–187.

Selten, J.P., Veen, N., Feller, W., et al. (2001). Incidence of psychotic disorders in immigrant groups to The Netherlands. *British Journal of Psychiatry* **78**: 367–372.

Sharpley, M., Hutchinson, G., McKenzie, K., and Murray, R.M. (2001). Understanding the excess of psychosis among the African-Caribbean population in England. Review of current hypotheses. *British Journal of Psychiatry Supplement* **40**: s60–s68.

Silove, D., Sinnerbrink, I., Field, A., Manicavasagar, V., and Steel, Z. (1997). Anxiety, depression and PTSD in asylum-seekers: Assocations with pre-migration trauma and post-migration stressors. *British Journal of Psychiatry* **170**: 351–357.

Silove, D., Steel, Z., McGorry, P., Miles, V., and Drobny, J. (2002). The impact of torture on post-traumatic stress symptoms in war-affected Tamil refugees and immigrants. *Comprehensive Psychiatry* **43**: 49–55.

Silove, D., Steel, Z., Susljik, I., et al. (2007). The impact of the refugee decision on the trajectory of PTSD, anxiety, and depressive symptoms among asylum seekers: A longitudinal study. *American Journal of Disaster Medicine* **2**: 321–329.

Steel, Z., Momartin, S., Bateman, C., et al. (2002). Psychiatric status of asylum seeker families held for a protracted period in a remote detention centre in Australia. *Australia and New Zealand Journal of Public Health* **28**: 527–536.

Steel, Z., Silove, D., Bird, K., McGorry, P., and Mohan, P. (2004). Pathways from war trauma to posttraumatic stress symptoms among Tamil asylum seekers, refugees, and immigrants. *Journal of Trauma Stress* **12**: 421–435.

Steel, Z., Silove, D., Phan, T., and Bauman, A. (2002). Long-term effect of psychological trauma on the mental health of Vietnamese refugees resettled in Australia: A population-based study. *Lancet* **360**: 1056–1062.

Sundquist, K., Johansson, L.M., DeMarinis, V., Johansson, S.E., and Sundquist, J. (2005). Posttraumatic stress disorder and psychiatric co-morbidity: Symptoms in a random sample of female Bosnian refugees. *European Psychiatry* **20**(2): 158–164.

Swinnen, S.G. and Selten, J.P. (2007). Mood disorders and migration: Meta-analysis. *British Journal of Psychiatry* **190**: 6–10.

Tang, S.S. and Fox, S.H. (2001). Traumatic experiences and the mental health of Senegalese refugees. *Journal of Nervous and Mental Disorders* **18**: 507–512.

Triandis, H.C. and Suh, E.M. (2002). Cultural influences on personality. *Annual Review Psychology* **53**: 133–160.

Turner, S.W., Bowie, C., Dunn, G., Shapo, L., and Yule, W. (2003). Mental health of Kosovan Albanian refugees in the UK. *British Journal of Psychiatry* **182**: 444–448.

Tweed, R.G. and Lehman, D.R. (2002). Learning considered within a cultural context: Confucian and socratic approaches. *American Psychology* **57**: 89–99.

Tweed, R.G., White, K., and Lehman, D.R. (2004). Culture, stress, and coping internally- and externally-targeted control strategies of european Canadians, East Asian Canadians, and Japanese. *Journal of Cross-Cultural Psychology* **35**: 652–668.

Weber, M. (1972). Ethnische gemeinschaftsbeziehungen. In M. Weber (Hrsg.) *Wirtschaft und Gesellschaft*, pp. 234–240. Tübingen: Mohr Siebeck.

Chapter 4

Post-migration and mental health: the Australian experience

Helen Herrman, Ida Kaplan, and
Josef Szwarc

Introduction

Inequities in health, avoidable health inequalities, arise because of the circumstances
in which people grow, live, work and age, and the systems put in place to deal with
illness. The conditions in which people live and die are, in turn, shaped by political,
social and economic forces.

(CSDH, 2008)

Mental health post-migration and its social determinants are topics of political
and social importance in many countries. In this chapter we consider post
migration experiences and mental health in its full sense, covering the spectrum from mental disorders to mental health and well-being. We consider the
mental health of people who have left their country of origin to reside in
another country, either as 'asylum seekers' who have asked the government to
recognize them formally as refugees and permit them to settle, or as recognized
refugees with permission to remain in the country of settlement.

We refer to the Australian experience over the last two decades to illustrate
several positive and adverse aspects of life post-migration. The Australian
experience is pertinent to the treatment of asylum seekers who arrive with or
without prior authorization, and the treatment of 'resettled refugees', people
selected in overseas locations by the government in consultation with the
United Nations High Commissioner for Refugees (UNHCR). Although the
number of asylum seekers in Australia has been relatively small their arrival
has provoked political and social controversy and harsh policies associated
with adverse effects on mental health. Examples include mandatory detention
for unauthorized arrivals, denial of employment rights and restriction of other
entitlements for many asylum seekers residing in the community, and the
granting of refugee status for temporary periods. There are similar policies

in place elsewhere in the world. In contrast, Australia has one of the world's largest resettlement programmes per capita and the government conducts and funds a number of programmes that aim to promote the physical, mental, and material well-being of resettled refugees. Those programmes include the provision of specialized counselling services and language tuition. In this chapter we consider the implications for mental health of several of these policies and programmes and their relevance to the experience of refugees and asylum seekers in other countries.

The social determinants of mental health

Mental health is described in various ways in an extensive literature, in terms of a positive emotion such as feelings of happiness, as a set of positive attributes that include the psychological resources of self-esteem and mastery, and as resilience or the capacity to cope with adversity (Kovess-Masfety, Murray, and Gureje, 2005). Mental health is defined by WHO (2007) as 'a state of well-being in which the individual realizes his or her own abilities, can cope with the normal stresses of life, can work productively and fruitfully, and is able to contribute to his or her community'. In this positive sense mental health has value as a personal and community resource.

Mental and physical health, and social and economic development are closely interrelated in all populations. Interventions that improve mental health may be expected to improve overall health, quality of life, and social functioning, benefits manifesting as better educational performance, greater productivity of workers, improved relationships within families, and safer communities (Herrman, Saxena, and Moodie 2005; Barry and Jenkins, 2007; Friedl, 2009).

Mental health can be improved through the promotion of health, the prevention of illness and disability, and the treatment and rehabilitation of those affected by mental illness. Activities and strategies can vary according to the type of improvement or outcomes sought but all are required and they complement one another. Mental health promotion refers to improving the mental health of everybody in the community, including those with no experience of mental illness as well as those who live with illness and disability. Like health promotion, mental health promotion involves actions that (1) support people to adopt and maintain healthy ways of life and (2) create living conditions and environments that allow or foster health.

Poor mental health is associated with socially disadvantaged and vulnerable groups of people with experience of poverty, discrimination, violence, and the denial of civil, economic, and social rights. The WHO's Commission on the Social Determinants of Health describes how together the structural determinants and conditions of daily life are responsible for a major part of health inequalities between and within countries (CSDH, 2008, p.1). The Commission relates the poor health of disadvantaged people to the immediate circumstances of their lives, their access to health care, schools, and education, their conditions of work and leisure, and their homes, communities, towns, or cities. In addition, the way that society is organized, the extent to which social interaction is encouraged, and the degree to which people trust and associate with each other are critically important determinants of health (CDSH, 2008; Lomas, 1998). The Victorian Health Promotion Foundation (VicHealth) has identified similar determinants of mental health, namely, the importance of social connections, freedom from violence and discrimination, and social participation (VicHealth, 2007; Walker, Verins, Moodie, and Webster, 2005). The civil, cultural, economic, political, and social dimensions of human rights underscore the need for action and involvement of a wide range of sectors in promoting mental health among vulnerable groups (Drew, Funk, Pathare, and Swartz, 2005).

In the case of refugees and asylum seekers, a similar analysis of determinants is warranted. Some are the legacy of pre-migration experiences and others are related to the legal, political, social, and economic context in which they and their families live in the post-migration situation. A review of the research worldwide identifies the role of enduring contextual factors before and after displacement as moderators of mental ill health among the world's refugees and asylum seekers (Porter and Haslam, 2005). Studies of asylum seekers also show that the context of a long asylum seeking process is associated with higher prevalence of psychopathology as well as lower quality of life, higher disability, and poorer physical health (Thomas and Lau, 2002; Laban, Komproe, Gernaat, and de Jong, 2008). Notably there is very little in the research literature about broader contextual factors such as the political environment and government policy as social determinants.

The following section provides a brief overview of factors affecting the mental health of refugees in their countries of origin, before their flight from persecution, and en route to the countries where they will seek asylum and permanent residence. The chapter then examines in turn the responses of the government, of service providers, and of civil society to asylum seekers and refugees in Australia. It describes how some responses have been detrimental to the mental health of asylum seekers and refugees, whereas others have been beneficial to their well-being.

Pre-migration factors affecting mental health

Having originated from conflict zones around the world, people from refugee backgrounds will have been exposed to a range of factors that have an adverse impact on their mental health. (US Committee for Refugees, 2001; Amnesty International, 2009) The lives of refugees have been characterized by extensive exposure to traumatic experiences such as political persecution, torture and other forms of violence, and human rights abuses. Protective factors such as relationships to significant caregivers have been disrupted by the death of family members and the systematic breakdown of family and community through rape and other atrocities. Protracted periods of displacement are characteristic. During displacement, populations have been deprived of adequate nutrition, health, education, and basic security. Refugees both originate from and seek asylum in some of the poorest countries in the world where lack of access to health care and education are long-term conditions. The experiences of refugees are therefore different from those of migrants who typically choose to leave their country and are increasingly selected by settlement countries for their skills and resources (see also Chapter 3).

There are several ways in which pre-arrival experiences and their effects persist long after arrival in a safe country, affecting some survivors for many years (Kinzie, Frederickson, Ben, and Karis, 1984; Simpson, 1993). The mechanisms for these long-term effects may operate at the individual, community, and societal levels. Mental symptoms and disorders that result from pre-arrival experiences of torture and traumatic experiences can interfere with meeting the challenges and demands of settlement. For example, post-traumatic stress disorder symptoms such as poor concentration and flashbacks can interfere with the important task of learning English (Allender, 1998). Similarly, social withdrawal associated with avoidance of fear-evoking situations or depression can serve as a barrier to survivors forming supportive relationships in the community or interacting with government, housing or employment authorities.

Other psychological mechanisms include the internalization of helplessness and loss of control (Kaplan and Webster, 2003), grief associated with the loss of family members, home, and community (Van der Veer, 1998; Kinzie, Boehnlein, and Sack, 1998), and guilt about family members remaining in difficult circumstances overseas (Jaques and Abbott, 1997).

In addition to affecting individual survivors, the refugee experience can undermine cohesion and supportive relationships within families and communities and these effects can persist well into the settlement period (Westermeyer, 1986). Effects can also persist across generations (Kuch and Cox, 1992; Estinger, 1973). The importance of family cohesion and continuity in relationships has long been recognized in the general body of psychological literature as having a major impact on functioning in emotional, cognitive, and social domains (Cook, Blaustein, Spinazzola, and van der Kolk, 2003). There is relatively little research on the effects on mental health of loss or history of instability in family relationships of people of refugee background. War-affected Lebanese children who experienced separation from their parents showed more depression than those without this experience (Macksoud and Aber, 1996), Other studies (Green, Korol, Grace, *et al.*, 1991; Punamaki, 2001) report that parental capacity and family cohesion are as important or more important than direct exposure to traumatic events in predicting the severity of post-traumatic stress reactions in young children.

It is also important to recognize the impact of pre-arrival experiences of violence, loss, and displacement on communities. Refugees who settle in Western countries can easily be thought of as belonging to a single community based on their country of origin. In fact there are multiple communities and often factions resulting from pre-arrival conflict. Furthermore, the aim of oppressive regimes is to destroy communities and most refugees have arrived from situations where the community has not functioned as such in a long time. They have been forced to occupy a position of dependence and their leadership has been dispersed. In many countries, weapons of violence such as rape have been used to deliberately destroy communities through destruction of the family (VFST, 1998).

Post-migration factors affecting mental health

Government policies

The response of governments to concerns about uncontrolled migration has highlighted the critical role of both government policy and the responses of civil society to fostering an environment that is either damaging or conducive to mental health. Several countries, including Australia, have adopted polices of deterrence including restrictive measures on persons seeking asylum (Silove, Steel, and Watters, 2000). In contrast, civil society in many countries has played a role in moderating restrictive policies and practices, due in part to the recognition of their adverse effects on mental health (Fazel and Silove, 2006). Understanding the social determinants of mental health is relevant to those developing public policies and programmes dealing with asylum seekers and refugees. It is important that they be aware not only of the need to provide services to address mental health problems arising from pre-migration experiences but also of the inadvertent impact that policies such as detention and denial of adequate welfare can have (also see Chapter 5).

Detention of asylum seekers

In 1986, the states comprising the Executive Committee (ExCom) of the UNHCR adopted a resolution expressing concern that many refugees and asylum seekers around the world were subject to detention (UNHCR).

according to ExCom, 'in view of the hardship which it involves, detention should normally be avoided' (UNHCR, 1986). Despite this, detention is common. Although there are significant differences between detention regimes, as in the legal frameworks and the conditions, there is substantial evidence that the very fact of detention, particularly for extended and uncertain periods, can be harmful to mental health. The case of Australia is a striking illustration.

In response to concerns about the possible arrival of large numbers of asylum seekers, in 1992 Australia introduced a policy of 'mandatory detention' of people who landed without authorization.[1] More than 15,000 unauthorized boat arrivals were detained in the period to the end of 2008, including many children (HREOC, 2004). People who are assessed as being refugees are promptly released but there is no time limit on detention and the process of finalizing applications can take years.

A recent review of studies on the effects of detention on mental health reported that detention is deleterious to mental health (Robjant, Hassan, and Katona, 2009). The extent of mental ill health was correlated with the length of time spent in detention (Sultan and O'Sullivan, 2001; Physicians for Human Rights and the Bellevue/NYU Program for Survivors of Torture, 2003; Eagar, Green, Jones et al., 2007). Immigration detention has been found to contribute to levels of PTSD (Ichikawa, Nakahara, and Wakai, 2006; Momartin, Steel, Coello, Aroche, Silove, and Brooks, 2006; Steel, Silove, Brooks, Momartin, Alzuhairi, and Susljik, 2006), depression (Ichikawa et al., 2006; Steel et al., 2006), and anxiety (Ichikawa et al., 2006).

Asylum seekers in the community

The Australian government has imposed a number of restrictions on the entitlements of certain asylum seekers residing in the community while their claims for recognition are resolved. These include prohibitions on working, denial of access to social security benefits and to free or subsidized medical treatment and medicine. The restrictions have left many asylum seekers destitute and reliant on charity, circumstances adverse to their physical and mental well-being. According to one Australian study, 'the conditions appear to be exacerbating pre-existing medical conditions and generating new ones. This is particularly the case in terms of mental health' (Network of Asylum Seeker Agencies, 2005).

---

[1] The policy applies to all people without visas, including those who entered the country with authorization and whose visas expired or were cancelled.

An inquiry into immigration detention and its alternatives conducted by a committee of Members of Parliament reported in 2009 that 'the harsh psychological burdens inflicted by long and indefinite periods of detention, as well restrictions on income, work and healthcare for community based… (applicants for asylum or other immigration visas)… is known to have harmful long term effects on all those involved' (Joint Standing Committee on Migration, 2009). The committee therefore recommended that the government ensure people awaiting resolution of their immigration status be provided with basic income assistance, health care, and permission to work. Following a lengthy review, in mid-2009 the government announced that it would introduce more flexible work rights arrangements for asylum seekers, which would also provide access to free or subsidized health care (Minister for Immigration and Citizenship, 2009).

Temporary visas

In order to discourage unauthorized asylum seekers, Australia in 1999 adopted a restrictive policy. If their refugee claims were accepted they would be granted temporary rather than permanent visas in the first instance and not permitted to sponsor family members to migrate to be reunited with them. In addition, their access to English language training and higher education was restricted.

The Australian policy was inappropriate according to the UNHCR. The concept of temporary protection of refugees was established 'as an exceptional emergency device to respond to an overwhelming situation, where there are self-evident protection needs, and little or no possibility to determine such needs on an individual basis in the short term' (UNHCR, 2000). Temporary protection regimes should not penalize refugees who arrive without proper documentation or otherwise discriminate between them, particularly when the refugees have been individually assessed as fulfilling the criteria of the Refugee Convention. Further, '(t)emporary protection granted following individual assessment should also not be an obstacle to the principle of family unity' (UNHCR, 2002a).

Australian refugees on temporary visas had sanctuary from persecution but the uncertainty of their status, ongoing separation from their families, and other factors such as a hostile media had deleterious effects on their well-being. A study comparing the mental health of refugees with temporary versus permanent visas found that the two groups had experienced similar levels of past trauma and persecution but the holders of temporary protection visas obtained higher scores on anxiety, depression, and PTSD symptoms (Momartin, Steel, Coello, Aroche, Silove, and Brooks, 2006).

A qualitative study on the long-term consequences of detention (Coffey, Kaplan, Sampson, and Tucci, 2010) reported that the temporary protection visa period effectively maintained people in a state of helplessness and hopelessness about the future and destroyed their identities as responsible family members. Following many representations by advocacy groups over an extended period, a new government in 2008 acknowledged the harmful effects of the policy and abolished it.

Family separation and reunification

Many refugees become separated from family members to whom they are attached when they flee from their countries of origin or during flight in search of safety. Separation may also be a consequence of the use of selection criteria for resettlement, when countries select 'families' based on definitions that are narrower in scope than the people with whom refugees are intimately connected.

Anxiety about the welfare of family members left behind in situations of danger and deprivation maintains a sense of helplessness and contributes to depression and long-term post-traumatic stress reactions (Rousseau, Mekki-Berrada et al., 2001; Lie, 2002). The impact on the individual's mental health can adversely affect their relationships and capacity for intimacy (VFST, 1998; Weine, Muzurovic et al., 2004). Conversely, the presence of family can be very beneficial to people who have survived traumatic experiences, by offering emotional, physical, and material support (Gorst-Unsworth and Goldenberg, 1998). There is also evidence that the presence of family helps people accomplish other settlement tasks (Shiferaw and Hagos, 2001; Bloch, 2002; Brahmbhatt, Atfield et al., 2007; Ong Hing, 2007).

UNHCR encourages countries to adopt a definition of family for the purposes of resettlement that respects 'culturally diverse interpretations of family members' and that includes 'persons who may be dependent on the family unit, particularly economically, but also socially or emotionally dependent' (UNHCR, 2008).

Australia's definition of the family unit at the point of selection for resettlement is broader than that of some other resettlement countries such as Canada and the USA though significantly narrower than the UNHCR model, for example by excluding people who are not related. In contrast, Canada's policy provides that 'those who do not meet the legal definition of a family member, but who are emotionally or economically dependent on the family unit may be included in the initial application for resettlement' (CIC, 2003).

Citizenship

Refugees are commonly keen to become citizens of the countries in which they have resettled because the rights and protections of that status provide a significant measure of security necessary to rebuild their lives. It is not surprising that they will look for 'political' security. Citizenship affords a sense of belonging and acceptance for people who have fled societies that rejected them.

In recent years a number of countries have made citizenship more difficult to acquire because of their concern that certain groups of immigrants are unwilling to adopt the values of the receiving society and want to retain separate identities. Some countries have adopted tests that require higher levels than previously of proficiency in the language of the resettlement country and assessments of knowledge of and commitment to the country's social and political values.

Australia imposed a new citizenship test in 2007 with a more demanding English language requirement and assessment of applicants' knowledge of Australian values, history, geography, economy, and other aspects. The government argued that the test was necessary to promote and encourage the integration of migrants from an increasingly diverse range of countries of origin. In the period leading up to the new test government ministers also expressed reservations about the long-standing commitment of the major political parties to the policy of multiculturalism. According to then Prime Minister Howard, maintenance of social cohesion was a key issue for Australia in the twenty first century, an issue which involved achieving a balance in questions of national identity and cultural diversity (Howard, 2006).

The new test was strongly opposed by many on a number of grounds, one of them being that the tougher language proficiency requirement was particularly difficult for refugees. For example, in the view of the Refugee Council of Australia, a peak organization of agencies involved with refugees:

> While many refugees are bilingual or multilingual, for some refugees learning English can be a very long and difficult process. There are a number of barriers that confront many refugees which distinguishes them from other migrants including: a limited or interrupted educational background due to armed conflict, forced displacement, the experience of flight and many years in refugee camps and countries of asylum; illiteracy or pre-literacy in their mother tongue which means that, while basic spoken English may be acquired over a period of time, complex English or functional written English may take many years to be attained; learning difficulties resulting from experience of torture and/or trauma.

> (Refugee Council of Australia, 2007)

Data on the implementation of the test confirmed the concerns of refugee advocates, showing that applicants who were refugees were far more likely to fail than other applicants (DIAC, 2009a). Following an independent review (Australian Citizenship Test Review Committee, 2008) the government announced that the test would be revised and, among other things, it would 'develop a citizenship course that will provide an alternative pathway to citizenship for refugees and disadvantaged or vulnerable migrants' (Australian Government 2008). A revised test was introduced in 2009.

Services

The health, education, and family service sectors play a crucial role in influencing whether the multiple and often complex needs of refugees and asylum seekers are responded to in a way that promotes mental health and well-being, prevents the development of mental health problems, and provides appropriate interventions when necessary (Department of Human Services, 2009). The service delivery area is also a traditional way in Australia of responding to disadvantage (Szoke, 2009). In Australia, national and state mental health plans have repeatedly called for improvements in service delivery noting the need for coordination across sectors and better responsiveness to needs at the individual, family and community levels. The role of government in providing funding and supporting strategies has been vital and in turn influenced from the ground up, by non-government and community based organizations. The following sections provide examples of services in Australia that have developed in response to the needs of refugees, most usually identified by NGOs that work closely with refugees and their communities. Strong advocacy, which has included representation on national committees aimed at promoting settlement outcomes and ongoing dialogue amongst government, non-government and community groups has led to the development of government funded programs that have grown in size over time.

Specialist services for survivors of torture and trauma

In Australia there is a network of eight agencies, one in each capital city, specialising in work with refugee survivors of torture and trauma (Forum of Australian Services for Survivors of Torture and Trauma, FASTT, 2006). As well as providing long term counselling, advocacy and complex case management to individuals and families, each agency has service capacity building programs to improve access to mainstream services, and community development programs to build the capacity of refugee communities. Training and consultations are provided to a range of health and community service professionals as Australian health and mental health care providers are not routinely trained to identify and deal with particular needs of refugees and asylum seekers. Agencies work with State and Federal governments through consultation and representation on advisory bodies to ensure that policies and services are responsive to the needs of refugees.

These specialist agencies are NGOs. Their services are based on a holistic approach to assisting refugee survivors of torture and trauma. Consequences of torture and trauma are physical and psychological, but responses are also needed to joblessness, homelessness and problems with bureaucracy and racism. Cross-cultural sensitivity is essential given the many different countries from which refugees arrive. Several principles are key to maximizing the benefits to service users (Aristotle, 1990). They include the commitment to genuine informed consent, to increasing the power that survivors have over their lives, to ensuring that service provision is guided by the service user and to respecting and reinforcing human rights as expressed in international standards.

The holistic philosophy of service provision is well exemplified in the practice of specialised one-to-one and family interventions by these services. While people can refer themselves or be referred by family members and professionals, most contacts result from outreach strategies specifically designed to make the specialist service known in a way which is de-stigmatising. An often-used strategy is to provide information sessions to community members in a highly accessible community based setting. The 'community' may be based on a common country of origin or based on a community of participants such as refugees attending adult English classes. The information sessions typically include psychoeducation about recognizing difficulties in everyday functioning that have significance for mental health. The terminology used is carefully considered and avoids mental health jargon. Information is also provided about other relevant services, namely primary care, emergency hospital services, legal services and generic settlement services. Representatives from one or more of those services usually participate in the planning and delivery of information. As a result participants identify themselves as requiring assistance and accessible means are provided for them to contact services immediately or at a later point. Service collaboration ensures multiple points of entry for specialised services as well as referrals back into other agencies.

The other key practice reflecting a holistic approach responsive to multiple needs is the use of a comprehensive psychosocial assessment approach. Current functioning is assessed in the various domains of learning, interpersonal behaviour, social networks, material circumstances, dealing with everyday tasks, physical health, trauma-specific psychological sequelae and personal goals. A comprehensive history is always taken to ensure an understanding of causes of problems. The approach is also family centred as it has long been recognized that the person presenting for assistance may be unaware of or reluctant to acknowledge the problems that spouses or children may be having. The approach allows for mutually agreed goals to be set and means, for example, that securing housing in a safe area can be as important a mental health intervention as counselling.

Health and settlement services for newly arrived refugees

Newly arrived families of refugee background characteristically experience multiple physical and mental health problems, alongside settlement stressors, which affect family functioning. Early intervention is valuable in facilitating access to services, treating physical health problems, responding to needs that would otherwise be detrimental to mental health and identifying people who are at risk of serious mental health problems

> A single mother, 30 years of age, had arrived from Sudan with two children 16 and 3 years of age. The mother's brother lived in Australia. The mother had a number of physical health problems including a vitamin D deficiency and a physical disability which limited her ability to walk. She presented as depressed and preferred not to see other people from Sudan. The 16-year-old had behavioural problems, teachers reporting that he was fighting with other children at school. The 3-year-old spent a lot of time with his uncle and family because of the mother's physical handicap. The torture and trauma history was undisclosed except for information that the woman's husband had been killed and that there was a long period of displacement. It was suspected that the youngest child was a child of rape.

This profile of a newly arrived refugee and her family is not atypical of people of refugee background who are eligible to receive settlement services under Australia's Integrated Humanitarian Settlement Strategy (IHSS), a national settlement program administered by Australia's Immigration department on behalf of the Australian government. The IHSS provides refugees settling in Australia with support and assistance during their first twelve months after arrival, through an integrated system of services that have links with other government and non-government services. Refugees receive assistance with securing long term rental accommodation, basic material goods to establish a household, information about and referral to mainstream services, referral for physical health assessment and if required, referral to specialised services dealing with psychosocial difficulties associated with the experience of torture and trauma.

For the woman described above, multiple needs were identified relatively soon after arrival and resulted in her referral to an NGO service, aforementioned as a specialist provider of torture and trauma services. This NGO provided counselling and advocacy interventions with a focus on restoring her ability to be an active parent to both children, and on her social isolation and depression. Other interventions managed by the service included liaison with the school, travel, help through a volunteer service, and referral to and follow up of disability support services. Physical health needs were addressed by the involvement of a refugee health nurse who maintained contact with the family to ensure access to primary health care services and maternal and child health care.

Refugee health nurses are an initiative of the Victorian state department of health (Department of Human Services, 2004). They are based in community health centres and have a health promotion role as well as provide direct service to clients, in their homes if required, including assistance with follow-up access to primary care services, allied health services, and hospital outpatient services. Clients who need assistance are identified by general practitioners who work in the community health centres or by any agency that is part of the IHSS programme.

Education Settings

Research and practice demonstrate the effectiveness of schools as key settings for the delivery of mental health promotion and early intervention strategies (Australian Health Promoting Schools Association, NHMRC, 1996). A number of school-based programmes have been developed in Australia that focus on children and adolescents with refugee backgrounds. They aim to promote mental health and identify children with existing mental health problems or those who are at risk of developing such problems. Schools have increasingly become aware that refugee students may not progress to completion of secondary education because of disrupted schooling prior to arrival in Australia, their difficulties in learning English and/or the pressure they face from families to perform at high levels while undertaking family duties.

School programmes involve one or more of the following components— referral to individual case workers for students and their families; group work in a classroom setting; homework clubs; professional development for teachers; research and policy advice to whole schools through participation in school committees, procedures and structures, and whole-of-school audits. A range of educational resources have been developed to raise awareness of refugee children and adolescents' educational needs, and they also provide information about classroom strategies and whole of school approaches (Bridging Refugee Youth and Children's Services (BRYCS), 2010). The extensive work conducted in this area mirrors that in the USA (Garbarino, Dubrow, Kostelny, and Pardo, 1992) and the United Kingdom (Rutter, 2003).

The strong recognition of schools as mental health settings and the abundant educational resources available are not sufficiently matched by implementation. Researchers and practitioners in the field have identified a number of strategies at the school and educational policy levels to enable sustainable responses but access to adequate funding resources is a constant challenge. Teachers have little time to implement strategies and this is a source of pressure for them. In addition, the education sector has limited capacity to respond to the needs of children with learning and behavioural difficulties as a result of developmental delays, traumatic events, family stresses, and/or disrupted schooling. This is a general problem, affecting also non-refugee children and adolescents with learning and behavioural difficulties often associated with social and economic disadvantage and family trauma.

Service coordination is crucial for children identified as having mental health problems or who are at high risk of developing such problems. In some metropolitan areas of major cities a mainstream child and adolescent mental health service has partnered with a school. In the absence of such partnerships, use of mental health services is extremely limited, the most common barriers being insufficient use of interpreters for communication, difficulties with travel, and fear associated with the notion of child mental health services. NGOs tend to fill the gap in service provision with their strengths in facilitating access to available services and through their engagement with families.

Another significant need in school-based mental health promotion is the insufficient involvement of families and communities (Rutter, 2003). Sanders and Epstein (1998) note many advantages of partnerships with parents. Expectations about performance can be aligned and parental fears about 'losing' their children to the dominant culture can be reduced. Parental engagement can also lead to facilitating improved conditions for learning and study at home and improved quality of life for families. Their inclusion also benefits the school and its teachers, promoting enlightened educational practice (Hamilton and Moore, 2003).

Family services

Community leaders have long expressed concern about tensions and conflict occurring in refugee families leading to family breakdown, intergenerational conflict, and social isolation (Mitchell, Kaplan, and Crowe, 2007) The stresses in families are caused or exacerbated by several factors: the changes in roles and relationships as a result of displacement and settlement; a breakdown of traditional family and community support systems (Gordon and Adam, 2005, Loar, 2004, Rousseau, Mekki-Berada, and Moreau, 2001; Simich, Este, and Hamilton, 2010; Sleiman, 2005); and the psychological legacy of trauma, which includes anxiety, post-traumatic stress disorder symptoms, depression, and guilt (Bashir, 2000; Rosenthal, Ranieri, and Klimidis, 1996; Weine, Muzurovic, and Kulauzovic, 2004).

Language and cultural barriers prevent family members from accessing services and programmes including structured support such as foster care, family mediation, and parenting programmes (Baasher, 2001; Coventry et al., 2002; Victorian Health Promotion Foundation (VFST), 2007; Cahill, 2005). In addition to such limitations in responsiveness by the mainstream family services, the barriers include poor understanding of the social and legal frameworks for service delivery, and refugee families feeling undermined by service responses that challenge expectations of family roles and behaviour.

An innovative project for increasing mainstream family services' responsiveness has been piloted in the Australian state of Victoria. It aims to create a network consisting of advisors from particular communities, in this case the Sudanese, Karen, and Afghan communities, representatives from the lead family service provider in the region, and representatives from other mainstream services such as child protection services and police. Network meetings take place monthly. Under the strategy, part-time qualified workers from the respective communities have positions in the mainstream services. The combination of the regular network meetings and the dedicated positions builds the capacity of the communities themselves to support families, increases the number of families who can have access to family services, and increases the capacity of participating agencies to respond effectively. Other network members have generated community-building activities to support the strategy.

In addition to improving the capacity of mainstream family services to respond to families with a refugee background, a number of community capacity-building strategies have been developed in Australia to strengthen family well-being. The following case study provides an example of a community development approach to promote family well-being and support families of refugee background. It is based on principles of empowerment and participation by refugee communities with assistance from an NGO.

Case study: two cultures one life

The largest refugee community to arrive in Australia in the period 2000–2005 was the South Sudanese. The Victorian Foundation for Survivors of Torture conducted extensive consultations to assess and review areas of need and identify the most appropriate focus for promoting mental health and well-being (Mitchell, Kaplan, and Crowe, 2006). Among the areas identified for focus were the need for a better understanding and participatory role in the Australian education systems, assistance in dealing with intergenerational conflict, and addressing the effects of war-related trauma. Leaders expressed the communal sadness over what had happened to their lives, a sense of a loss of their cultural and personal identities, the destruction of their plans for the future, and guilt at leaving loved ones behind in difficult circumstances. Certainly the natural feeling of responsibility for families overseas meant that most of the community members were sending money to them, thereby contributing to the poverty experienced during settlement.

Working in partnership with community leaders and stakeholders, programmes were developed and conducted for education, parenting, and trauma. The initial programme consisted of three weekend workshops attended by 30–35 community leaders. Programme content included the cultural and legal frameworks in Australia relevant to parenting and family relationships. Workshops were structured in a way to move through a process of

awareness raising and sharing of South Sudanese practices and values and Australian practices and values and generation of solutions based on those discussions. To ensure implementation of the strategies generated in the workshops, community sub-committees were
established to achieve goals in the areas of education, parenting, and trauma. The education
sub-committee developed in partnership with VFST a schools training package, initiated
and conducted community consultations with schools, and co-facilitated education information sessions with teachers in schools and with their community in community forums.
The intergenerational subcommittee organized and contributed to conducting weekend
parent-youth groups. The trauma sub-committee elected to nominate community leaders to
receive training in working with the effects of trauma and loss in the context of family
mediation.

Civil society

In Australia as elsewhere, the arrival of asylum seekers and refugees has evoked
mixed responses from members of the receiving society. Some have actively
welcomed the new arrivals, by providing material aid, legal assistance, and
language tuition, and inviting them to participate in social, religious, cultural,
and sporting activities.[1] At the initiative of the Refugee Council of Australia,
community groups and individuals, local authorities are encouraged to become
'Refugee Welcome Zones' and formally declare their commitment to welcom-
ing refugees and enhancing cultural and religious diversity in their areas.
Seventy one authorities had declared themselves to be Refugee Welcome Zones
at mid-2009.

Other members of society have responded negatively, expressed either
rhetorically (e.g. letters to media), politically (e.g. support for politicians who
advocate harsh policies), or through conduct directed at individuals and
groups (e.g. abusive language; violence; discrimination in access to housing
and employment). The hostility that asylum seekers and refugees encounter
personally or collectively harms their well-being. A review of research on self-
reported racism and health found a link between self-reported discrimination
and depression and anxiety and a probable link with a range of other mental
health and behavioural problems (Paradies, 2006).

The Australian Government and a number of agencies in Australia support
a variety of activities to counter racism and other forms of intolerance. For
example, the Australian Government provides funds to community-based

---

[1] Australian examples are Asylum Seeker Resource Centre, www.asrc.or.au; Asylum
Seeker Project, Hotham Mission, www.hotham.mission.org.au; Fitzroy Learning
Network, www.fitzroylearningnetwork.org.au; Rural Australians for Refugees,
www.ruralaustraliansforrefugees.org.au.

organizations 'to address issues of cultural, racial and religious intolerance by promoting respect, fairness, inclusion and a sense of belonging for everyone' (DIAC, 2009b; Victoria Dept of the Premier and Cabinet, 2005). The VicHealth strategy for mental health and well-being includes the prevention of ethnic and race-based discrimination and promoting respect for diversity (VicHealth, 2009).

Conclusions

Refugees flee because they have endured terrible events in countries of origin, in the course of their flight, and in the places where they seek temporary shelter. That pre-migration experiences such as violence, imprisonment, and profound deprivation may adversely affect mental well-being even after people have arrived in places of safety seems unsurprising. The importance of post-migration factors in fostering mental well-being or compounding the adverse effects of previous experiences is receiving increasing attention. More research is required to identify and understand the determinants of mental health post migration and to evaluate the impact of policies and interventions.

A growing body of robust evidence indicates that the mental health of refugees, whether asylum seekers or recognized refugees, is affected not only by what occurred before they arrived or their individual vulnerabilities but also by how they are treated by government, service providers, and civil society in the countries where they seek to settle. As illustrated in Australia, a wide range of health and non-health decisions made by governmental and non-governmental actors affect the mental health of asylum seekers and refugees by determining their access to services, their capacity to meet basic needs and participate economically, and whether they encounter social exclusion or inclusion, discrimination, or tolerance. The participatory processes that empower people of refugee background to have their needs and rights met are also relevant to their mental health.

All sectors in the settlement country may be influential in establishing an environment that is supportive or damaging. Clinicians have an important role in the treatment and prevention of illness for individuals. They may also have important roles as advocates to other health and non-health service providers on behalf of individual clients and as advocates on behalf of the population of asylum seekers and refugees generally.

There are compelling humanitarian and human rights grounds for settlement countries to protect and promote the mental health of asylum seekers and refugees by addressing the spectrum of determinants that have significant effects both positively and negatively. Such action is also in the national interest.

Positive mental health is an important facilitator of successful settlement and integration and fosters the economic, social, and cultural contribution of the new arrivals for the benefit of the whole community.

References

Allender, S.C. (1998). Adult ESL learners with special needs: Learning from the Australian perspective, National Centre for ESL Literacy Education, ERIC Clearinghouse.

Amnesty International. (2007). The state of the world's human rights. http://thereport. amnesty.org/en retrieved June 23.

Australian Citizenship Test Review Committee. (2008). Moving forward...Improving pathways to citizenship – a report by the Australian citizenship test review committee, Commonwealth of Australia, Canberra.

Australian Government. (2008). "Government response to the report" http://www. citizenshiptestreview.gov.au/content/gov-response/.

Australian Health Promoting Schools Association. (2003). A national framework for health promoting schools retrieved June 24 2009 from http://www.ahpsa.org.au/files/ framework.pdf.

Baasher, T.A.(2001). Islam and mental Health. *Eastern Mediterranean Health Journal* 7(3): 372–376.

Bashir, M. and Bennett, D. (Eds.). (2000). *Deeper Dimensions – Culture, Youth and Mental Health.* Sydney: Transcultural Mental Health Centre.

Barry, M. and Jenkins, R. (2007). *Implementing Mental Health Promotion.* Edinburgh: Churchill Livingstone Elsevier.

Bloch, A. (2002). Refugees' opportunities and barriers in employment and training. DWP research report 179. Department for Work and Pensions, Leeds.

Brahmbhatt, K., Atfield, G., Irving, H., Lee, J. and O'Toole, T. (2007). *Refugees' Experiences of Integration: Policy Related Findings On Employment, ESOL and Vocational Training.* Birmingham: University of Birmingham.

Bridging Refugee Youth and Children's Services (*BRYCS*), (2010). Multilingual School-Related Resources for Refugee Families. www.brycs.org/highlighted-resources.cfm?schools&dist=9

Cahill, D. (2005). The conundrum of globalization. *Australian Mosaic* 12(4): 6–11.

CIC (2003). IP 3: In Canada processing of convention refugees abroad and members of the humanitarian protected persons abroad classes part 1 (General). Toronto, Citizenship and Immigration Canada.

Cook, A., Blaustein, M., Spinazzola, J., and van der Kolk, B. (Eds.). (2003). Complex trauma in children and adolescents: National Child Traumatic Stress Network. Complex Trauma Task Force. Retrieved from http://www.nctsnet.org/nccts/nav.do?pid=ctr_rsch_prod.

Coffey, G.J., Kaplan, I., Sampson, R.C., and Tucci, M.M. (2010). The meaning and mental health consequences of long-term immigration detention for people seeking asylum Reference. *Social Science and Medicine.* 70: 2070–2079.

Coventry, L., Guerra, C., Mackenzie, D., and Pinkney, S. (2002). *The wealth of All Nations: Identification of strategies to assist refugee young people in transition to independence.* Australian Clearinghouse for Youth Studies for the National Youth Affairs Research Scheme.

CSDH (2008). *Closing the gap in a generation: health equity through action on the social determinants of health.* Final Report of the Commission on Social Determinants of Health. Geneva, World Health Organization.

DHS (2008). Refugee health and wellbeing action plan 2008–2010: current and future initiatives. Melbourne: Department of Human Services.

DIAC (2009a). Australian Citizenship Test Snapshot Report – April 2009, Department of Immigration and Citizenship, Canberra.

DIAC (2009b). http://www.harmony.gov.au/ (retrieved 24 April 2009 http://www.citizenship.gov.au/_pdf/cit-test-snapshot-apr-09.pdf, retrieved 25 June 2009.

Drew, N., Funk, M., Pathare, S., and Swartz, L. (2005). Mental health and human rights. In H. Herrman, S. Saxena and R. Moodie (Eds.), *Promoting Mental Health: Concepts, Emerging Evidence, Practice,* pp. 89–108. Geneva: WHO.

Eager, K., Green, J., Jones, L. *et al.* (2007). The health of people in Australian detention centres–health profile and ongoing information requirements. Australia: Centre for Health Service Development, University of Wollongong.

Estinger, L. (1973). A follow-up study of the Norwegian concentration camp survivors' mortality and morbidity. *Israel Annals of Psychiatry and Related Disciplines* 2: 199–209.

Fazel, M. and Silove, D. (2006). Detention of refugees. *British Medical Journal* 332: 251–252.

Friedl, L. (2009). *Mental health, resilience and inequalities.* Copenhagen: World Health Organization 2009.

Garbarino, J., Dubrow, N., Kostelny, K., and Pardo, C. (1992). *Children in danger. Coping with the consequences of community violence.* San Francisco: Jossey-Bass.

Gordon, R. and Adam, M. (2005). *Family Harmony: Understanding family violence in Somali and Eritrean communities in the Western Region of Melbourne.* Women's Health West, Melbourne, Victoria. www.whwest.org.au/docs/familyharmony05.pdf.

Gorst-Unsworth, C. and Goldenberg, E. (1998). Psychological sequelae of torture and organised violence suffered by refugees from Iraq. *British Journal of Psychiatry* 172(1): 90–94.

Green, B., Korol, M., Grace, M., *et al.* (1991). Children and disaster: Age, gender and parental effects on PTSD symptoms. *Journal of the American Academy of Child and Adolescent Psychiatry* 30: 945–951.

Hamilton, R.J. and Moore, D. (2003). *Educational Interventions for Refugee Children Theoretical Perspectives and Implementing Best Practice.* London and New York: Routledgefarmer.

Herrman, H., Saxena, S., and Moodie, R. (eds.). (2005). Promoting mental health: Concepts, emerging evidence, practice. A report from the World Health Organization Department of Mental Health and Substance Abuse in Collaboration with the Victorian Health Promotion Foundation (VicHealth) and The University of Melbourne. Geneva: World Health Organization.

Howard (2006). John Howard's Australia Day Address to the National Press Club [January 25, 2006]http://www.australianpolitics.com/news/2006/01/06-01-25_howard.shtml, retrieved 25 June 2009.

HREOC (2004). A Last Resort? The National inquiry into children in immigration detention, Australian Human Rights Commission, Sydney.

Ichikawa, M., Nakahara, S., and Wakai, S. (2006). Effect of post-migration detention on mental health among Afghan asylum seekers in Japan. *The Australian and New Zealand Journal of Psychiatry* 40 (4): 341–346.

Jaques L. and Abbott, L. (1997). Resettlement disrupted. Effects of having a family member in a conflict zone. In B. Ferguson, and D. Barnes (Eds.), Perspectives on Trans-Cultural Mental Health. Culture and Mental Health. Current Issues in Trans-Cultural Mental Health, pp. 68–76, NSW, Australia: Trans-cultural Mental Health Service.

Joint Standing Committee on Migration. (2009). Immigration Detention in Australia – Community-Based Alternatives to Detention, Commonwealth of Australia, Canberra 2009.

Kinzie, J.D., Boehnlein, J. and Sack, W.H. (1998). The effects of massive trauma on Cambodian parents and children. In Danieli, Y. (Ed.), *International Handbook of Multigenerational Legacies of Trauma*, pp. 211–220. New York: Plenum Press.

Kinzie, J.D., Fredrickson, M.D., Ben, R., Fleck, J., and Karis, W. (1984). Post traumatic stress disorder among survivors of Cambodian concentration camps. *American Journal of Psychiatry* 141: 644–650.

Kovess-Masfety, V., Murray, M., and Gureje, O. (2005). Evolution of our understanding of positive mental health. In H. Herrman, S. Saxena and R. Moodie (Eds.), *Promoting Mental Health: Concepts, Emerging Evidence, Practice* 35–46, Geneva: World Health Organization.

Kuch, K. and Cox, B. J. (1992). Symptoms of post traumatic stress disorder in 124 survivors of the Holocaust. *American Journal of Psychiatry* 149: 337–340.

Laban, C.J., Komproe, I.H., Gernaat, H.B.P.E., and de Jong, J.T.V.M. (2008). The impact of a long asylum procedure on quality of life, disability and physical health in Iraqi asylum seekers in the Netherlands. *Social Psychiatry and Psychiatric Epidemiology* 43: 507–515.

Lie, B. (2002). A 3-year follow-up study of psychosocial functioning and general symptoms in settled refugees. *Acta Psychiatrica Scandinavica* 106: 415–425.

Loar, L. (2004). Making Tangible Gains in Parent-Child Relationships with Traumatized Refugees. *Intervention* 2(3): 210–220.

Lomas, J (1998). Social capital and health—implications for public health and epidemiology. *Social Science and Medicine* 47(9): 1181–1188.

Macksoud, M.S. and Aber, J.L. (1996). The war experiences and psychosocial development of children in Lebanon. *Child Development* 67(1): 70–88.

Minister for Immigration and Citizenship (2009). Budget 2009–10 – New Directions in Detention http://www.minister.immi.gov.au/media/media-releases/2009/ce01-budget-09.htm, retrieved 20 June 2009.

Mitchell, J., Kaplan, I., and Crowe, L. (2007). Two Cultures: one Life. *Community Development Journal* 42: 282–298.

Momartin, S., Steel, Z., Coello, M., Aroche, J., Silove, D., and Brooks, R. (2006). A comparison of the mental health of refugees with temporary versus permanent protection visas. *Medical Journal of Australia* 185: 357–361.

Network of Asylum Seeker Agencies. (2005). Seeking Safety, Not Charity: A Report in Support of Work-Rights for Asylum-Seekers on Bridging Visa E http://safetynotcharity.victas.uca.org.au/downloads/Nasavic_BVE_Report_Final.pdf, retrieved 25 April 2009.

Ong Hing, B. (2007). Promoting family values and immigration. *House judiciary subcommittee on immigration*. Washington, DC.

Paradies, Y. (2006). A systematic review of empirical research on self reported racism and health. *International Journal of Epidemiology* 35: 888–890.

Physicians for Human Rights and the Bellevue/NYU Program for Survivors of Torture (2003). From Persecution to Prison: The Health Consequences of Detention for Asylum Seekers. http://physiciansforhumanrights.org/library/report-persprison.html.

Porter, M., and Haslam, N. (2005). Predisplacement and post displacement factors associated with mental health of refugees and internally displaced persons: A meta-analysis. *JAMA: Journal of the American Medical Association* 294: 602–612.

Punamaki, R.L. (2001). From childhood trauma to adult well-being through psychosocial assistance of Chilean families. *Journal of Community Psychology* 29(3): 281–303.

Refugee Council of Australia (2007). Submission to the Senate Legal and Constitutional Affairs Committee Inquiry into the Australian Citizenship Amendment (Citizenship Testing) Bill, published in Senate Standing Committee on Legal and Constitutional Affairs (2007) Inquiry into the Australian Citizenship Amendment (Citizenship Testing) Bill 2007, Parliament of Australia, Canberra.

Robjant, K., Hassan, R., and Katona, C. (2009). Mental health implications of detaining asylum seekers: systematic review. *The British Journal of Psychiatry* **194**: 306–312.

Rosenthal, D., Ranieri, N., and Klimidis, S. (1996). Vietnamese adolescents in Australia: Relationships between perceptions of self and parental values, intergenerational conflict, and gender dissatisfaction. *International Journal of Psychology* **31**: 81–91.

Rousseau, C., Mekki-Berrada, A., and Moreau, S. (2001). Trauma and extended separation from family among Latin American and African refugees in Montreal. *Psychiatry* **64**(1): 40–68.

Rousseau, C. and Drapeau, A. (2003). Are refugee children an at-risk group?: A longitudinal study of Cambodian adolescents. *Journal of Refugee Studies* **16**(1): 67–81.

Rutter, J. (2001). *Supporting refugee children in 21st century Britain: a compendium of essential information.* Stoke-on-Trent: Trentham Books.

Sanders, M.G. and Epstein, J.L. (1998). International perspectives on school-family community partnerships. *Childhood Education* **74**: 340–342.

Shakeh, M., Zachary, S., Marianio C., Jorge, A., Derrick, M. S., and Robert, B. (2006). A comparison of the mental health of refugees with temporary versus permanent protection visas. *Medical Journal of Australia* **185**(7): 357–361.

Shiferaw, D. and Hagos, H. (2001). Refugees and progression routes into employment. London, Refugee Council/Pan London Refugee Training and Employment Network.

Silove, D., Steel, Z., and Watters, C. (2000). Policies of deterrence and the mental health of asylum seekers. *Journal of the American Medical Association* **284**(5): 604–611. DOI:10.1001/jama.284.5.604.

Simich, L., Este, C., and Hamilton H. (2010). Meanings of home and mental well-being among Sudanese refugees in Canada. *Ethnicity and Health* 1–14.

Simpson, M.A. (1993). Traumatic stress and the bruising of the soul. In J.P. Wilson and B. Raphael (Eds.), *International Handbook of Traumatic Stress Syndromes*, pp. 667–684, New York: Plenum Press.

Sleiman, D. (2005). Perspectives on new arrival African Humanitarian Entrants in the city of Whittlesea, July 2005. http: www.vicnet.net.aw/ciwwhit

Steel, Z., Silove, D., Brooks, R., Momartin, S., Alzuhairi, B., and Susljik, I. (2006). Impact of immigration detention and temporary protection on the mental health of refugees. *British Journal of Psychiatry* **188**: 58–64.

Sultan, A. and O'Sullivan, K. (2001). Psychological disturbances in asylum seekers held in long-term detention: A participant–observer account. *Medical Journal of Australia* **175**: 593–596.

Szoke, H. (2009). Recognising resilience and rights. paper presented at centre for public policy conference, values and public policy, fairness, diversity and social change. Melbourne.

Thomas, T. and Lau, W. (2002). Psychological well being of child and adolescent refugees and asylum seekers: overview of major research findings of the past ten years. www.humanrights.gov.au.

UNHCR (1986). Detention of refugees and asylum-seekers, No.44 (XXXVII) – Conclusion adopted by the Executive Committee on the International Protection of Refugees, United Nations High Commissioner for Refugees, Geneva.

UNHCR (2000). Complementary forms of protection: Their nature and relationship to the International Protection Regime" – EC/50/SC/CRP.18.

UNHCR (2002a). UNHCR Regional Office for Australia, New Zealand, Papua New Guinea and the South Pacific, Temporary Protection, Discussion Paper No.2 – 2002.

UNHCR (2002b). Refugee Resettlement: An International Handbook to Guide Reception and Integration, Melbourne.

UNHCR (2008). Challenges and Opportunities in Family Reunification, Annual Tripartite Consultations on resettlement. Geneva, United Nations High Commissioner for Refugees.

UNHCR (2009). Asylum Level and Trends in Industralised Countries, www.unhcr.org/statistics.

United States Committee for Refugees and Immigrants, U.S. Committee for Refugees World Refugee Survey, 2001.

Victorian Health Promotion Foundation (VFST) (2007). *Raising Children in Australia - resources for early childhood services working with parents from African Backgrounds.* Melbourne. VFST www.foundationhouse.org.au/resources/publications_and_resources.htm

Victoria Dept. of the Premier and Cabinet (2005). *A fairer Victoria : creating opportunity and addressing disadvantage.* Melbourne: Dept. of Premier and Cabinet.

Victorian Foundation for Survivors of Torture (VFST). (1998). *Rebuilding Shattered Lives.* Melbourne: Author.

VicHealth (2003). Promoting the Mental Health and Wellbeing of New Arrival Communities. Learnings and Promising Practices, Victorian Health Promotion Foundation, Melbourne.

VicHealth (2007). More than Tolerance: Embracing Diversity for Health: Discrimination Affecting Migrant and Refugee Communities in Victoria, Its Health Consequences, Community Attitudes and Solutions – A Summary Report Victorian Health Promotion Foundation, Melbourne.

VicHealth (2009). http://www.vichealth.vic.gov.au/en/Programs-and-Projects/Mental-Health-and-Wellbeing.aspx, retrieved 25 June 2009.

Weine, S., Muzurovic, N., Kulauzovic, Y. *et al.* (2004). Family consequences of refugee trauma. *Family Process* 43(2): 147–160.

Walker, L., Verins, I., Moodie, R., and Webster, K. (2005). Responding to the social and economic determinants of mental health: a conceptual framework for action. In: Herrman, H., Saxena, S., and Moodie, R. (Eds.), *Promoting Mental Health: Concepts, Emerging Evidence, Practice*, pp. 89–108. Geneva: WHO.

Westermeyer, J. (1986). Migration and psychopathology. In L. Williams and J. Westermeyer (Eds.), Refugee Mental Health in Settlement Countries, New York: Hampshire Publishing.

Wilkinson, R. and Marmot, M. (2003). *Social Determinants of Health: The Solid Facts.* 2nd edition. Geneva: World Health Organisation.

Chapter 5

Psychiatric diagnoses and assessment issues for refugees and asylum seekers

Kamaldeep Bhui and Nasir Warfa

Psychiatric diagnosis and coherent understanding

Psychiatric diagnosis is founded upon listening to the patient's words and communications of distress, and trying to assign meaning and clinical significance to the content, and to the form and flow of speech (DSM-IV-TR, 2000). Additional behavioural changes and altered states of consciousness and functioning contribute to an overall diagnostic judgement (DSM-IV-TR, 2000). Psychopathological studies have radically altered our understanding of mental distress, helping refine diagnostic categories; for example, these have created distinctions between psychotic and non-psychotic conditions, and affective and non-affective psychoses, varieties of common mental disorders, and, more recently, post-traumatic disorders (Bhugra and Bhui, 2007).

Another recent trend in psychiatric practice and research is to recognize co-morbid states, and that mental illness may be pheno-typically expressed on a continuum rather than discrete categories. Categories are still preferred by many to make it easier to decide who is and who is not in need of clinical treatment, on the basis of constellations of symptoms, affect, and expressions of distress, and social, cultural, and historical information about changes in functioning (Kleinman, 1987). This is a complex task taking account of subtle emotional states, as well as constellations of the characteristics mentioned earlier. Yet, whatever diagnostic systems are put in place, there is always a challenge to them over time, as more scientific knowledge about mental disorders emerges (Summerfield, 2008). Thus, consecutive versions of ICD and DSM express the evolving culture of psychiatric practice, based on expertise found among clinicians, and developed following field trials and research.

The application of standard (ICD and DSM) diagnostic processes in psychiatry among refugees and asylum seekers is even more challenging given the complex social and healthcare needs of this group (Warfa *et al.*, 2006).

The experience of multiple pre-migration traumatic events coupled with the acculturation difficulties they face in the host countries make refugee groups particularly vulnerable to some psychiatric disorders with particular aetiologies (Berry, 1991; Arcia *et al.*, 2001; Bhui *et al.*, 2003). For instance, our recent study with Somali refugees and asylum seekers living in the UK showed that a significant number of this community have high levels of psychiatric illnesses (Bhui *et al.*, 2006) but their psychiatric care needs are not often diagnosed or assessed correctly until they develop more severe and chronic mental disorders (McCrone *et al.*, 2005). Several factors contribute to the poor management of mental distress among refugee populations. Clinicians often complain that these groups do not speak adequate English and therefore are difficult to understand, undermining diagnostic precision and judgements about the severity of their psychological distress.

It is known, although occasionally disputed, that the content of expressions of distress for any one diagnostic group does vary across language groups, and across national and international contexts; linguistic idioms of distress and ways of explaining distress and misfortune differ by cultural groups, some perhaps assigning significance to supernatural forces, or failure to adhere to religious prescriptions, or to social deviance (Warfa, 2007). Clinicians are, therefore, right to illustrate the impact of poor language and cultural communications and/or misunderstandings on the identification and treatment of mental illness found among refugees and asylum seekers. Degrees of misdiagnosis may occur but never be detected, recognized or remedied, but explained away as inevitable given the complexity in diagnosis across cultures. Complexity certainly arises from language differences, but also partly because of refugee patients' specific cultural expressions and idioms of health and illness; for example, somatization of psychological symptoms, perhaps symbolizing physical injury, sites of torture, or metaphorical idioms of distress involving bodily symptoms. All of these factors contribute to poor precision in the diagnosis of mental disorders and psychiatric co-morbidities among refugee patients, many of whom have urgent treatment needs (Bhui *et al.*, 2006a). Clinicians have professional and ethical responsibilities for the care they provide for all their patients. Not offering accurate mental health assessments to refugee patients partly because of their complex care needs or allowing their psychiatric conditions to deteriorate to the point of complete mental breakdown, be it unintentionally or otherwise, would be seen as a failure to abide by the very essence of medical ethics.

Given the under-diagnosis and limited mental health service utilization of asylum seekers and refugees who are at high risk of severe mental disorders (McCrone *et al.*, 2005), we suggest that the standard psychiatric diagnostic processes should be revisited to include the specific psychiatric needs of refugees and asylum seekers. The cultural issues of any one national, regional or linguistic, or religious group should not be lost. For example, by giving attention to the issues of language barriers, we propose the concept of 'coherent understanding' as key. We propose the term 'coherent understanding' to reflect how refugee patients' individual and cultural expressions of distress, their complex historical experience and world view, their personality constellation, and their interpersonal impacts are all taken in by the clinician to form a coherent set of explanations and judgements about the nature of an illness, its prognosis and the potential treatments. The clinician will have varying degrees of confidence in the diagnosis, and in the plan for treatment. Does this always mean equal levels of proficiency and confidence with refugee populations? We propose not, but rather than relegate these doubts, these should be located within the diagnostic judgements, almost as a degree of certainty, with a back-up plan should the proposed treatment or diagnostic judgement not show benefit.

Therefore across language barriers, not only are the words and their semantic halo of uncertain significance to a health professional whose cultural and language background differs, but the task of 'coherent understanding', irrespective of ethnic matching, is itself challenged by differences in common points of reference, shared historical worlds, theories of mind and madness. The pathological significance of certain phenomena varies across cultures and religious groups. For instance, a refugee or an asylum seeker from Tibet or Nepal with strong convictions in Buddhist philosophy would not necessarily see hopelessness as pathology but an experience to embrace (Boisen, 1960). Paranoia may also be appropriate amongst victims of physical violence or discrimination, or amongst people who have been tortured by the authorities in their countries. In a forthcoming article (Warfa et al., 2010b), we reported the narratives of many asylum seekers and foreign nationals who were exposed to extreme violence including rape, repeated rape, anal penetration with foreign objects, amputations of male/female genitals, and being forced to engage in sexual violence against family members. Mental health professionals may not always be familiar with these types of pre-migration traumatic life experiences of refugees and asylum seekers, with some implications for under-diagnosing their psychiatric illnesses and thus prolonging suffering. To this end, the management and diagnosis of the psychological needs of such vulnerable groups would require extra care, patience, and sensitivity. Moreover, delusions of possession may be difficult to discern if a supernatural locus of control is the norm for a group, or is part of a culturally sanctioned process of recovery; for example, Muslim asylum seekers may attribute any experience of delusions of possessions to the will of Allah. Refugee and asylum seeking patients who have strong convictions in religion and spirituality do not normally come forward for psychiatric treatment at early stages and instead may resort to religious services or sometimes exorcism to cope with delusions of possession (Bhavsar and Bhugra, 2008). This may explain the low pattern of service utilization by asylum seekers and refugees with severe mental disorders (McCrone *et al.*, 2005). In such cases, mental health practitioners may particularly find it challenging to deal with patients who present both religious delusions and/or culturally sanctioned over-valued ideas. Bhavsar and Bhugra (2008) illustrated the crucial role which religious delusions and rituals play in the management, diagnosis, and treatment of patients with delusions. Crucially, discussing refugee patients about their spiritual and religious needs during the consultation process may lead to better diagnostic outcomes and thus improved recovery. It is one frame of reference about the patient that can be explored and understood, amongst others; for example, country and town of origin, family structure, preferred leisure, illness experiences, and popular folk beliefs about illness and recovery.

Similarly, hallucinations can vary in their modality and content; for example, visual hallucinations are thought to be more common amongst people with psychosis in low-income countries. What of altered states of consciousness as a means of dealing with extreme distress? Should these always be thought of as having an organic aetiology or accepted as being more common in some cultural groups? Many of these issues are commonly discussed in relation to culturally isolated and unique populations as if their unusual symptoms are a consequence of developmentally and geographically unique trajectories. Although exotic descriptions of psychopathology were common during early expeditions to discover new peoples and their minds, such a point of reference is unlikely in the modern globalized world; telecommunication networks ensure that people are not so culturally isolated and unique. It is unlikely that communications of distress cannot be understood. Yet, there is a more subtle impact of the cultural environment on judgements about illness severity, familiarity of symptom expressions, and expectations of recovery and intervention. So symptoms profiles seem to vary across national groups, and over time; people incorporate common technologies or belief systems at particular historical periods into their idioms of distress, and specifically into delusions and hallucinations. Hysteria is now uncommon in the developed world, but probably it is becoming less common in the developing world, possibly as a consequence of industrialization. Culture-bound syndromes have been largely relegated to artefact, but probably are evidence of a lack of 'coherent understanding'. As the world's cultures become more similar, so disorders previously thought to be culturally bound seem familiar; common features are extracted and identified and expressed in universal language in diagnostic revisions.

However, to dismiss cultural variations is also not correct. There are plenty of examples of disorder (Koro, Latah, eating disorders), which are understood best as cultural elaborations of physiological phenomena. Do these really need different diagnostic categories depending on how common the form and content are in a particular society? Is PTSD a disorder only in developed, high-income, and peaceful countries? In fact, several epidemiological studies established that pre-migration trauma is a risk factor for not only PTSD but also depression and suicide among refugees and asylum seekers, regardless of geographical variations (Robertson *et al.*, 2006, see Figure 5.1; Silove *et al.*, 2007; Pedersen *et al.*, 2008). Although PTSD will be common among refugees and asylum seekers and in conflict zones, the diagnosis and treatment of personality disorders may prove challenging when considering cross-cultural and language groups (including but not exclusively refugee groups), not only as personality traits might be understood as being culturally determined and defined by national norms, but judgements about deviance are so linked to culturally normed such that it is likely such judgements are imprecise unless the cultural points of orientation are shared by the assessor and the patient. Perhaps that is why some studies show a low prevalence of personality disorders among African Caribbeans, for example.

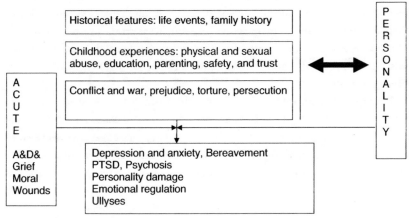

Fig. 5.1 Life course influences and mental disorder.

Unique diagnostic issues among refugees and asylum seekers

The issues discussed so far might be found in any text of cultural psychiatry. Refugees and asylum seekers present unique diagnostic challenges partly because of the combination of pre-migration traumatic life experiences and post-migration social problems. The issues of pre- and post-migration life difficulties can affect diagnosis as refugee patients would require more time and resources for a thorough mental state examination and history taking. Furthermore, they may be refugees from countries in which mental illness is stigmatized, or in which there is extreme poverty, and very poor educational opportunities. These environments are likely to include less formal child safety protections, and so unsafe and risky situations may be more likely. These predispose to adult psychiatric disorders. Early childhood experiences, including sexual and physical abuse, and emotional neglect are all known to impact adversely on resilience, employment, and mental health outcomes in adulthood. Although this information can be gathered at initial assessment, the characteristics of the country of origin, and common social and societal problems will need some understanding. Early family and kinship structures may also differ between societies and so, again, assumptions about family constitution, parental absence, and adverse childhood experiences should be put to one side and the issues explored with an open mind during a first assessment. These early influences may lead to at-risk psychological states in the form of particular personality attributes and disorders, which will at least predispose to other forms of mental illness and at the same time present vulnerabilities to exposure to other forms of risk. For example, child soldiers arise in a particular context of a breakdown in the social fabric of war-torn countries. Children may be involved in committing atrocities, witnessing them, or being victim to them and then having to manage the consequences, yet they remain children. This may lead them onto a path of significant psychological damage, substance misuse, with difficulty overcoming powerful affective states with which they have grown up.

Therefore, the symptom and diagnostic profile of refugees and asylum seekers is likely to reflect these experiences. In our 2006 census of all psychiatric inpatient units in London, we found that refugees and asylum seekers were under-represented in psychiatric wards, whereas refugees' illnesses challenged staff because of the complexity of the care package required (Bhui *et al.*, 2006b). This highlights the psychiatric processes associated with refugees and asylum seekers and how their unique care needs challenge existing mental health services. Being caught in a war-torn situation and being victim to persecution, torture, and corruption will all lead to a particular breakdown in trust and confidence in authority and in securing a safe environment (Steel *et al.*, 2002). Physical and mental scars may distort the experience, but damage to a spiritual or moral coherence in the world will be far more difficult to overcome, perhaps leading to fundamental shifts in the personality structure and functioning of people.

Paradoxically, it is likely that it is the most resilient and able who escape these situations as asylum seekers, primarily into neighbouring countries, but also further afield to higher-income countries, some with managed programmes of processing refugees and some not. Nonetheless, despite this selection effect, significant emotional strain appears to be common but does not always lead to significant psychiatric or psychological disorders; indeed most studies emphasizing the pathological outcomes are not population based and appear to take convenience samples, but then erroneously attribute the findings to populations of refugees in general. One theory is that when the most resilient refugees are exposed to numerous social problems in the host countries, the thresholds of their resilient nature are put to the test (Warfa *et al.*, 2006). For example, Silove *et al.*, (2000) linked the elevated levels of mental health problems among asylum seekers with the host countries' new immigration policies of deterrence, stating that:

> Concerns about uncontrolled migration have encouraged host countries to adopt policies of deterrence in which increasingly restrictive measures are being imposed on persons seeking asylum...In several countries, asylum seekers living in the community face restricted access to work, education, housing, welfare, and, in some situations, to basic health care services...allegations of abuse, untreated medical and psychiatric illnesses, suicidal behaviour, hunger strikes have been reported.
>
> (Silove *et al.*, 2000)

In other words, the unfair treatment of asylum seekers might have weakened their resilient nature to control or cope with the experience of maladjustment and extreme social adversity. This may make diagnostic judgements amongst this group much more problematic, as the aetiology has to be located in the domestic immigration and host response to the pre-migration risk factors. (See also Watters, 2001.) Diagnosis is meant to guide treatment. How can a diagnosis address genocide, torture, or unjust immigration policy?

The social fabric of diagnostic dilemmas

So what are the diagnostic dilemmas? To begin with, more traumatic experiences may be overstated to lead to PTSD, especially when it is known that this diagnosis carries special significance for governments to conclude harm has been caused, and a medical condition now exists, which should be considered amongst the extenuating circumstances when decisions on refugee status are made. Some services and organizations, indeed, run services specifically for victims of trauma and for people with varieties of PTSD syndromes; for example, the Medical Foundation for the victims of torture and violence.

Such services are also a neat way of suggesting that the needs of refugees are met more widely, in a more convenient and familiar manner, using a conventional model of treatment that is evidence based. The treatment does not address the tear in moral fabric or the trust in a just world, but specifically targets such expressions as a cognitive distortion or a symptom rather than a reality-based judgement.

It is known that some asylum seekers themselves wish to see a doctor rather than another specialist, just to ensure medical reports can be provided at an opportune moment, and legal teams seek out diagnosis of PTSD as part of building a case for granting refugee status. This contributes to ongoing debate about the over-medicalization of refugee experiences. For example, PTSD has been described as a social construct rather than a useful psychiatric diagnosis (Summerfield, 2008). Nevertheless, it is now accepted (and widely agreed by clinicians working with refugees and asylum seekers around the world) that those who experienced mass violence, ethnic conflicts, and traumatic events have greater levels of unmet needs and therefore are more vulnerable to mental disorders such as PTSD and depression (Warfa et al., 2006). It this within this context that psychiatrists and psychologists emphasize the recognition and early diagnosis of the psychosocial needs of refugees and victims of torture and mass violence.

On the other hand, multiple social, humanistic, and psychological needs are difficult to manage, so can sometimes be medicalized in order to provide an optimistic framework for intervention, a framework that does not have to constantly struggle with the moral and social injustice that accompanies conflict, war, and asylum. Health services cannot change the past, nor impact on international conflict.

Having a testimonial of atrocities, and a detailed account of life events, may well be therapeutic and helpful. It may also be a distraction from the everyday struggles that some face. Addressing these daily hassles, securing social support, finding good schools and safe environments for children, ensuring adequate housing and food for families, surviving discrimination are all higher on the agenda of refugees than dealing with common mental disorders or common states of psychological distress. Perhaps dealing with these social issues, by way of a 'social fabric diagnosis', is more important to the person's journey to recovery and well-being. This is particularly challenging for clinicians who are not aware of the holistic social and healthcare needs of refugees and asylum seekers.

Mental disorders can be very disabling and impair function and can culminate in chronic disability and suicide in the most severe cases. Providing intervention of these disorders only, removed from the 'social fabric diagnosis' and intervention, is likely to fail. Highly important is the co-morbidity issue. Co-morbid states are more common among refugees and asylum seekers (Bhui *et al.*, 2006) and this makes a definitive and confident diagnosis and management plan less effective. For example, the management of personality disorder, one consequence of early trauma, or even intense trauma in later life, may differ from that of pure schizophrenia in terms of the degree of engagement or assertiveness in treatment. If the two conditions are co-morbid (schizophrenia and personality disorder), addressing the psychosis without addressing the PD or vice versa may lead to persistent symptoms, which might be seen as treatment resistance, or non-compliance and thereafter undermine the clinician's notion of a coherent understanding of the patient's illness experience. It is known that PD diagnoses are uncommon in refugee groups (as well as in some ethnic communities), contrasting with diagnosis of psychosis. A key question is if they are uncommon amongst these refugee and ethnic communities or under-recognized. Co-morbid personality damage, substance misuse, and Axis I disorders are likely therefore to pose special challenges among asylum seeker and refugee populations where the skills and tools for precise assessment may be undermined because of linguistic, theoretical, philosophical, and practical challenges.

Finally, legal systems operate differently in different countries and impose particular restrictions, which may have differential impacts on risks of mental disorder and on the management of psychiatric services. So we know forced unemployment, unmanaged asylum, and delays in reaching a detention decision all contribute to a higher risk of mental disorder. And yet, in the face of cultural confusion in communication, and the concerns about malingering or over-medicalization, a psychiatric diagnosis may be the only credentials to refugee status, yet denied to some individuals. Despite the utility of a diagnosis to support the granting of refugee status, the assignation of the diagnosis itself is emphasized too much, to the neglect of the web of communications within which the diagnosis is located, and the narrative of the patient's dilemmas. Loss is a common experience among asylum seekers and refugees: loss of homeland, the murder of relatives, family, children, and parents; loss of familiar environments and loss of self concepts, which may boost social status, and the loss of employment and dignity associated with working (Warfa *et al.*, 2010a). These losses can serve to undermine resilience, and thus different types of bereavement are common and may complicate clinical presentations.

In summary, among refugees, especially those who have witnessed atrocity or have been tortured, there is a fractured sense of a just and social world in which there are places of safety and in which they have a place. The homeland is no longer what it was, the new land is not what was expected, battles are fought on a daily basis with public services, legal and immigrant agencies, and all whilst nursing social and emotional wounds, which in some instances lead to severe mental illness, including depression, psychosis, and suicide. The historical, social, moral, and developmental fabric of a psychiatric diagnosis has long been forgotten, and needs to be recaptured.

The plight of refugees is an instance in which the limitations of our categories and diagnostic judgements become evident, especially if these are used dispassionately and without proper consideration of where asylum seekers are coming from, and where they are going to, and what they face in their journeys. Here, we are lacking a conceptual and practical framework for making such diagnostic judgements in routine clinical practice in a systematic and consistent manner. What mental health practitioners require is adjustments to the diagnostic processes and assessments in refugee mental health to include the complex and multi-dimensional profile of their health and social care issues and psychiatric co-morbidities. We propose notions of 'coherent understanding' and 'social fabric diagnosis' as a way of beginning to capture the distress experienced by refugees and asylum seekers. Practitioners struggle with this. Although diagnostic classifications permit notation of social factors, and personality issues, the universality of the intended classification does take away from a more personalized experience, and a more person-centred diagnostic formulation. Cultural formulations have been recommended in DSM to include attention to cultural identity, explanatory models, and transference and counter-transference issues. The limitations of assessment, the confidence of diagnostic judgements, or of coherent understanding when arriving at a diagnosis, need to be noted. How does one capture the social fabric diagnosis? Psychiatrists from the Psycho-pathological and Psychosocial Assistance Service (SAPPIR) in Barcelona, have described the common symptoms that most immigrants present when attending the centre and have called it *Chronic and Multiple Stress Syndrome* in immigrants (or *Ulysses syndrome*) (Achotegui, 2002). They liken the risky journey that immigrants pursue to the odyssey of the mythical Greek character in his long voyage through the Mediterranean. Immigrants affected by this syndrome present depressive symptomatology with atypical characteristics, where depressive symptoms are mixed with anxious, somatoform, and dissociative symptoms. It is proposed that a new category is necessary, a mixture of PTSD and adjustment disorders. Even this does not capture the social context, and the damage to the socially secure world including attachments, notions of safety and security, and appropriate risk taking to lead to greater well-being. The parallels with Ulysses are more telling of the experience of refugees and asylum seekers that they continue to try and survive and make progress in a society, but are forever held back and continue not to progress in their desire to become established citizens. We are short of empirical research, which follows refugees through these journeys, and are in need of conceptual and diagnostic frameworks that permit such notions to be accommodated.

References

Achotegui, J. (2002). *La depresión en los inmigrantes: una perspectiva transcultural* Barcelona: Mayo.

American Psychiatric Association. (2000). Diagnostic and statistics manual of mental disorders. Washington, DC: APA.

Arcia, E., Skinner, M., Bailey, D., and Correa, V. (2001). Modes of acculturation and health behavior among Latino immigrants to the u.s. *Social Science and Medicine* **53**: 41–53.

Berry, J.W. (1991). Understanding and managing multiculturalism. *Psychology and developing Societies* **3**: 17–49.

Bhavsar, V. and Bhugra, D. (2008). Religious delusions: finding meanings in psychosis. *Psychopathology* **41**(3): 165–172. Review.

Bhugra, D. and Bhui, K. (2007). *Textbook of Cultural Psychiatry*. Cambridge University Press.

Bhui, K., Mohamud, S., Warfa, N., Craig, T., and Stansfeld, S. (2003). Cultural adaptation of mental health measures: Improving the quality of clinical practice and research. Editorial. *British Journal of Psychiatry* **183**:184-6.

Bhui, K., Craig, T., Mohamud, S., *et al.* (2006a). Mental disorders among Somali refugees: Developing culturally appropriate measures and assessing sociocultural risk factors. *Social Psychiatry and Psychiatric Epidemiology* **41**(5): 400–408.

Bhui, K., Audini, B., Singh, S., Duffett, R., and Bhugra, D. (2006b). Representation of asylum seekers and refugees among psychiatric inpatients in London. *Psychiatric Services* **57**(2): 270–272.

Boisen, A. (1960). Out of the *Depths: An Autobiographical Study of Mental Disorder and Religious Experience*. New York: Harper.

Kleinman, A. (1987). Anthropology and psychiatry. The role of culture in cross-cultural research on illness. *British Journal of Psychiatry* **151**: 447–454.

McCrone, P., Bhui, K., Craig, T., *et al.* (2005). Mental health needs, service use and costs among Somali refugees in the UK. *Acta Psychiatrica Scandinavia* **111**(5): 351–357.

Pedersen, D., Tremblay, J., Errázuriz, C., and Gamarra, J. (2008). The sequelae of political violence: Assessing trauma, suffering and dislocation in the Peruvian highlands. *Social Science and Medicine* **62**(2): 205–217.

Robertson, C.L., Halcon, L., Savik, K., Johnson, D., Spring, M., *et al.* (2006). Somali and Oromo refugee women: trauma and associated factors. *Journal of Advanced Nursing* Dec **56**(6): 577–587.

Silove, D., Steel, Z., and Watters, C. (2000). Policies of deterrence and the mental health of asylum seekers. *Journal of American Medical Association* **284**: 604–611.

Silove, D., Steel, Z., Susljik, I., *et al.* (2007). The impact of the refugee decision on the trajectory of PTSD, anxiety, and depressive symptoms among asylum seekers: A longitudinal study. *American Journal of Disaster Medicine* **2**(6): 321–329.

Steel, Z., Silove, D., Phan, T., and Bauman, A. (2002). Long-term effect of psychological trauma on the mental health of Vietnamese refugees resettled in Australia: a population-based study. *Lancet* **360**(9339): 1056–1062.

Summerfield, D. (2008). How scientifically valid is the knowledge base of global mental health? Analysis. *British Medical Journal* **336**: 992–994.

Warfa, N. (2007). Culture and the Mental Health of African Refugees: Somali help seeking and healing in the UK and USA. In K. Bhui and D. Bhugra (Eds.) *Culture and Mental Health: A Comprehensive Textbook*. London: Hodder Arnold.

Warfa, N. and Bhui, K. (2003). Refugees and mental healthcare. *Psychiatry*, Special topics, 2(6): 26.

Warfa, N., Bhui, K., Craig, T., *et al.* (2006). Post-migration residential mobility, mental health and health service utilization among Somali refugees in the UK: A Qualitative Study. *Health and Place* **12**: 503–515.

Warfa, N., Bhui, K., Watters, C., Craig, T., Mohamud, S., and Curtis, S. (2010a). Migration experiences, employment position and psychological distress: A cross-national comparative study of Somali immigrants. (Unpublished Manuscript).

Warfa, N., Izycki, K., Jones, E., and Bhui, K. (2010b). Descriptions of torture and sexual violence among asylum seekers and foreign nationals detained in the UK. (Unpublished Manuscript).

Watters, C. (2001). Emerging paradigms in the mental health care of refugees. *Social Science and Medicine* **52**: 1709–1718.

Chapter 6

Complex mental health problems of refugees

Daya Somasundaram

Introduction

Home is a place of safety and sanctuary and the bonds to soil and village are powerful. It represents the identity and closeness of the family in a familiar environment. The neighbourhood and community provide the points of reference, the daily rhythm and meaning to existence. So leaving one's home, pulling out one's roots from familiar surroundings, relationships, and way of life is always stressful. Added to the disruption of these ties, the migrant must deal with negotiating the hurdles, complex procedures, regulations, and officials that govern national and international movement and have to adapt to a new country, society, and culture.

Many refugees and asylum seekers fleeing war, famine, and natural disasters have had to face persecution, the destruction and devastation of homes and villages, and the loss of loved ones on top of the trauma of being uprooted and cast away from all that is familiar. Refugees often have to depend on others for their basic needs, seeking shelter with relations and friends or in refugee camps. These temporary arrangements with crowded conditions, inadequate shared facilities, poor sanitation, lack of privacy, and other privations can become extremely stressful with conflicts, loss of self-esteem and dignity, and feelings of helplessness and dependency especially if prolonged (Raphael, 1986). Disruption of social network leads to what Erikson (1976) called '*loss of communality*'. The social fabric of relationships, support, and meaning is torn asunder leaving people unprotected and alone. These changes are likely to contribute to a sense of rootlessness and alienation from both the new culture and the old one. Family problems can arise due to separations, death, injuries, misunderstandings, lack of space due to overcrowding, and trauma in members.

While the migratory process may appear to be as simple as applying for a visa online and taking a plane to the host country, visa procedures can be complicated, frustrating, and time-consuming. Some immigration procedures can be extremely humiliating and culturally insensitive. For example, in Cambodia for the mandatory medical check-up for obtaining the visa for migration by the embassy designated European doctor, applicants had to strip completely and wait for their turn. Although this may have seemed innocuous to a Western person, it led to many potential applicants being a source of stories, discussion, and rumours in the local community. Even when not humiliating, policies of lengthy and mandatory detention of asylum seekers significantly contribute to mental health problems. Detainees often found the long detention in Australia triggered memories of past traumatic experiences and were more stressful and difficult to bear than the traumatic experiences including detention and torture that they had undergone in their home country. They had felt that at long last, they had left all the past behind and reached safety only to have to face further detention and the possibility of being sent back (Fazel and Silove, 2006; Steel and Silove, 2001 - see Chapter 4).

Most developed countries encourage immigration of skilled workers who can make a positive contribution to the economical development while restricting asylum seekers and refugees. People and families in robust health, highly motivated, and skilled in the ways of the modern world may migrate for economic reasons, to better themselves or settle down in a hospitable environment. Sometimes referred to as the *healthy immigration effect*, these skilled immigrants are generally healthier and enjoy a better self-perceived sense of well-being than native-born persons and refugees and asylum seekers. However, the health advantage tends to erode over time and disease patterns converge on those of the host population (Tse and Hoque, 2006).

The differentiation into skilled migrant, refugee, and asylum seeker categories is from the perspective and need of the new country (also see Ruiz and Bhugra elsewhere in this volume). As noted elsewhere, the reasons for moving are many—from the planned, voluntary migration for economic betterment to coercive eviction or fleeing for fear of persecution or death. Fleeing refugees with marketable skills may find it easier to apply for and be accepted through normal visa procedures and pathways, whereas asylum seekers face the hazards of risky journeys, the uncertainty of their application being rejected and forced return to their home country. Those in the new country may also have migrated at different times for similar or diverse reasons and be in varying stages of assimilation and acculturation to a host culture or form a separate community.

Many studies have found an increased incidence of psychosis in certain migrant communities compared to both the host and home country (e.g. Odegaard, 1932; Thomas *et al.*, 1993; Sharpley *et al.*, 2001;) leading to the hypothesis of '*migration psychosis*' among immigrants. While this has been attributed to the stresses of migration, acculturation, discrimination, and settlement difficulties, there is also the possibility that people who are prone to mental illness are more likely to migrate (Murphy, 1973). According to this hypothesis, people with personality abnormalities, prodromal illness, or those 'exported' by family are more vulnerable, having sensitive and neurotic traits, poor tolerance, resilience, and coping skills and so may be the first to flee the outbreak of hostilities and threats in their home community. Although difficult to disprove, the hypothesis is undermined by more recent studies that show that the health of recent immigrants is often better than that of their counterparts in the host population (Ministry of Health, 2006; Rasanathan, Ameratunga, and Tse, 2006; Takeuchi *et al.*, 2007). However, this may reflect only those migrating under the skilled or business categories. The health of refugees and those coming for family reunification show much poorer health status. For example, in the UK, they are found to suffer from such physical conditions as malnutrition; communicable diseases like tuberculosis, hepatitis, and HIV/AIDS; and physical injuries from war and torture; as well as depression, anxiety, and PTSD (Wilkinson, 2007).

If chosen for refugee status by the new country, then arrival and the process of acculturation, adaptation, or assimilation are part of readjustment. These processes can manifest with increased levels of suicide, homicide, substance abuse, interpersonal conflict, and aggression and a variety of psychological and psychosomatic health problems (Berry, 1990). Classically four basic outcomes have been described (see Table 6.1). These processes are helpful in understanding the ways in which communities settle down. From a mental health point of view, those integrating with the host community while maintaining ties with their home culture, the goal of multiculturalism, is the best outcome. Those in the marginalized category, rejecting the host way of life while distancing themselves from their home community become alienated and alone. Few become distrustful, suspicious, and paranoid. People who hold fast to their old ways and community, refusing to change and adapt to the new social ecology, tend to separate themselves into small enclaves, clannish groups with children

Table 6.1 Berry's model of acculturation and assimilation (Berry, 1990)

	Maintain home culture Yes	Maintain home culture No
Participation with host Yes	Integration	Assimilation
Participation with host No	Separation	Marginalization

growing up with confused identities. Those who assimilate fully, being absorbed into the local culture, lose their old identity, moorings, and relationships.

Patel and Stein (2007) provide an outline of the key risk factors experienced by refugees in settling into host countries:

- *Marginalization and minority status:* as a minority, refugees often face racial discrimination, restricted employment opportunities, and social suppression by the mainstream community, which can lead to low self-esteem and depression. Refugees are seldom a homogenous group as there can be many ethnic groupings, some of whom are marginalized even in their home country.

- *Socio-economic disadvantage*: often it is the social and economic inequities in the home country and socio-economic opportunities for advancement that cause migration in the first place. Migrants may belong to a lower class, caste, tribe, or suppressed ethnic group that faces social and economic hardships at home. This is particularly so in the rigid, hierarchical, segmented social structures found in some traditional cultures. Some children may have experienced poverty and malnutrition that will have had a profound impact on their development. Migrants may thus arrive in an impoverished state, in poor health, and with children who perform poorly in educational settings. In the host country too, refugees find themselves at a socio-economic disadvantage, having lower incomes and social status. Those coming from a high socio-economic status in their home country may find the reduction in status as migrants profoundly humiliating and difficult to bear. For example, a person who had been a respected professional back home may have to drive taxis, do demeaning labour work to survive or remain unemployed on social welfare. Bhugra and Ayonrinde (2004) have pointed out that discrepancy between expectations, aspiration, and tachievement can result in poor self-esteem and frustration, leading to depression.

- *Lack of family and social support*: separations within family and extended family, loss of community support, lack of religious and cultural practices, rituals, and worship has been described as cultural bereavement (Eisenbruch, 1991) (also see Chapter 15 by Wojcik and Bhugra in this volume).

- *Adaptation to the new culture*: difficulties with secondary language proficiency, education, employment, housing, visa status, exploitation in the labour market and decline in social status are some of the stress factors that consistently make adaptation an onerous process. Phenomena of 'culture shock' may need to be overcome. Those migrating from very different backgrounds, particularly of a traditional or deprived variety, will find the ways of the new world they face perplexing, difficult to understand, demanding, and stressful. Sometimes there is a clash of values, priorities, and meaning.

- *Age and gender*: some age groups such as the elderly are particularly at risk. They may initially be more reluctant to leave home to which they would have stronger ties; find the migration process more strenuous, adaptation into the host country well nigh impossible; and have more physical health problems. Intergenerational conflict would be common, though migrating families may find the grandparents useful for childcare, and a treasure house of traditional values and knowledge. Some may insist on their own reverse migration back to the old country. Children, adolescents, and youth, particularly second generation, may grapple with excessive demands from traditional parents; intergenerational conflicts; changing identity crisis caught between that of the host country and their ethnic belonging; and educational and employment endeavours making them more prone to depression, risky behaviour, and perhaps, suicide (Rasanathan *et al.*, 2006; Lau and Thomas, 2008). Those undergoing adolescent crisis (Juang, Syed, and Takagi, 2007; Rasanathan *et al.*, 2006), without one or both parents, without language skills and poor peer support are at an incre ased risk (Lau and Thomas, 2008). Unaccompanied children, as has been shown for Korean adoptees in America (Hubinette, 2007), could experience difficulties in their foster home.

+ Females who head families (Smith, 2006), come as brides (Thai, 2007), enter the labour market (Smith, 2006), and those coping with disruptive family dynamics may face serious difficulties due to changes in gender roles and gender role expectations and consequently may decompensate.

Families

The family is central to traditional 'collectivistic communities'. Families tend to think and act as a unit. There are strict hierarchical roles and obligations that emphasize harmony and support to each other during difficulties. The individual submerges his or her 'self' within the nuclear and extended family dynamics. In individualistic cultures, importance is given to the rights, views, needs, and desires of the individual; he or she is privileged even at the expense of the family and community. Migrating families have to make the transition to the more 'individualistic' system in host mainstream societies of the Western world that emphasize emancipation from the family. As a result 'Refugee immigrant families experience feelings of social and cultural isolation and struggle to function as family systems, especially when considering gender issues, intergenerational factors, and the process of acculturation and assimilation as related to family dynamics. Moreover, the immigrant families struggle within various ecological social systems outside the family system, including the educational, physical and mental health, economic, and political systems' (Kawamoto and Anguiano, 2006).

The recommendations for providing 'Culturally Competent Services' in a Royal College of Psychiatrists' publication gives pride of place to the family (see Box 6.1). The family can be a source of support and help in the treatment process of clients as well as a cause of problems. The adjustments in the family may well create further problems in settlements. The traumatized person often also contributes to the pathological family dynamics:

Case study one

B. was a middle-aged man who had migrated with his family several years ago as a refugee. He had undergone severe trauma in his home country, including detention, torture, and witnessing gruesome events of deaths and destruction. He was a loving father to his children but had difficulties with his wife who with the children had adapted better to the host culture. He had ongoing problems with PTSD and depression, for which he abused alcohol and prescription drugs. Under the influence of alcohol he met with a road traffic accident and suffered a fractured arm and some brain damage. This added pain and weakness of the arm and cognitive deficiency, particularly memory difficulties, to the earlier symptoms. Although well educated and intelligent, he was on a disability pension due to his physical and mental incapacity. The immigrant family also had the perennial economic and housing problems. Despite all these, he had given up alcohol and was making considerable progress in his treatment when he received news that his brother and sister-in-law had been killed by a rival tribe as a revenge for his having escaped. The surviving children and grandmother (client's mother) had escaped to a neighbouring country and were living in a refugee camp in terrible conditions. He felt directly responsible and terribly guilty. There was an immediate relapse and exacerbation of his symptoms. He hired a migration lawyer and went through the complicated process of trying to sponsor the orphaned children and his mother but the application was rejected. The lawyer demanded more money to appeal but was pessimistic about the possibilities. On leaving the lawyer's office, he appeared to have gone into a fugue and wandered the streets during the rainy night to turn up at home the next morning in a dishevelled state. His wife was understandably (according to him) furious and in the ensuing argument he had hit her. She called the police and he was put on a restraining order, which left him homeless on the streets. He desperately wanted to get back to his family but was prevented by the legal and social system that had now been activated by domestic violence. He attempted suicide and was admitted to hospital. He was discharged to a temporary lodge and had to be admitted again after taking alcohol and another suicide attempt.

Once the issue of domestic violence had been triggered, the Western healthcare system worked to separate the family members, ostensibly to protect the wife and children. But for this patient, the support and help of the family was the one thing necessary for recovery. The possibility of eventual successful suicide was high. Significantly, the perpetrators back home have succeeded in reaching him in the safety of the host country, to destroy the very basis of his family life. When these were pointed out to him and his current condition discussed with a view of imparting insight and motivation to regain access to his children, he started to show unusual resilience for the first time, struggled to get his life reorganized, ventured to learn English, and start working and help other inmates in the lodge where he was staying. Where he had been completely dependent on his wife for his care and manifested with illness behaviour and substance behaviour, the current turn of events gave the impetus for recovery.

Case study two

Ms H was a middle-aged widow with two sons whose husband had been murdered back home for political reasons. She herself had undergone considerable trauma and hardship in escaping with her children that continues in frequent re-experiencing as flashbacks and nightmares. PTSD and depressive symptoms are prominent in her mental state. She is illiterate and suffers from a variety of physical and mental health problems for which she is under treatment from a variety of medical systems (GP, Respiratory, ENT, Gynaecology, Eye, and Psychiatry). She suffers from severe asthma, which becomes exacerbated by different stresses including her family dynamics. She then is taken by ambulance to hospital but refuses to stay there for more than a day as the children go hungry when she is not there to cook for them. They would come and hang around the hospital or wander the streets. She was on several types of medications, inhalers, nebulizer, and oxygen at home. She has put on weight, becoming obese, further aggravating her arthritic and other physical conditions. She also accesses several services including social welfare (disability pension), housing, legal, education, NGOs, community, and others with whom she has multiple appointments and meetings, many of which she misses. She hardly understands all these procedures and is unable to get around to the different places. Yet, she is supposed to be following English and driving classes. At home she had problems with both children. The eldest, at 16 years, appears to be going through an adolescent crisis and externalizes the stress through aggression and violence. He breaks all kinds of expensive items at home including the TV, computer, slams things as he walks back and beats up his younger brother. He leaves home and does not come back for long periods or nights. At school too he has constant problems with classmates, hitting them and getting into trouble. He does not respect the mother, often scolding her in 'filth' and once reported her to police saying she was not giving them food. She says he is completely out of her control. The younger one tends to internalize his problems, becomes withdrawn, sad, biting his fingers. Both have counsellors and are being followed up by adolescent and child mental health. The home life is very emotional, stormy, and unpredictable. They do not mix with other families, tend to withdraw from social life, isolate themselves, not participating in any of the cultural or religious activities of their community, and have no social support. However, they are in constant contact with their home network through the telephone. Recently, news of the death of her brother-in-law in a car accident has upset the family functioning further. Again, the legacy of killing the father has set in motion the abnormal family dynamics.

The abnormal family dynamics, aggravated and sustained by the mother struggling with her own trauma, loss, and physical illnesses, influenced other family members to more maladaptive behaviour patterns. When treating individual clients, there is a need to look at how best we can address the family as a unit and find support for them. However, the Western family therapy approach with a modular session with all family members in room with the therapist may not work. A holistic integral approach, working with available family members, addressing their various needs and relationships as well as the family dynamics, finding and mobilizing support systems is important. In a healthy, supportive family environment, members would recover and may not need individual treatment. It is useful to involve the family from the outset of treatment by involving them in the initial history and assessment, encouraging their contribution and point of view. They could also be invited to sit in with the clients when appropriate in the regular sessions (mothers with young children should be encouraged to bring them and they could play or come and go from the outer room) and be given specific tasks, such as giving medication or massage, as well as used as co-therapists.

Interventions

Clients with complex needs will need a multidisciplinary team to address their problems in an integrated, holistic way. Simple medication and/or counselling will not be sufficient in a majority of cases. However, preventive public health measures and early intervention can provide very timely help before problems become complicated. Many of the difficulties are interrelated and feed into each other. Breaking the vicious cycle early or giving the necessary information or basic self-help steps could be crucial. For example, many clients need information about what services are available, how to best access them and networking with the services to provide the links for the clients before they become bewildered, frustrated, and depressed. Initially, they may need interpreters and social workers or befrienders to help them find their way around. Culture brokers may be required. Basic and simple educational and informational material in the language of the client like pamphlets, posters, or media announcements on such issues as services, how to access them, common stress and psychosocial problems, dos and don'ts can be made available at common meeting places. Points of contact like social services and primary healthcare facilities should be culturally competent and sensitive (Box 6.1). Language is often a problem and skilled interpreters should be available. The role and function of the interpreter can be vital (Tribe and Raval, 2003). However, some interpreters could be problematic, particularly if from the same community, as sensitive clients may want to preserve confidentiality or the interpreter may inadvertently influence the relationship in subtle ways. Workers, including health staff, should become aware of cultural issues, preferences, sensitive areas, fears and concerns, variety of problems, possible solutions, referral pathways and common ethnic idioms, expressions and cultural nuances. Positive attitudes; an openness, warmth, and friendliness; and skills in dealing with multicultural clients and issues are essential. Refugees with complex problems will need socio-economic and legal assistance to deal with asylum applications, housing, employment, and other day-to-day and settlement issues. Often these pressing needs have to be attended to before meaningful

Box 6.1 Culturally competent service (Patel and Stein, 2007)

- The family is usually the preferred point of intervention. Understanding family structure and dynamics will be helpful in service delivery.

- Be aware that individuals from minority groups will be struggling with the demands and ideals of at least two cultures.

- Be aware that individuals will make choices, life decisions, and treatment decisions based on cultural forces.

- Appropriate pieces of cultural knowledge should be incorporated into day-to-day clinical practice and policy making.

- Cultural competence will involve working closely with natural informal network of a particular minority, for example local religious leaders or spirit healers.

- Cultural competence extends the concept of self-determination to the whole minority community, so minority groups should be encouraged to participate on boards and serve in the administrative team and be recruited to staff in the mental health teams at all levels.

- Cultural competent services should practise equal and non-discriminatory policies. Responsive and special outreach services for particular minority groups may also be helpful.

Source: Patel, V. and Stein, G. (2007)

psychotherapy can be started. Sometimes when these basic problems are sorted out, refugees may regain their self-esteem and functionality and no longer need specific psychological help.

Health professionals should familiarize themselves with culture specific conditions and presentations, idioms of distress, emic and etic categories, and provide a more broad therapeutic service. Using assessment tools developed in one culture blindly in another will lead to problems in diagnosis and also in acceptance of any interventions. Thus understanding cultural belief systems and explanatory models are important in interpreting complaints and developing a trusting relationship and rapport. Active listening, attention to body language, and cultural and gender sensitiveness are important parts of communication skills. Referral for specialized care for those with severe problems like traumatization, depression, psychosis, and substance abuse will need to be done. It is being increasingly recognized that clients with complex mental health problems need a multidisciplinary, holistic, long-term approach that addresses their physical, psychological, economic, sociocultural and spiritual needs (Table 6.2). The WHO definition of health gives a good framework to conceptualize multidisciplinary interventions that would address their complex needs (see Table 6.2):

> Health is a state of complete physical, mental, (family), social and (spiritual) well-being, and not merely an absence of disease or infirmity.
>
> World Health Organisation (WHO)

The spiritual dimension has been put forward at various WHO fora but has not been formally accepted yet. On the other hand spirituality forms a key part of social and psychological make-up of the individual.

Innovative, new approaches effective for preventive and therapeutic use at the individual and community levels for a range of physical and mental health problems include traditional cultural practices. These include traditional techniques from Yoga and Buddhism. These produce profound muscular and physiological relaxation and mental tranquillity that are useful in treating anxiety disorders, somatization, and physical conditions that are aggravated by stress like hypertension, asthma, and diabetes. Mindfulness Based Cognitive Therapy (MBCT) has been found effective for a number of common mental disorders including recurrent and chronic depression (Baer, 2006).

In our local practice, breathing techniques, repetition of words, muscular and mental relaxation, mindfulness, and meditation were distilled out of the traditional practices after close study (Somasundaram, 2002). In addition, traditional massage was used where indicated to induce states of relaxation. The appropriate traditional methods were selected depending on the religion, culture, needs, and outlook of the patient: see Box 6.2.

As mental distress in traditional cultures is often experienced and expressed in somatic terms, it will benefit from interventions structured initially in physical terms (Bracken, Geiller, and Summerfield, 1995; Kirmayer, 1996). These practices are especially helpful for somatoform disorders where there is abnormal preoccupation with the body. The exercises will help to divert the attention away into more healthy body awareness. Other conditions like anxiety, depression, PTSD, and culture bound syndromes that manifest through somatic complaints will also be helped by these practices. At the psychological level, these methods produce a state of relaxation countering states of arousal, anxiety, and tension.

These techniques have also proven helpful for torture survivors with musculoskeletal pains and a distorted body image due to the systematic infliction of excruciating pain and injury. Similarly in landmine victims and others with amputation experiencing phantom limb problems, these methods can be used to help restore a feeling of wholeness. For certain culture bound syndromes

Table 6.2 Dimensions of health

Dimensions of health	Causes	Symptoms	Diagnosis	Interventions
Physical	Physical injury, infections, epidemics	Pain, fever, somatization	Physical illness, psychosomatic, somatoform disorders	Drugs treatment, physiotherapy, relaxation techniques, massage
Psychological	Shock, stress, fear – terror, loss, trauma	Tension, fear, sadness, learned helplessness	ASR, PTSD, anxiety, depression, alcohol and drug abuse	Psychological first aid, psychotherapy, counselling, relaxation techniques, CBT
Family	Death, separation, disability	Vacuum, disharmony, violence	Family pathology, scapegoating	Family therapy, marital therapy, family support
Social	Unemployment, poverty, war	Conflict, suicidal ideation, anomie, alienation, loss of communality	Parasuicide, suicide, violence, collective trauma	Group therapy, rehabilitation, community mobilization, social engineering
Spiritual	Misfortune, bad period, spirits, angry gods, evil spells, Karma	Despair, demoralization, loss of belief, loss of hope	Possession	Logotherapy, rituals, traditional healing, meditation, contemplation, mindfulness

Box 6.2 Traditional methods which may be helpful

1 Breathing exercises (*Pranayamam, Anapana Sati, or mindful breathing*)

2 Muscular relaxation (*Shanthi or Sava Asana, mindful body awareness, Tai Chi*)

3 Regular repetition of words

   a. Hindus – *Jappa: Pranava mantra, 'OM'*;

   b. Buddhists – Pirit or chanting: *Buddhang Saranang Gachchami*;

   c. Islam – Dhikir, *Tasbih: Subhanallah*;

   d. Catholic Christians – *Rosary, prayer beads:* the Jesus prayer (*Jesus Christ have mercy on me*)

   e. Cambodia – *Keatha, angkam: Puthoo*; Vietnamese – *Mophit*

   f. Scientific – T.M.

4 Meditation (*Dhyanam, Contemplation, Samadhi, Vipassana*)

5 Massage: *Ayurvedic* or *Siddha* oil massage and the Cambodian, *thveu saasay*

like *Dhat syndrome* (semen loss anxiety) in South Asia and idioms of distress like *che kabal (headache)* in Cambodia or *Perumuchu (chronic, sighing respiration)* in Tamils, these cultural methods in assessments were useful. In the long-term management of alcohol and drug abuse, Yoga and/or mindfulness was introduced as a means of changing life styles.

The benefits of these originally spiritual practices are not confined to producing relaxation. When methods are culturally familiar, these tap into past childhood, community, and religious roots and thus release a rich source of associations that can be helpful in therapy and the healing process. Mindfulness and meditation draw upon hidden resources within the individual and open into dimensions that can create spiritual well-being and give meaning to what has happened. Although these techniques do no formal psychotherapy, they may accomplish what psychotherapy attempts to do by releasing cultural and spiritual restorative processes.

Conclusions

Migrants may initially appear robust and resilient. However, vulnerable groups like refuges, asylum seekers, those coming for family reunion, elderly, women, unaccompanied children, second and later generations may have developed a variety of mental health problems. Qualitative research may help delineate the needs and problems faced by the refugees. Culture sensitive services, family approaches, and traditional methods may help ameliorate the complex difficulties faced by refugees.

Acknowledgement

The University of Adelaide, particularly the Glenside Campus and Barr-Smith Library, provided excellent facilities to carry out the literature survey and collaborative work to produce this paper. The Scholar Rescue Fund based in New York bestowed the fellowship and timely assistance to leave the disturbed northern province of Sri Lanka to find respite in Adelaide, Australia. STTARS in Adelaide and the clients who come there are the real source of much material discussed here.

References

Baer, R. (2006). *Mindfulness-Based Treatment Approaches: Clinician's Guide to Evidence Base and Applications*. Amsterdam: Academic Press.

Berry, J.W. (1990). Acculturation and adaptation: Health consequences of culture contact among circumpolar people. *Arctic Medical Research* **49**: 142–150.

Bracken, P.J., Geiller, J.E., and Summerfield, D. (1995). Psychological responses to war and atrocity: The limitations of current concepts. *Social Science and Medicine* **40**: 1073–1082.

Bhugra, D. and Ayonrinde, O. (2004). Depression in migrants and ethnic minorities. *Advances in Psychiatric Treatment* **10**: 13–17.

Eisenbruch, M. (1991). From post-traumatic stress disorder to cultural bereavement: Diagnosis of Southeast Asian Refugees. *Social Science and Medicine* **33**: 673–680.

Erikson, K.T. (1976). Loss of communality at Buffalo Creek. *American Journal of Psychiatry* **135**: 300–305.

Fazel, M. and Silove, D. (2006) Detention of refugees. *British Medical Journal* **327**: 251–252.

Hubinette, T. (2007). Asian bodies out of control: Examining the adopted Korean existence. In R.S. Parrenas and L.C. Siu (Eds.), *Asian Diasporas*, pp. 177–200, Stanford: Stanford University Press.

Juang, L.P., Syed, M., and Takagi, M. (2007). Intergenerational discrepancies of parental control among Chinese American families: links to family conflict and adolescent depressive symptoms. *Journal of Adolescence* **30**: 965–975.

Kawamoto, W.T. and Anguiano, R.V. (2006). Asian and Latino immigrant families. In B.B. Ingoldsby and S.D. Smith (Eds.), *Families in Global and Muliticultural Perspective*, pp. 209–230, Thousand Oaks, California: Sage Publications.

Kirmayer, L.J. (1996). Confusion of the senses: implications of ethnocultural variations in Somatoform and Dissociative Disorders for PTSD. In A.J. Marsella, M.J. Friedman, E.T. Gerrity, and R. M. Scurfield (Eds.), *Ethnocultural Aspects of Posttraumatic Stress Disorder*, pp. 131–163, Washington DC: American Psychological Association.

Lau, W. and Thomas, T. (2008). Research into the psychological well-being of young refugees. *International Psychiatry* **5**(3): 60–62.

Ministry of Health (2006). Asian Health Chart Book 2006. Wellington: Ministry of Health.

Murphy, H.D. (1973). Migration and mental health. In C. Zwingmann and M. Pfister-Ammende (Eds.), An *Appraisal of Uprooting and After*, New York: Springer-Verlag.

Odegaard, O. (1932). Emigration and insanity: A study of mental disease in Norwegian born population in Minnesota. *Acta Psychiatrica et Neurologica Sacandinavica, Supplement No. 4.* Quoted by Patel and Stein (2007).

Patel, V. and Stein, G. (2007). Cultural and international psychiatry. In G. Stein and G. Wilkinson (Eds.), *General Adult Psychiatry*, pp. 782–810, London: Royal College of Psychiatrists.

Raphael, B. (1986). *When Disaser Strikes.* London: Hutchinson.

Rasanathan, K., Ameratunga, S., Chen, J., *et al.* (2006). *A Health Profile of Young Asian New Zealanders Who Attend Secondary School: Findings from Youth 2000.* Auckand: University of Auckland.

Sharpley, M.S., Hutchinson, G., Murray, R.M. and Mckenzie, K. (2001). Understanding the excess of psychosis among the African-Caribbean population in England. A review of current hypothesis. *British Journal of Psychiatry* **178**: s60–s68.

Smith, S.D. (2006). Global families. In B.B. Ingoldsby and S.D. Smith (Eds.), *Families in Global and Muliticultural Perspective*, pp. 3–24, Thousand Oaks, California, USA: Sage Publications.

Somasundaram, D.J. (2002). Using traditional relaxation techniques in healthcare. *International Medical Journal* **9**: 191–198.

Steel, Z. and Silove, D. (2001) The mental health implications of detaining asylum-seekers. *Medical Journal of Australia* **175**: 596–599.

Takeuchi, D.T., Zane, N., Hong, S., *et al.* (2007). Immigration-related factors and mental disorders among Asian Americans. *American Journal of Public Health* **97**: 84–92.

Thai, H.C. (2007). My mother fell in love with my-xuan first: arranging 'traditional' marriages across the diaspora. In R.S. Parrenas and L.C. Siu (Eds.), *Asian Diasporas*, pp. 85–104, Stanford: Stanford University Press.

Thomas, C.S., Stone, K., Osborn, M., Thomas, P.F., and Fisher, M. (1993). Psychiatric morbidity and compulsory admission among UK-born Eurpoeans, Afro-Caribeans and Asians in central Manchester. *Bristish Journal of Psychiatry* **163**: 91–99.

Tribe, R. and Raval, H. (2003). *Working with Interpreters.* Hove: Brunner-Routledge.

Tse, S. and Hoque, M.E. (2006). Healthy immigrant effect – triumphs, transience and threats. In S. Tse, E. Hoque, K. Rasanathan, M. Chatterji, R. Wee, S. Garg, and Y. Ratnasabapathy (Eds.), *Prevention, Protection and Promotion.* Proceedings of the Second International Asian Health and Wellbeing Conference, November 11, 13–14, (pp. 9–18). Auckland, New Zealand: University of Auckland.

Wilkinson, G. (2007). Psychiatry in general practice. In G. Stein and G. Wilkinson (Eds.), *General Adult Psychiatry*, pp. 747–781, London: Royal College of Psychiatrists.

Chapter 7

International refugee policy

Sean Cross, Jim Crabb, and Rachel Jenkins

Introduction

The way in which refugees and asylum seekers are dealt with in terms of policy is complex. By their very definition, refugees and those seeking such a status routinely cross international borders. As such the policy framework, within which all who work in this area must operate, is constructed at several levels—at the level of regional or local government dealing with acute needs; at the level of the nation state; by supra-national structures such as the European Union (EU); and at a global level through the auspices of the United Nations (UN). The political motivation at each of these levels will vary, for example with the UN taking a much wider politically cosmopolitan approach as opposed to nation states, which may be perceived as acting in their own narrower best interests.

This chapter will attempt to further the understanding of the interplay between policy construction and practical outcome by steering a story through the history of refugee policy making. As such it will be divided into several sections. It will initially give a historical overview and then take a more detailed look at recent events using the example of the UK within Europe as a model of one Western nation's response to recent refugee developments. We will look at the legal framework that has evolved in the UK through a variety of Acts of Parliament. These have been adopted to deliver policies in response to events from the post Cold War world to the realities of the early part of the 21st century and allow a picture of how the cosmopolitan aspiration of the original ideas for dealing with refugees often come into conflict with national self interest. Finally, the chapter will end by looking at some concrete policy examples of dealing with mental health issues in a variety of acute refugee settings.

Historical overview

International mechanisms for the management of refugees were initially attempted in the years following the First World War in Europe. This was due to the large number of displaced persons on the continent after the fighting ended due to the collapse of the defeated powers. However, it was not until after the Second World War that a greater commitment to the ideas of a liberal institutional framework was accepted, of which the following are the most important parts.

The 1951 Convention Relating to the Status of Refugees

The 1951 Convention forms the basis of international law relating to refugees. It sets out the rights of those who claim asylum and the responsibilities of nations granting the asylum. It enshrined a principle of *non-refoulement*, meaning that individuals should not be forced to return to the area from which they have fled. 'Article One' still forms the basis on which individual signatory nation states determine claimants' status. According to the Convention, which provides no definition for the term 'asylum seeker', a refugee is defined as follows.

> A person who is outside his/her country of nationality or habitual residence; has a well-founded fear of persecution because of his/her race, religion, nationality, membership in a particular social group or political opinion; and is unable or unwilling to avail himself/herself of the protection of that country, or to return there, for fear of persecution(UN, 1951).

The 1967 Protocol

In 1967 a Protocol extending to the Convention was agreed (UN, 1967). Thereafter a fully global obligatory legal system took shape such that the same rights and protection under the United Nations were granted to refugees beyond Europe. This occurred at the height of the Cold War, when movement of people was far less than today. It is therefore only since its aftermath in the 1990s that the principle of *non-refoulement* of individuals from across the world has been tested. So far 146 states have signed the Convention and Protocol.

Other important elements

A major additional legal framework exists in the ECHR or European Convention on Human Rights (Council-of-Europe, 1950). This was fully incorporated into UK law as recently as 1998 when the Human Rights Act was adopted (Crown, 1998). Articles 3, 5, and 8 of the ECHR in particular form the basis of claims by asylum seekers at appeal in the UK. A more thorough attempt at defining and outlawing causes for refugee flight has been attempted in instruments such as the Convention Against Torture (UN, 1987); however, it is the original Convention which continues to form the basis of intra-state responsibilities in the world.

Table 7.1 Definitions of terms

Term	Definition
Refugee	A generic term to describe all people forced to move; however, legally these are individuals who meet certain criteria: an international border must have been crossed and status confirmed.
Asylum seeker	Refers to individuals who flee and who make a claim to refugee protection under law, but whose status has yet to be determined. Almost universally a Western construct.
Internally Displaced Person (IDP)	Refers to individuals often experiencing the same problems as refugees, but legally describes those who have not crossed an international border.

Definitions

Confusion over terminology when discussing different groups is common. The differences are technical and legal rather than intrinsic to the individuals themselves—Table 7.1. These have already been described in Chapter 1.

Contemporary international players in policy work and practise

The agency founded to work in this area was the United Nations High Commission for Refugees (UNHCR). Established on 14th December 1950 by the UN General Assembly, it has a mandate to lead and coordinate international action to protect refugees and to resolve refugee problems worldwide. Headquartered in Geneva, it has a staff over 6,000 in 116 countries and publishes regular updates on the number of individuals of concern that it believes fall within its remit worldwide.

As guardians of the international conventions as well as active participants in managing the plight of some refugees, the UNHCR has a history of political engagement in both source and host countries. Its importance can be seen in its leadership, which has seen two former European Prime Ministers Ruud Lubbers and Antonio Gutteres as High Commissioner over the last decade. The extent to which the international body has influenced the UK debate can be seen in several ways. Its liberal-institutionalist post-Second World War founding and history makes its approach one that sees it often at variance with state-based attempts at heightened control.

In assessing the pressures that policy, whether instigated at a national or supra-national level, faces, a discourse analysis can be done using internet-based search engines. Data from two UK newspapers, the *Guardian*—a left of centre broadsheet and the *Daily Mail*—a right of centre tabloid, will be used to demonstrate a variety of points.

Table 7.2 *Guardian* and *Mail* searches for mention of UNHCR in asylum stories[1]

	Guardian	Daily Mail
Search term 'asylum'	11154	849
Search term 'UNHCR' or 'UN'	718	16
Percentage of stories with 'UN' or 'UNHCR' mentioned	**6.4%**	**1.8%**

The UNHCR's influence on the discourse within the UK reveals difference in how often the organization is mentioned at all. As can be seen in Table 7.2, in all stories it occurs infrequently. This may be interpreted as evidence for the issues being seen as 'national' rather than global.

The higher proportion of stories in the *Guardian* linking asylum and the UNHCR can be explained perhaps in terms of the manner of reporting. It is also a matter of the views of the two newspapers, with the *Mail* seeing the issue as a more internal concern. Interventions by the UNHCR on matters concerning the UK are common. Many press releases use gentle and encouraging language most notable when the UK has actively involved itself in resettlement programmes such as with Liberians in 2003 (UNHCR, 2003) or the tripartite arrangement on voluntary repatriation negotiated between the UK, the Afghan government, and the agency (UNHCR, 2002a).

However, direct confrontation and criticism do occur. A UNHCR press release from 2002, responding to the Yarls Wood asylum detention centre fire, expressed concern about the mixing of 'bona fide refugees' with those who had failed the process (UNHCR, 2002b). Other more vociferous examples in the UK include an intervention to criticize the restricted access to legal advice (Guardian, 2003a); defending the current 1951 framework as 'relevant and timeless' in response to Prime Minister Tony Blair's expressed belief that it was 'completely out of date'(Guardian, 2003b); expressing opposition to operational matters such as deportation plans of Somali asylum seekers (Guardian, 2005a); or even intervening in the UK's internal general election campaign when the UNHCR criticized the Conservative Party opposition platform of quotas and withdrawal from the 1951 Convention (Guardian, 2005b).

After the cold war—a UK and European policy response

The end of the Cold War, for obvious political reasons, saw the start of the most recent global increase in those seeking asylum. Six major pieces of

[1] Searches conducted of *Guardian* and *Mail* internet search archives on 2nd February 2007.

legislation have been passed by the UK parliament since 1993. The other major development has been that of increased European cooperation in this area but even now it remains nascent, with an aspiration for a fully integrated and coordinated policy in 2010. A summary of each of the new laws in the UK follows below. A number of themes are evident and will be discussed after they have been laid out. Excellent and detailed descriptions of different Western nations' responses are available (Gibney, 2004).

Asylum and Immigration Appeals Act (1993)

This was the first major piece of legislation since the 1970s and since asylum had become a major political issue across Europe. In particular, the numbers of people fleeing the growing conflicts in the Balkans gave cause for concern and this appeared to be a move of pre-emption rather than reaction. It was not until this point that the 1951 Convention was fully incorporated into UK law as prior to this, immigration officers and adjudicators simply had to 'take account' of the Convention when making decisions. The Act also reinforced the welfare responsibilities of local authorities, although its main thrust was a restrictive appeal procedure.

Asylum and Immigration Act (1996)

The last Act addressing this issue made by John Major's government continued the move to restriction. An increase in asylum claims preceded its passing into law; mostly as a result of the Balkan wars. Employment rights were curtailed and benefits and housing support for asylum seekers were also made harder to achieve. A framework for removal of asylum claimants to safe third countries was also laid down.

Immigration and Asylum Act (1999)

The White Paper from the UK Home Office (Ministry of Home Affairs) from which this was drawn, spoke of an alliterative 'fairer, faster and firmer' approach (HO, 1998). Approximately 40% of the asylum seekers in the UK in 1998 and 1999 came from Europe—mostly Kosovo, and a core part of the Act attempted to discriminate between those who were seen as genuine and those who were not. To this end, asylum was again linked with immigration in general. The Act sought to streamline administrative processes as well as extend the powers of border guards. Increased penalties for clandestine entrants including higher carrier liabilities were introduced and successive avenues of appeal were curtailed. In addition a more controlled approach to welfare assistance occurred. A statutory emphasis of the difference of asylum seekers to any other citizens was permitted as responsibility shifted from the local authority to central government with the founding of the National Asylum Support System (NASS). Taking these responsibilities away from local authorities fits with a securitization process in which serious, important security matters are not left as the responsibility of local government. Support 'in kind' was championed with ideas such as vouchers instead of money. This would subsequently not succeed.

Two further developments were incorporated. An increase in the powers of immigration officers enabled them to work more often without the presence of police officers and the operational management of detention centres was covered, even if they were eventually to play a far smaller role that originally anticipated.

Despite what was seen as a tightening of the procedures, the subsequent three years, 2000–2002, saw the largest number of asylum seeker applications demonstrating perhaps the severe difficulties a single nation state has in developing isolated policy to a global issue. This time also marked a shift away from European to Asian/Middle Eastern claimants.

A Common European Asylum Policy—1999, Tampere and beyond

At the same time as the UK addressed the issue of asylum, a second track of management was being established at a European level. Ratification of the Amsterdam Treaty of 1998 led to immigration and asylum taking on increased importance supra-nationally. However, at the Tampere in Finland the Justice and Home Affairs summit of the Finnish presidency in 1999, all 15 member states expressed a wish to form a 'Common European Asylum policy' (European-Council, 1999).

The countries of the EU re-affirmed their commitment to the principle of asylum and an avoidance of a 'Fortress Europe' approach. Whilst a unified policy approach aimed to create minimum standards across the Union, it also aimed to avoid 'asylum shopping' from one state to another. One popular news study showed that in the year 1999–2000, asylum seekers were dealt with very differently across the EU as demonstrated in Table 7.3 below (BBC, 2001).

The Tampere agreement outlined a series of minimum standards representing at best a skeletal framework that was successfully adopted 5 years later. It included minimum standards for an EU-wide temporary-protection regime, reception conditions for asylum seekers, eligibility criteria for those given the status of refugees and others in need of international protection, and minimum standards for procedures to determine or withdraw refugee status.

Regulations were also established to determine which state would be responsible for examining an asylum application lodged in an EU member state by a

Table 7.3 Comparison of asylum statistics from six EU members from 1999–2000

Country	UK	Germany	Holland	France	Belgium	Austria
Applications (2000)	97,860	78,760	43,890	38,590	42,690	18,280
Recognition of asylum seeker status 1999	72.5%	13.5%	15.6%	19.3%	32.4%	56.6%
Percentage granted refugee status	12.1%	11.3%	2.5%	19.3%	32.4%	41.7%

third-country national that became known as the Dublin II Regulation. A fingerprints database was set up and a European Refugee Fund and other financial instruments supporting EU asylum systems and initiatives were established.

The consolidated *acquis* dealing with asylum after the incorporation of the Treaty of Amsterdam stretches, as of December 2006, to four Council Directives, ten Council Decisions and five Regulations from the Council, Commission, and Parliament. Taking the issue forward at a European level has been affected by the uncertainty as a result of the internal institutional difficulties brought about by the Dutch and French rejection of an EU Constitution and the subsequent institutional difficulties that have arisen.

The Europeanization of the issue in the development of the Common European Asylum Policy at once seems to make sense and contradict the thrust of the UK government wishing to exercise a heightened level of control over the issue. There have been two main assessments of this move towards a greater European position on the matter of asylum (Geddes, 2003). The 'losing control' hypothesis argues that in the advancement of, for want of a better word, 'globalization' or at least greater interdependency, has resulted in an inevitable erosion of state-based responsibility in this area. Alternatively an 'escape to Europe' hypothesis sees this move as in fact a reassertion of state-based control power but one step removed from the state itself thus avoiding the domestic political and legal constraints. Whichever way it is viewed, it is the case that in the continent that gave a raison d'etre for the original Convention, a re-internationalization is taking place.

Nationality, Immigration and Asylum Act (2002)

In the UK, 80,315 asylum seekers were registered in 2002—the second highest annual figure of the decade. This Act was also the first piece of specific asylum legislation after the World Trade Centre attacks of 9/11 and coincided with the number of claimants from the Middle East growing to 22%. In addition to general immigration issues it also included citizenship themes such as the introduction of citizenship ceremonies in which an individual must take an oath and pledge and have a greater understanding of what are circumscribed 'British values'.

In addition, an extension of the powers of detention and removal was granted, along with a further tightening of the mechanisms by which appeal procedures could be launched. These restrictions included certification of clearly 'unfounded' claims, those claims that could have been appealed earlier, introduction of statutory closure dates, and the use of a statutory review process in an attempt to prevent lengthy and costly judicial reviews. The funding of a voluntary assisted return programme was confirmed and an extension of trafficking offences was put in place.

Asylum and Immigration (Treatment of Claimants, etc.) Act (2004)

This Act came within two years of the previous legislation and at a time when asylum continued to register as a major political concern. However, the figures showed a downward trend with 49,405 claimants for 2003 and 33,690 for 2004.

The Act created new and extended criminal offences aimed at traffickers. Treatment of claimant provisions also included believability guidelines to detect genuineness and credibility. They advised that certain 'behaviour' could be interpreted as designed to conceal information or mislead and that it was appropriate to take it into account when determining status. In addition, further alterations of housing rights were mandated as well as the abolition of entitlement to back payments of benefits to those eventually found to be genuine refugees. Further powers were also granted to immigration officers such as taking fingerprints at the beginning of an enforcement process.

The appeals procedures were again tightened including the merging of the immigration and asylum systems into a single tier of appeal after which further limited onward appeal was possible. These measures proved particularly controversial with restrictions in appeals most vociferously opposed by the judiciary. An extension of provisions on removal to safe third countries also occurred.

Immigration, Asylum and Nationality Act (2006)

This received Royal assent just twenty months after the previous Act. Two documents that the government had published formed its basis. These were 'Controlling Our Borders: Making Migration Work for Britain' (HO, 2006) in which asylum again is reiterated as a migration rather than obligation phenomenon and 'Confident Communities in a Secure Britain', the Home Office

Strategic Plan document for the years 2004–2008 (HO, 2004). Acknowledging the impact on wider societal community relations, the move is toward granting asylum seekers a temporary status within the country and to keep the country of origin under review. Use of electronic tagging for failed asylum seekers, continued use of detention centres for those classified as failed, and speedier removal of the same are the main thrusts.

Several themes emerge through these new laws including a general response of increasingly restrictive practices by policy makers to the increased numbers seeking entry to the UK. All the Acts above continue to conflate asylum with immigration, so that it is seen as a migration phenomenon requiring migration policy responses rather than as an obligation act as envisioned in the original Convention. All the Acts have outcomes, whose legitimacy may be understood as a result of securitization with policies on border control, citizenship, regulations on the manner of asylum claims, and treatment of those deemed to have failed the process with tighter control. In addition, all push towards a consistent outcome of fewer asylum claims granted.

However, currently the population of concern for the UNHCR is at its highest and stands at over 30 million—see Table 7.4. This charts figures from the past 2 decades and shows that the largest rise in numbers occurred in the early 1990s coinciding with the end of the Cold War. A significant jump also occurred in 2006, accounted for by improved mechanisms for collecting data on a wider range of people of concern, in particular IDPs. Although the number of 'refugees' then falls throughout the 1990s, the numbers of those for whom the organization has cause for concern remains stable and high, reflecting the serious ongoing problem of forced migration of internally displaced persons. The UNHCR's work involves not only intervention and advocacy but also the practical management of refugee camps and the organization of direct resettlement programmes such as transporting individuals from one country to another. As can be seen later, the majority of people of concern are in Asia and Africa, with the largest recent groups of concern being Iraqis, Afghans, Sudanese, and citizens of the Democratic Republic of Congo—in line with recent geo-political expectations.

Health policy in practise

Large-scale populations on the move bring with them major difficulties as any population has basic needs. In a situation in which political structures are absent and service provision non-existent, the basic health requirements of internally displaced people becomes of paramount importance. Access to food, water, shelter, accommodation, livelihood, health care, and general public services, all tend to be lacking when on the move or when living in

Table 7.4 UNHCR numbers of refugees and people of concern 1990–2006

Year	Refugees	Total population of concern
1990	14,773,000	
1991	17,369,000	
1992	16,855,000	
1993	17,838,000	
1994	16,326,000	
1995	15,574,000	
1996	14,896,000	
1997	13,357,000	20,047,000
1998	12,015,000	20,124,700
1999	11,480,000	20,821,000
2000	11,687,000	20,006,100
2001	12,129,000	20,028,900
2002	12,116,000	20,892,500
2003	10,549,000	17,101,300
2004	9,680,000	19,518,400
2005	9,559,100	20,751,900
2006	9,877,707	32,861,285

temporary accommodation (IDMC, 2007; Forced-Migration, 2008). A complicating factor remains the original precipitant for the mass movement. Natural disasters, famines, wars, or political persecution mean that the population on the move is already one in significant need. Coordination of help has had a chequered history and in 1992 the Inter-Agency Standing Committee (IASC) was founded, which describes itself and its role as 'a unique inter-agency forum for coordination, policy development and decision-making involving the key UN and non-UN humanitarian partners. The IASC was established in response to United Nations General Assembly Resolution 46/182 on the strengthening of humanitarian assistance. General Assembly Resolution 48/57 affirmed its role as the primary mechanism for inter-agency coordination of humanitarian assistance. The lead is often taken by the international bodies but negotiating authority and jurisdiction can often be difficult.'

Assessment of the impact on mental health of individuals involved in any mass movement can be thought of as occurring at one of three levels:

1) Mental illness present in the population prior to any flight
Although exact prevalence rates vary across countries, mental illness is present in every population. Therefore in any population on the move will be those

who have psychotic disorders (approximately 1%); common mental illnesses such as depression or anxiety (between 5 and 20%); personality disorders (up to 5%); or those with learning disabilities or epilepsy (up to 5%). Many of these conditions will be treated outside of a hospital setting but for those who are in-patients, any sudden necessary move may be devastating.

2) Aggravation of existing conditions by the need of flight

The chaos of the flight will disrupt not only access to medications but also familial, social, and important cultural structures used in the management of many of them, worsening the likelihood of continued appropriate management.

3) New cases of mental health problems as a direct consequence of the situation

These include not only the trauma of the actual flight itself but also the many cases of those who subsequently experience problems as a result of war or even torture. The psychiatric literature is filled with vociferous debates on the validity of diagnoses such as post-traumatic stress disorder (PTSD). The medicalization of stress and trauma and their management have been criticized as being essentially a Western construct (Summerfield, 1996b). This debate has informed a number of different approaches to psychosocial interventions with refugees (Summerfield, 1996a) (Mollica *et al.*, 2002). It has also been argued that such policy decisions can divert resources away from physical health care and material needs (Richters, 1998).

Each of these levels of mental health problems should be seen as applying an extra level of vulnerability to an already vulnerable population group. Each will have to deal with general health issues too. Gastrointestinal infections remain a major source of morbidity, not only on the move but also within the relative safety of camps. It is estimated that a cholera outbreak killed 50,000 Rwandan refugees in camps inside Zaire during the first weeks of July 1994 (Goma-Epidemiology-Group, 1995). Health services for displaced populations need to span primary care and treatment through to more prevention-based strategies such as clear sanitation, clean water, vector control, health education, immunization programmes, as well as direct monitoring and treatment. Communicable disease management may bring further difficulties in host countries when a significant at-risk population moves from a high- to a low-disease-risk area, provoking an adverse host population reaction due to a perception that a disproportionate amount of healthcare resources are required. However, attempts at facing this difficulty by screening and quarantine of displaced populations in the UK has not only been shown to be stigmatizing but also ineffective (Coker, 2003).

Data on HIV in refugee camps is scarce; however there is thought to be an association between forced migration and infection. Factors believed to influence this include increased poverty, reduced social/familial ties, increased sexual violence, and increased socioeconomic vulnerability presumably leading to prostitution/sexual exploitation. Displaced populations will need to have access to family planning, HIV testing and treatment.

Traditionally in situations of forced migration, external policy resources have been focused on emergency food supplies, but it is recognized that malnutrition is also a risk in the longer term. Particularly vulnerable are the elderly, children, and households with a female head. This was demonstrated by studies amongst Kurdish refugees from Iraq in 1991, in which families headed by women were significantly more malnourished (Cahill, 1999). In Rwandan refugee camps in eastern Zaire, one month after the influx of July 1994, the prevalence of acute malnutrition was 18–23% (Goma-Epidemiology-Group, 1995).

Further at risk groups

Women, children, and the elderly tend to be overrepresented in these groups, particularly when fleeing war. Displaced women are at an increased risk of sexual violence and a lack of reproductive health and maternal health can lead to additional health risks (IDMC, 2007). Though it may be true that the majority of hardships of forced migration fall on women, it is also damaging for them to be seen as being helpless victims. This perception has been criticized for resulting in interventions that are imposed upon women without their participation and leadership in policy design, implementation, monitoring, and evaluation (Lindsey, 2001; Turner, 2001).

Displaced children are denied education and often have to work to survive. This raises the possibility of exploitation and familial separation. In addition to the psychological damage this can inflict, it makes children vulnerable to forced recruitment to military groups in such places as Chad, Columbia, Sudan, Myanmar, and Sri Lanka (IDMC, 2007). Significant proportions of new HIV infections also occur in the 10–24 age group, with sexual exploitation thought to be one of the main mechanisms of spread (UNICEF, 2000). Even when reaching the safety of Western settings, there have been controversial policy interventions directed at children. In Australia, a practice of detention of some children in asylum facilities was pursued for some time and vehemently opposed by some in academic psychiatry (Silove, 2002).

Attempts at international policy responses to these challenges have resulted in the Convention on the Rights of the Child, which set international norms for the recognition and observance of children's rights (UN, 1989). The three key principles are:

1 the best interests of the child must be observed;

2 non-discrimination must be observed to assure that all children have the right to be treated equally; and

3 children must have the right to participation.

The health needs of the elderly are frequently neglected despite the high rate of existing disease and physical frailty of this population. In some situations, such as Kosovo, it was argued that elderly people were more at risk for under-nutrition than young children (Salama *et al.*, 2001).

Some refugee camps last for many years, and this longevity brings its own sets of problems, with unemployment, high alcohol consumption, gender violence, high birth rates, and impaired access to education and health care on a long-term basis, all aggravating rates of mental disorders. There are often also difficulties living alongside the host populations, and enhanced environmental degradation caused for example by the need for domestic firewood.

Intervention strategies

The complexities and difficulties of dealing with many of these issues were highlighted by the Inter-Agency Standing Committee, which brings together a large number of multinational agencies in an attempt to coordinate responses to international crises. In a report called 'IASC Guidelines on Mental health and Psychosocial support in emergency settings', a four-level 'pyramid' of interventions to ensure mental health is described (IASC, 2007).

Level 1 Basic services and security—these affect all concerned and emphasize the importance of food security, basic nutrition, water and sanitation availability, and shelter in ensuring adequate mental health.

Level 2 Community and family supports—this highlights a smaller number who are able to maintain their own mental health and well-being if access to certain family and social resources are maintained. Services such as family tracing and unification, assisted mourning and communal healing ceremonies, mass communication, and constructive coping methods, youth and women's networks are all suggested.

Level 3 Focussed non-specialized supports—for a smaller number of people who may require interventions at an individual or family level by trained and supervised workers who may not necessarily have years of training or experience. Examples highlighted at this level include community workers providing emotional and livelihood help to survivors of violence.

Level 4 Specialized services—for the smallest number of people who, despite the interventions mentioned so far, require further help. The presence of a pre-existing mental illness or subsequent development of one would result in the necessity for specialized services. However, even though this population is a small percentage of the whole, the epidemiological prevalence rates can mean that large numbers can still be affected.

In practice, since even in non-emergency situations, the prevalence of common mental disorders is at least 10% in adults and 10% in children, and that of psychosis is 0.5–1%, it is clear that the involvement of primary care will be essential, and therefore training and supervision is required with referral of the most complex cases to specialist services if they exist and if they are accessible.

Outside of the emergency setting

Policies that attempt to provide help to those who make it to a Western nation can be divided into similar levels of intervention. There are important differences though. It is often stated that the population who make it into the West are those who show the greatest resilience and fortitude. Negotiating long journeys across continents, often mixed up with people smugglers, requires significant fortitude. This tends, although not completely, to exclude the most vulnerable from such a journey. As such the asylum seeker population making it to the West are mostly young and male. Those with pre-existing severe mental illnesses tend also to be excluded. Basic essential needs are addressed even if at a minimal standard, such as through the NASS in the UK, and therefore the focus of service provision tends to be at a higher level and at those who have developed mental health problems as a result of some aspect of their experience.

However, a comprehensive review of the literature found that in order to benefit fully from the UK healthcare system, refugees and asylum seekers needed many steps to be taken, which included access to primary care with full permanent registration; information about health services; appropriate and comprehensive health assessments including mental and physical health; adequate access to translation, interpreting, and advocacy services in appropriate languages; adequate and appropriate responses to mental health problems; access to specialist services for survivors of torture and organized violence; and advice and information on health promotion (Feldman, 2006). Many of these can be seen as extensions of the level 2 family and community support services in the IASC report from earlier. As can be seen from the earlier review of legislation, few of these items were focussed upon in any of the Acts or policy statements in the UK.

Conclusions

The framework within which policy is produced to address refugee and asylum seeker mental health is complex. The global Conventions provided the original levels of obligation and duty and continue to attempt to be enforced by the agencies that arose. Historical events over the last two decades have resulted in an increase in numbers of those fulfilling criteria for being at risk. However, the response from many Western nations has been one of restriction and, as can be seen from the example of the UK, an increased conflation of the duties of asylum with immigration in general. In dealing with mental health problems—whether in the context of the West in those who have negotiated their way across boundaries, or in the chaos of large-scale groups on the move—we see a number of important elements needing to be considered. Basic physical health needs together with more complex interventions are needed no matter where the individual ends up. Coordination of these responses has been attempted by the IASC in emergency settings. There also needs to be more coordinated international policy response to long-term refugee settings in low- and middle-income countries.

In Western settings, where a small proportion of the world's total refugee population eventually arrive, responses are often provided by a mix of statutory and voluntary sector interventions.

References

(1993) Asylum and Immigration Appeals Act. *ISBN 0105423939*.

(1996) Asylum and Immigration Act. *ISBN 0105449962*.

(1999) Immigration and Asylum Act. *ISBN 0105633992*.

(2002) Nationality, Immigration and Asylum Act. *ISBN 0105441021*.

(2004) Asylum and Immigration (Treatment of Claimants, etc) Act. *ISBN0105619043*.

(2006) Immigration, Asylum and Nationality Act. *ISBN 0105613061*.

BBC (2001). Europe's soft touch?. BBC News, 4th September 2001. *http://news.bbc.co.uk/1/hi/uk/1524588.stm*

Cahill, K.M. (1999). *A Framework for Survival: Health, Human Rights, and Humanitarian Assistance in Conflicts and Disasters*. New York: London: Routledge.

Coker, R. (2003). Migration, public health and compulsory screening for TB and HIV. London: Institute for Public Policy Research.

Council-of-Europe (1950). Convention for the Protection of Human Rights and Fundamental Freedoms. Registry of the European Court of Human Rights.

Crown (1998). Human Rights Act. *ISBN 0105442984*.

European-Council (1999). European Council Conclusions 'Tampere European Council' 15th–16th October 1999.

Feldman, R. (2006). Primary health care for refugees and asylum seekers: a review of the literature and a framework for services. *Public Health* **120**: 809–816.

Forced-Migration (2008). http://www.forcedmigration.org/guides/fmo030/

Geddes, A. (2003). *The Politics of Migration and Immigration in Europe*. London: Sage.

Gibney, M.J. (2004). *The ethics and politics of asylum: liberal democracy and the response to refugees*. Cambridge: Cambridge University Press.

Goma-Epidemiology-Group (1995). Public health impact of Rwandan refugee crisis: what happened in Goma, Zaire, in July, 1994? Goma Epidemiology Group. *Lancet* **345**: 339–344.

Guardian (2003a). UN attacks plan to limit legal aid for asylum seekers. 1st September 2003, *The Guardian*.

Guardian (2003b). UN chief chides Blair for slating convention. 29th October 2003, *The Guardian*.

Guardian (2005a). UN condemns return of Somalis. 12th June 2005, *The Guardian*.

Guardian (2005b). UN says Tory plans will boost flow of asylum seekers. 20th April 2005, *The Guardian*.

HO (1998). Fairer, Faster, Firmer – A Modern Approach to Immigration and Asylum. *The Stationary Office*.

HO (2004). Confident Communities in a Secure Britain. UK Home Office Strategic Plan document for the years 2004–2008.

HO (2006). Controlling our borders: making migration work for Britain. UK Home Office.

IASC (2007). IASC Guidelines on Mental Health and Psychosocial.

Support in Emergency Settings. Inter-Agency Standing Committee (IASC) Geneva: IASC.

IDMC (2007). Internal Displacement Global Overview 2007.

Lindsey, C. (2001). Women Facing War. ICRC Study on the Impact of Armed Conflict on Women. IN http://www.icrc.org/web/eng/siteeng0.nsf/d268e7e7eea08ab74125675b003 64294/5bd0956e8c9593cfc1256b66005efee9? (Ed. *OpenDocument Geneva: ICRC, 2001*).

Mollica, R.F., Cui, X., McInnes, K., and Massagli, M.P. (2002). Science-based policy for psychosocial interventions in refugee camps: a Cambodian example. *Journal of Nervous and Mental Disorders* **190**: 158–166.

Richters, A. (1998). Sexual violence in wartime. Psycho-sociocultural wounds and healing processes: The example of the former Yugoslavia. In P.B.A.C.P. (Eds.) *Rethinking the Trauma of War*. London: Free Association Press.

Salama, P., Buzard, N., and Spiegel, P. (2001). Improving standards in international humanitarian response: the Sphere Project and beyond. *Journal of the American Medical Association* **286**: 531–532.

Summerfield, D. (1996a). The impact of war and atrocity on civilian populations: basic principles for NGO interventions and a critique of psychosocial trauma projects. London: Relief and Rehabilitation Network Overseas Development Institute, 1996.

Summerfield, D. (1996b). The psychological legacy of war and atrocity: the question of long-term and transgenerational effects and the need for a broad view. *Journal of Nervous and Mental Disorders* **184**: 375–377.

Turner, S. (2001). Vindicating masculinity: the paradoxical effects of empowering women in a refugee camp. In M.L.A.A.A. (Eds.) *The Refugee Experience. Psychosocial Training Module, Vol. 1 (2nd edn)*. Oxford: Refugee Studies Centre, University of Oxford, 2001.

UN (1951). Convention relating to the Status of Refugees.

UN (1967). Protocol Relating to the Status of Refugees.

UN (1987). Convention Against Torture.

UN (1989). Convention on the Rights of the Child.

UNHCR (2002a). Afghanistan, UK and UNHCR sign voluntary repatriation agreement. UNHCR Press Releases, 12th October 2002.

UNHCR (2002b). UK: Yarlswood detention centre fire. UNHCR Briefing Notes, 15th February 2002.

UNHCR (2003). UK gets wide support for UNHCR resettlement scheme for vulnerable refugees. UNHCR News stories, 4th Sept 2003.

UNICEF (2000). State of the World's Children 2000. New York: UNICEF.

Chapter 8

Dealing with cultural differences

Pedro Ruiz, Susham Gupta, and
Dinesh Bhugra

Introduction

Although reasons for seeking refuge and asylum are many, the underlying principles of assessment remain broadly the same. It is a good clinical practice to
seek details of personal experiences. Cultural patterns of distress need to be
explored to ensure that any intervention is appropriate and both useful and
acceptable to facilitate therapeutic engagement between patients and clinicians.
Not only are healthcare systems multi-cultural and multi-disciplinary, they also
differ according to social policy, cultural expectations, and resources allocated.
Healthcare beliefs will be another factor in managing illness episodes. However,
other components of assessments need to be recognized and remembered. In
this chapter we highlight some of the key principles. Arguably in any civilized
society, health care for all is a must, although response and attitudes towards
refugees and asylum seekers will mould response and access to services.

Culture, cultural identity, and mental illness

We know that cultural factors are crucially influential in maintaining the
mental health of individuals in various ways. These factors can have precipitat-
ing, perpetuating, pathoplastic, as well as pathoprotective effects (Tseng *et al.*,
2004). Particularly for refugees and asylum seekers, these factors may have
additional import in the assessment and diagnosis of mental illness. Thus cultural competence and awareness are vital both for delivery of care and for public
health in a multi-cultural society as well as at the individual clinical–patient
interaction level (Gupta and Bhugra, 2009). Cultural competence is at the core
of good clinical practice.

Assessment

In most cultures there will be a broad heterogeneity of cultures and people and
that will bring with it issues of language, beliefs, religious values, and attitudes,

which will determine both help-seeking and pathways people follow into health care. It is essential for clinicians to be aware of the principles that they may use in understanding cultural differences, which might exist between themselves and their individual patients and how this might affect the assessment processes.

A thorough assessment has at its core a therapeutic encounter, which has a degree of openness in the exchange of views and exploration of symptoms and experiences. The clinician must, in the first instance, listen carefully and then, if need be, acknowledge any lacunae in their knowledge of culture and its components and also how their own culture impacts upon their own values and responses. This could require repeated and lengthy interviews with patients and their families. This will almost certainly allow the clinicians to familiarize themselves with cultural values and beliefs if they were not already aware of these factors. It will also allow corroboration of history and may well improve the quality of the assessment. The place and purpose of the assessment will differ depending upon the reasons for assessment and urgency—for example, it could be in the outpatients clinic or in a police station. A community or outpatient assessment may differ greatly in nature and duration and corroboration with one being held in an in-patient unit for a patient compulsorily detained. Principles of assessment for clinicians are illustrated in Table 8.1.

The idioms of distress will influence the presentational styles and attitudes to help-seeking.

Table 8.1 Principles of assessment (after Gupta and Bhugra, 2009)

◆ Awareness of one's personal competencies

◆ Awareness of one's own limitations in knowledge and experience

◆ An unprejudiced neutral but sympathetic approach

◆ Exploration of the patient's and family's competency, strengths, skills, and limitations regarding language, new country, etc.

◆ Explore the culture, their concept of mental health, and expectations of the therapeutic encounter

◆ Explore the linguistic skills early and then decide not to use family members, especially children, as interpreters.

◆ Appropriate preparation of advice and guidance to interpreters

◆ Know and build on the strengths, skills, and weaknesses of the interpreters

◆ Access cultural factors, acculturation, acculturative stress, and explanatory models (see Table 8.2).

Table 8.2 Assessing explanatory models—questions to ask the patient about their illness

- What are the symptoms that the patient has presented with?
- What is their significance: personal, familial, and cultural?
- Are they pathological as defined by the culture or by the individual?
- What terms are used to explain these by the patient and/or their carers?
- What do others—i.e. the community or culture—call them?
- What do they see as the causative factors?
- What do they think the outcome is likely to be?
- Why did they appear now?
- How do they affect the patient and their carers?
- How do they affect others widely around them?
- How serious is the problem?
- What course is likely?
- What do they fear most about their symptoms?
- What treatment, if any, will help? If so, what sort?
- Who should provide it?

Communication

Even though most of the communication is non-verbal, relative emphasis on verbal and nonverbal communication will vary between cultures. Awareness of a sense of personal space and notions of privacy, physical and eye contact, gestures, idioms of distress, and other non-verbal communications is very important as they form a significant part of the therapeutic interaction and in forming a rapport and understanding and making sense of the psychopathology.

History taking

While taking a history, some of the additional features that clinicians must be aware of are as follows.

Linguistic difficulties—Patients whose first language is not English may find it more difficult to describe, explain, or communicate their problems for various reasons, most of which are cultural. Friends and relatives (especially those more proficient in English and/or with greater level of acculturation) may assist communication of psychopathologies. However, this approach is not without drawbacks. In some settings, patients who are being interviewed in their second language may well hide symptoms of thought disorder, and also these difficulties may not be given the same prominence as the clinician may err towards caution and blame these on linguistic skills. Furthermore, stigma towards mental illness by the family and others may influence the interpreter's explanation of events. If interpreters are to be used, the clinician must ensure that they are well trained and able to interpret accurately rather than just transliterate, especially when dealing with emotions. Clinicians should be trained to work with interpreters and instruct them accordingly (Gupta and Bhugra, 2009).

Adverse life events—The impact of life events will vary across cultures and the way these influence individuals will be affected by social support and cultural emphasis placed on these. For example, the significance of the loss of a pet in the UK may not have the same impact on people in other cultures. Even the effects of migration will vary depending on circumstances leading to migration; and the personality of the migrants, degree of cultural dissonance, and level of acculturation may act as mediating factors. A flexible enquiring style will be more helpful in establishing normative stress (which can be confirmed by talking to the family and others in the community as well) and the exact impact of such life events.

Explanatory models—Kleinman (1980) described the need to be aware of how patients interpret their symptoms, the way they describe them and how they seek help (see Table 8.2). Metaphors for describing psychological distress and symptoms often differ between cultures: in the UK 'I am gutted' and in Punjabi 'my heart is sinking' represent similar feelings of depression and anxiety, and although neither expression is truly somatic, the physical description plays a role in explanation of the real experience. If the explanatory models of patient and clinician vary, which may well be true if the clinician focuses on only biological symptoms, it will become difficult to find common ground that can lead to proper diagnosis, rational discussions on intervention, and therapeutic adherence.

Pitfalls in mental state examination

While carrying out the standardized mental state examination, clinicians must be particularly aware of some of the following (for further details see Bhugra and Bhui, 1997; 2007):

Behaviour—Some behaviours are culturally sanctioned in certain circumstances (e.g. speaking in tongues, possession states). These must be evaluated carefully. Both the behaviour and the responses to it by the family and cultural group will allow the clinician to explore further without alienating the patient. Unusual or odd behaviour that is not clearly understandable is too often regarded by psychiatrists as evidence of pathology without attention to the cultural context. Such behaviour may also be adaptive or coping.

Thoughts—It might be difficult to assess abnormal contents or forms of thoughts. Interpreters and relatives may be able to provide some clue. However, as already mentioned, if interviewed in their secondary language, the patient may be able to withhold information and hide thought disorder.

Delusions—although the definition of delusions includes abnormal experiences which can not be understood in the cultural context, often this could be misdiagnosed by clinicians. The form and context of delusions will be determined by culture, education, and socioeconomic status, e.g. beliefs in magic spells. Delusional beliefs are not pathognomonic of psychiatric conditions. Therefore, clinicians must always consider alternative explanations for a patient's beliefs, rather than simply assuming that these are delusional. Confirmation from other members of cultural groups will enable the clinician to reach an appropriate diagnosis. It can be argued that if the family brings the patient to the clinician, they have already decided that the experiences and behaviour of the patient are pathological.

Hallucinations—young people from a lower socioeconomic background are more likely to report hallucinations (Mukherjee *et al.*, 1983). Other factors include religious affiliation. Mukherjee *et al.* (1983) found that in the US, 20% of those who belonged to the Church of God showed a prevalence of hallucinations compared with none of the Jewish faith. As in the case of delusions, an understanding of the cultural context is essential and should be taken into account before defining hallucinations as pathological. It is important to bear in mind the possibility of abnormal bereavement, post-traumatic, dissociative factors, which may be more common in refugees and asylum seekers. The use of illicit substances such as khat or cannabis, the use of which may vary between cultures, although normative and culturally acceptable, may well contribute to psychotic symptoms.

Cognition

Assessment of memory and other cognitive impairments can be potentially a significant problem among migrants in general but more so in refugees and asylum seekers and should be considered in the context of linguistic and educational backgrounds. Use of standard tools which are not culturally specific may over-estimate impairment. There have been some efforts at developing culture-specific tools but their use is still limited. Assessment by clinicians from the same background or use of experienced interpreters can improve outcome. It is important to take into account the level of functioning and not just outcomes of scales to determine the nature and progression of memory-related problems. In understanding the cognitive schema related to depression, the role of culture and definitions of the self can not be underestimated.

Additional factors that are important for understanding the therapeutic encounter include experiences of individual and institutional racism, altered levels of social support, and alienation due to cultural or personal factors. Perceived or real racism will alter the way the healthcare system is seen and the way help is sought. Threat to the immigration status, such as fear of deportation, may influence presentation and also affect therapeutic adherence.

Cultural identity

Every individual has multiple identities. These have multiple meanings and values. Our identities are influenced by how we see ourselves and how we see others seeing us. These multiple identities may change when the context changes. For example, a male student at a university while lecturing other students is a male lecturer. On finishing his activity his identity shifts back to being a student, but his maleness does not change necessarily. Similarly, a refugee may be a patient in the clinic but a father, son, or brother outside, a breadwinner and husband; and these identities change with the context. Some aspects of identity are visible, such as gender, race, and biological features; but others may remain hidden, such as sexual orientation. Religious identity may become visible only if certain symbols reflecting a religious proclivity are worn, such as a turban or a cross. Identity by and large remains a social construct. This raises serious issues about how migrants and refugees are seen and understood in the new culture. Every individual develops a sense of identity, which is usually multi-dimensional. However, there is a hierarchy within this complex sense of individuality. This may differ from how others view the person. A Hispanic female doctor who is a mother of three working in New York may be identified by her various roles by others; but when asked, she might identify herself primarily as a good Catholic. A sense of identity starts to develop from an early age by virtue of one's gender and associated physical and psychological make-up, as well as one's social and cultural environment. Some features of identity may come naturally or instinctively, while others are attributed and then accepted (see Bhugra and Gupta, 2010). These forms may not always fit well together and could bring about conflict within oneself especially when they differ from societal expectations. This has a great bearing on one's mental health and if unresolved may cause a significant amount of continuing personal and social distress, especially among refugees and asylum seekers. On the other hand, this could also give a person a strong sense of individuality and resolve. Once formed, the main sense of self remains generally intact while other aspects evolve reflecting changes occurring in one's personal life and aging process. Cultures will determine to some extent whether its members are ego-centric or socio-centric.

Religion continues to play a central part on the social, personal, and spiritual part of many people's lives. Religious identity is both less overt and not biologically determined. Persons belonging to a certain religion may choose to express themselves in such a way (e.g. dress codes) that may distinguish them from others. Within a religious community this may be a way of conveying a sense of cohesion and identity. However, people often attribute possible religious backgrounds by identifying people's physical features or distinctive names. These may be used as a way of discriminating people both overtly and covertly, as is more important in populations with ethnic and religious diversity and conflict.

Culture identity is integrated in one's sense of self from one's upbringing, family, peers, education, society, art, literature, folk tales, etc. This process goes on most of one's lifetime. Culture not only influences the cognitive schema but also moulds the way one thinks of oneself and sees others. It is also important in the way people deal with interpersonal relationships. There is no doubt that culture defines people and distinguishes them from others by their social behaviour, religious beliefs, clothes, cuisine, entertainment, arts (high culture), etc. Cultures can also overlap at various levels—e.g. students from various ethnic backgrounds attending a certain college may feel that the culture of their college and their identity as a student in that institution is far more relevant. Cultural identity highlights a person's uniqueness. Cultural identity, its preservation and differences, especially in a multicultural setting and in a more globalizing world, can potentially bring about conflicts and contribute to mental health problems.

Sexual identity

Gender and sexual identities are at the core of one's understanding of oneself. Gender awareness develops relatively early and is both biologically and socially reinforced. Gender identity has an influence on sexual identity, which developed in late childhood and adolescence when one starts to relate to others in a sexual and emotional context. Sexual orientation is determined by the level of sexual attraction to either or both sexes. Non-concordance of sexuality with the norm can often cause anxiety, especially in cultures with less accepting attitudes towards alternative sexualities.

Many aspects of one's identity are fluid and influenced by one's interaction with the outside world. With an increasingly globalized world and the growth of electronic media and information technology (i.e. the internet), there is unprecedented interaction between people of various cultures and identities. Though this can bring about better awareness and understanding of other cultures, it might also lead to possible conflict within one's own existing sense of self. This is especially true for those from non-Western cultures, as the globalized culture is primarily Western. Internet sites such as 'Second Life' are being used to develop parallel lives, which provide distraction and an idealized existence. Furthermore, the internet is being used increasingly to learn about illnesses and medicines and side effects, thereby changing the nature of the doctor–patient relationship (see Jones *et al.*, 2010).

Some principles of management

Several chapters in this book have described in detail management issues. Here we propose to highlight only some of the key principles.

The main goal of treatment is for the patient to get better, but this improvement may be sought in the context of functional improvement only rather than getting rid of symptoms. Thus, there may well be a discrepancy between the patient's and doctor's treatment goals. The treatment and its consequences may well differ across different cultures and different generations. An open and honest discussion is required.

As mentioned earlier, the management of psychiatric problems is determined by a number of social, political, and economic factors. Clinicians must understand the context of help-seeking and the location of the encounter. Often health professionals may be the only source of support and contact with the new society. Such a place may be the only forum where they can express their distress. For refugees and asylum seekers this may well be the last resort.

Indigenous therapies: using indigenous models (e.g. religious models of therapy in India) or folk tales (in the form of Cuento therapy for Puerto Rican children in the US) may well be more acceptable in some settings and may provide some advantages, especially when combined with more evidence-based therapies. The clinician's attitude and style are likely to influence therapeutic encounter and therapeutic relationship. Some cultural groups may prefer the therapist to be directive, whereas others may see the therapist as a collaborative partner. The clinician may need to change their management approaches accordingly.

Ethnic matching: although some believe it is preferable for patients to see therapists from the same ethnic or cultural background, research data for the effectiveness of this approach are lacking. The therapist may still be seen by the patient as 'one of them' by virtue of his or her professional background and will also appear to have the power to detain the patient or write a supporting letter to get their social security or stay sorted. Thus a subtle dynamic may appear that could affect therapeutic alliance. Patients may be more wary of clinicians from the same culture and other minority cultures, as this may be seen as more stigmatizing or that the culture or the community is being let down. A narrow definition of ethno-specific services can deepen existing problems of cultural integration both of patients and of the health system and society in general.

Diet and related factors: Dietary patterns, fasting, and religious taboos will contribute to difficulties in treatment adherence. Factors such as height and weight vary across ethnicities and can contribute to altered metabolism, thus producing more side effects with lower dosages. Religious or dietary taboos will also influence therapeutic adherence.

Complementary therapies: Traditional/herbal remedies (e.g. cumin, St John's Wort) may be taken without the clinician being aware of the interaction. Many such remedies are metabolically active and may contain metals such as lead, mercury, or antimony, and other components may interact with prescribed medication.

Other factors such as smoking, stress, prescription patterns, and individual personality factors may all play a significant role, and the clinician must explore these.

Conclusions

In this chapter, we addressed most of the key principles related to the challenges faced by refugees and asylum seeking populations. In this context, the cultural differences, cultural identity, and the mental illnesses that affect these refugee populations and asylum seeking groups need to be understood well and addressed.

The key principles related to the clinical evaluation and assessments are essential with respect to this patient population. Likewise, explanatory models related to clinical assessments are of major relevance in these population groups. All aspects of the clinical assessment such as communication, history taking, linguistic difficulties, adverse life events, explanatory models, challenges with the mental state examination, behaviour observations, thought abnormalities, cognitive deficits, and cultural identity must be all carefully taken into consideration.

References

Bhugra, D. and Bhui K.S. (1997). Cross-cultural competencies in psychiatric assessment. *British Journal of Hospital Medicine* **57**(10): 492–496.

Bhugra, D. and Bhui, K. (2007). *Textbook of Cultural Psychiatry*. Cambridge: Cambridge University Press.

Bhugra, D. and Gupta, S. (2010). Culture and its influence on diagnosis and management. In C. Morgan and D. Bhugra, *Principles of Social Psychiatry* (2nd ed). Chichester: Wiley-Blackwell.

Gupta, S. and Bhugra, D. (2009). Globalization, economic factors and prevalence of psychiatric disorders. *International Journal of Mental Health* **38**(3): 53–65.

Jones, K., Woollard, J. and Bhugra, D. (2010). Modern Social Networking and Mental Health. In C. Morgan and D. Bhugra (eds) *Principles of Social Psychiatry* (2nd ed). Chichester: Wiley-Blackwell.

Kleinman, A. (1980). *Patients and Healers in the Context of Culture: An Explanation of the Borderland between Anthropology, Medicine and Psychiatry.* Berkeley CA: University of California Press.

Mukherjee, S., Shukla, S., Woodle, J., Rosen, A., and Olarte, S. (1983). Misdiagnosis of schizophrenia in bipolar patients: A multi-ethnic comparison. *American Journal of Psychiatry* **140**: 1571–1574.

Tseng, W.S., Griffith, E.H., Ruiz, P., and Buchanan, A. (2004). Culture and psychopathology in the forensic context. In A. Feltaus and H. Sab (Eds.) *The International Handbook of Psychopathic Disorders and the Law* Volume II, Laws and Policies, pp 473–488, Chichester: John Wiley and Sons Ltd.

Chapter 9

Therapeutic skills and therapeutic expectations

Pedro Ruiz

Introduction

The conceptualization of 'therapeutic skills' and 'therapeutic expectations' is rapidly changing all over the world. The traditional application of therapeutic skills is no longer based on the 'psychodynamic model' or the 'socio-rehabilitation approach'; nowadays, a more advanced biopsychosocial model is the one that most often prevails around the world; however, we must also be fully aware that this model is also very much impacted by 'culture', 'race', and 'ethnicity' (Ruiz, 2004).

Understanding culture-bound syndromes

At the core of the therapeutic skills and therapeutic expectations worldwide nowadays is the understanding and addressing of culture-bound syndromes (Ruiz, 1995; 1998). Some experts in the field of cross-cultural psychiatry question the veracity of culture-bound syndromes, as well as clinical acceptance and treatment (Bhugra, *et al.*, 2007). Despite these clinical and historical concerns with respect to these culture-bound syndromes, their current relevance and role in clinical, educational, and investigational efforts is well accepted by most experts in the field of cross-cultural psychiatry worldwide, especially in the Americas, Asia, Australasia, and Africa, as well as in most regions of Europe and the Middle East.

In this context, racial, ethnic, and cultural manifestations such as religions, traditions, beliefs, myths, values, interpersonal relation patterns, modes of production, languages, socioeconomic philosophies, coping styles, modes of adaptations, and the like all play a role in the clinical manifestations of symptoms, both physical and psychological, and also help construe the culture-bound syndromes. The full understanding of these unique cultural manifestations will certainly lead to the appropriate or inappropriate diagnostic considerations, therapeutic interventions, and adherence or non-adherence to

(Alarcon and Ruiz, 1995). Obviously, culture and cultural ramifica-
116 ffect every aspect of an individual's life, including the way that health
ıd illness are perceived by patients, as well as the doctor-patient relationships, and the health-seeking behaviour of patients. Thus, a thorough knowledge of these cultural factors and ramifications will certainly offer physicians,
psychiatrists, and other health and mental health professionals a unique understanding and view of the patient's conceptualization of their illness, and also a
better opportunity to ensure treatment compliance and, therefore, a better
chance to secure a cure from the afflicting illness, whether it be physical or
psychological in nature (Ruiz, 1985). To ignore or be insensitive to the cultural
manifestations of patients' illnesses, whether they be physical or psychological,
will certainly lead to misunderstanding between patients and physicians/pro-
fessionals, as well as frustration both for patients and physicians/professionals.
It might certainly also lead to the stretching of the majority culture, mostly
represented by physicians/professionals, into the minority culture, mostly
represented by patients; worse, in many occasions it can also lead to the unin-
tended harm of the patient.

Among the most worldwide accepted culture-bound syndromes are those
that appear in Appendix I of the Diagnostic and Statistical Manual of Mental
Disorders, 4th Edition (DSM-IV) (American Psychiatric Association, 2004).
Although it is not intended to describe them individually in this chapter, for
the benefit of the readers we can enumerate them; they are as follows:

- Amok
- Ataque de Nervios
- Bilis or Colera (also Muina)
- Bouffee Delirante
- Brain Fag
- Dhat
- Falling-Out, Blacking-Out or Blackout
- Ghost Sickness
- Hwa-byung or Wool-hwa-byung
- Koro
- Latah
- Locura
- Mal de Ojo or Evil Eye
- Nervios
- Pibloktoq or Artic Hysteria

- Qi-gong Psychotic Reaction
- Root Work
- Sangue Dormido or Sleeping Blood
- Shenjing Shuairuo or Neurasthenia
- Shen-K'uei in Taiwan or Shenkui in China
- Shin-byung
- Spell
- Susto, Fright or Soul Loss
- Taijin kyofusho
- Zar.

Other cultural-bound syndromes not noted in the DSM-IV, but observed frequently in the worldwide literature are (Ruiz, 1985; Ruiz and Bhugra, 2008):

- Caida de la Mollera
- Empacho
- Malgri or Territorial Anxiety
- Possession
- Rokjoo
- Puerto Rican Syndrome (synonymous with Ataques de Nervios)
- Shinkeishitsu Neurosis
- Shuk Yang, Shoo Yong or Suo Yang.

As the globalization process increases and also spreads out from country to country, the knowledge and sensitivity vis-à-vis the culture-bound syndromes will become more important and relevant; this importance and relevance will not only apply to psychiatrists and other mental health professionals, but to all physicians and health care professionals as well.

Acquiring cultural competency

During the last decade, the concept of 'cultural competence' has become not only important, but a relevant clinical requirement as well. In this respect, new and highly regarded texts and/or educational and training tools have become available to the field of psychiatry and mental health at large not only in the United States, but worldwide as well (Mezzich, *et al.*, 1996; Canino and Spurlock, 2000; Constantine and Sue, 2005; Ruiz, 2000; Lim, 2006; Bhugra and Bhui, 2007; Bhui and Bhugra, 2007; Munoz, *et al.*, 2007; Ruiz and Primm 2009).

What is unique and relevant in this respect is that all the major organizations that have an impact in the curriculum and practice of psychiatry and mental health in the United States have incorporated in their accreditation and certification processes all the important clinical issues pertaining to the role of culture and/or cultural competence in their requirements for accreditation and certification guidelines as, for instance, the American Board of Psychiatry and Neurology, Inc (ABPN) and the Accreditation Council for Graduate Medical Education (ACGME). These key decisions on their part have also impacted other organizations such as U.D. State Licensing Boards, Psychiatric and Mental Health Professional Associations' Continuing Medical Education Programs, etc. In this context, all accredited psychiatric residency training programmes in the United States currently incorporate in their clinical and didactic curriculums all relevant issues pertaining to the attainment of 'cultural competence'.

These positive advances in the field of cross-cultural psychiatry at large, not only in the United States but across the world as well, will in turn have appositive outcomes with respect to the quality of care offered to psychiatric/mental patients in all regions of the world. These positive outcomes are essential and crucial to the field of psychiatry and mental health at large. Quality of care, coupled with comprehensive access and parity of care as well as humane care, must be the number one priority for all professionals working in the field of psychiatry and mental health across the world. Investigational and educational efforts should also be directed to achieve new and better models of care thus positively impacting on the quality of care offered and rendered to psychiatric/mental patients. The achievement of these objectives and goals is fully intertwined to the ideal 'therapeutic skills' sought by all psychiatrists and mental health professionals practising worldwide. Likewise, 'therapeutic expectations' should not only be of the highest quality, but should also be shared both by psychiatric/mental patients and psychiatrists as well as other mental health professionals. Once these objectives and goals are achieved, not only in highly industrialized and developed countries but in all countries across the world as well, we will know that we secured fairness and justice for those who suffer from mental illnesses and psychiatric disorders.

Conclusions

In this chapter, we first described the status of 'therapeutic skills' and 'therapeutic expectations' in the field of psychiatric and mental health at large. In so doing, we underline the relevance and importance of including all manifestations of culture vis-à-vis mental health and mental illness; we also integrated all relevant factors pertaining to 'ethnicity' and 'race' within the core foundation of 'culture'. These three terms were also defined for clarification and clarity purposes. Secondly, we addressed the role of migration in relation to mental health and mental illness. In this context, we also addressed the recent and current impact of the globalization process, which is occurring, nowadays, in all regions of the world within the context of migration and the acculturation process. Next, we described and reviewed the United States immigration process, as a way of using it as a case model from which we could advance theoretical and practice examples across the world. Disparity issues pertaining to health and mental health care were also extensively discussed, with emphasis on ethnic, racial, and gender related disparities; also, attention was given to key factors such as access to care, parity of care, and humane care, within the context of the health and mental health delivery system that currently prevails in the United States.

Subsequently, we focused on the unique role of culture-bound syndromes as they relate to the diagnosis and treatment of psychiatric disorder and mental health conditions across the world. Enumeration of the most frequent and common culture-bound syndromes was provided in order to enhance the opportunities for further expansion of educational knowledge in this regard. Finally, the concept of cultural competence was examined, as a way of providing a strong foundation for the understanding and utilization of this concept in the daily practice of psychiatric care and mental health care with patients from different ethnic, racial, and cultural backgrounds. This concept has become very important and relevant worldwide as the globalization process impacts all regions of the world.

Hopefully, the topics addressed and discussed in this chapter will increase the therapeutic skills of psychiatrists and other mental health professionals in their quest to enhance their diagnostic armamentarium and their desire to provide a higher quality of psychiatric and mental health care to their psychiatric/mental patients; additionally, it is also anticipated that psychiatrists and other mental health professionals will be able to enhance their therapeutic expectations, as well as the therapeutic expectations of their patients, based on the knowledge and information provided in this chapter.

References

Alarcon, R.D. and Ruiz, P. (1995). Theory and practice of cultural psychiatry in the United States and abroad. In J. M. Oldham and M. B. Riba (Eds.) *Review of Psychiatry* **14**, pp. 599–626, Washington DC: American Psychiatric Press Inc.

American Psychiatric Association (2004). Diagnostic and Statistical Manual of Mental Disorders, 4th Edition, Washington DC: American Psychiatric Publishing.

Bhugra, D., Sumathipala, A., and Siribaddana, S. (2007). Culture-bound syndromes: a re-evaluation. In D. Bhugra and K. Bhui (Eds.) *Textbook of Cultural Psychiatry*, pp. 141–156, Cambridge: Cambridge University Press.

Bhugra, D. and Bhui, K. (2007). *Textbook of Cultural Psychiatry*, Cambridge: Cambridge University Press.

Bhui, K. and Bhugra, D. (2007). *Culture and Mental Health: A Comprehensive Textbook.* London: Hodder Arnold.

Canino, I.A. and Spurlock, J. (2000). *Culturally Diverse Children and Adolescents: Assessment Diagnosing and Treatment*, 2nd Edition. New York: The Guilford Press.

Constantine, M.G. and Sue, D.W. (2005). *Strategies for Building Multicultural Competence in Mental Health and Educational Settings.* Hoboken, NJ: John Wiley and Sons.

Lim, R.F. (Ed.). (2006). *Clinical Manual of Cultural Psychiatry.* Washington DC: American Psychiatric Publishing.

Mezzich, J.E., Kleinman, A., Fabrega, H. Jr, and Parron, D.L. (1996). *Culture and Psychiatric Diagnosis: A DSM-IV Perspective.* Washington DC: American Psychiatric Press.

Munoz, R., Primm, A., Ananth, J., and Ruiz, P. (2007). *Life in Color: Culture in American Psychiatry.* Chicago: Hilton Publishing Company.

Ruiz, P. (1985). Cultural barriers to effective medical care among Hispanic–American patients. *Annual Review of Medicine* **36**: 63–71.

Ruiz, P. (1995). Cross cultural psychiatry – Foreword. In J. M. Oldham and M. B. Riba (Eds.) *Review of Psychiatry* Volume 14, pp. 467–476, Washington DC: American Psychiatric Press.

Ruiz, P. (1998). New clinical perspectives in cultural psychiatry. *Journal of Practical Psychiatry and Behavioral Health* **4**: 150–156.

Ruiz, P. (2000). *Ethnicity and Psychopharmacology.* Washington DC: American Psychiatric Publishing.

Ruiz, P. (2004). Addressing culture, race and ethnicity. *Psychiatric Annals* **34**: 527–532.

Ruiz, P. and Bhugra, D. (2008). Introduction to the special issue on psychiatry in Asia. *International Review of Psychiatry* **20**(5): 405–408.

Ruiz, P. and Primm, A.B. (Eds.). (2009). *Disparities in Psychiatric Care: Clinical and Cross-Cultural Perspectives.* Philadelphia: Lippincott Williams and Wilkins.

Chapter 10

Treatment goals and therapeutic interactions

J. David Kinzie and J. Mark Kinzie

Introduction

Case study one

Mohammed is a 22-year-old man from Iraq who was first seen in the Intercultural Psychiatric Program four months after arriving in the United States. He was a student in Iraq and his family was prominent in the community. His family had been threatened because of their religion. His older brother was kidnapped and killed despite the family paying a ransom. One night, Mohammed was walking home with friends when they encountered a road block with armed men. The men asked their religion. Mohammed tried to guess the men's religion, but guessed incorrectly. He was beaten and shot. His friends were killed. Mohammed feigned death. When they threw him on a pile of bodies, he let out a noticeable gasp. One of the men subsequently stabbed him on the left side of his head and left him for dead. Later, American troops came across the pile of bodies. Fearing the pile to be booby trapped with a bomb, they shot at it with guns. Mohammed was shot in the stomach. He physically recovered in a hospital. He and his family spent a short time in Syria before coming to the United States. On presentation, Mohammed was hopeless and said that he should have died not his friends. He had traumatic reminders of the past whenever he saw violence on television or saw the police. He had nightmares every night about the shooting. He felt flat and numb, as if a wall now separated him from the rest of the world. He was constantly on alert for his safety and could not relax. He had exaggerated startle response. Although not actively suicidal, he reported that life was not worth living. He has residual weakness on the right side of his body and walks with a limp as a result of being stabbed in the head.

According to the United Nations High Commissioner for Refugees in the year 2007, there were 16 million refugees throughout the world. In addition, there were 26 million internally displaced persons from conflicts and 25 million internally displaced persons from natural disasters. Overall, this gave 67 million refugees and internally displaced persons (UNHCR, 2007). Multiple studies of refugees who have been resettled in third countries have documented multiple traumas they have endured and the greatly increased psychiatric symptoms. These various studies include, selectively, those from Southeast

Asia (Beiser and Hou, 2001), Cambodians in the United States (Carlson and Rosser-Hogan, 1993), Bosnian refugees in the Netherlands (Drozdek, 1997), Ethiopian refugees (Fenta *et al.*, 2004), Somali, Afghan, and Iranian refugees (Gerritsen *et al.*, 2006), Somali and Oromo refugees (Jaranson *et al.*, 2004), and Vietnamese refugees in Norway (Hauff and Vaglum, 1994). Many of these studies have included long-term follow-up of refugees and continue to show multiple psychiatric and social problems. An example is a study of Cambodian refugees in Long Beach, California (Marshall *et al.*, 2005). A large review of mental disorders among 7000 refugees resettled in Western countries (Fazel *et al.*, 2005) found that 9% were diagnosed with post-traumatic stress disorder (PTSD) and 5% with Major Depressive Disorder. It was found that refugees were about ten times more likely to have PTSD than age-matched general populations in these countries.

The Intercultural Psychiatric Program, formerly the Indochinese Psychiatric Program, at Oregon Health and Science University in Portland, Oregon, has treated refugees for over thirty years. Over this time, we have treated several thousand refugees and currently have 1200 in treatment. Our experience in this is reflected in this report. Our sample includes Southeast Asians (Vietnamese, Cambodians, Lao, Mien), Africans (particularly Somalis and Ethiopians of Oromo and Amharic tribes), Bosnians, Russians, Guatemalans, and El Salvadorans from Central America, Kurdish and Farsi speakers from Iran and Afghanistan, Arabic speaking patients predominantly from Iraq, and, more recently, refugees from Burma (Kinzie *et al.*, 1980; Kinzie and Manson, 1983; Kinzie, 1986). We will review our work and that of others. The primary symptoms and social problems of refugees, a treatment approach to these patients, problems, and future directions will also be addressed.

Review of the symptoms

In our experience evaluating 487 recent refugees from multiple cultures, we have found that 65% had PTSD or PTSD plus depression. Twenty one percent had just depression and an additional 12% had pure schizophrenia or other psychosis, often associated with depression.

Post-traumatic stress disorder

As most authors have found, traumatized patients from war-torn, ethnic cleansing, and violent countries have experienced massive trauma and subsequently suffer from PTSD. Our studies have found that this existed early on among Cambodians (Kinzie *et al.*, 1984). Subsequently, our research indicated that it is extremely common in all Southeast Asian refugees (Kinzie *et al.*, 1990).

Presenting symptoms are often poor sleep, nightmares, intrusive thoughts, and irritability with sometimes aggressive actions.

Case study two

Rukia is a 35-year-old Somali mother of four children who was first seen eight months after arriving in the United States. Rukia was living in Mogadishu with her mother and family. The men of the house were out on business when men with guns came into the house demanding money and jewellery. Her mother tried to stop them. She was forcibly raped in front of the family by the men. She was then shot in the head by one of the men. Rukia has vivid memories of her mother's brain tissue and blood splatter onto the floor. The men then tried to rape Rukia. She resisted and was pushed into the kitchen fire, which contained boiling oil for frying. She covered her face, but badly burned the back of her hands and neck. The next morning the surviving family escaped without burying their mother. The family spent eight years in a refugee camp in Kenya before coming to the United States. Even now, Rukia has nightmares of that traumatic night every night. The image of her mother being shot and her brain tissue on the floor is one that she is unable to get out of her head. The scars on her hands and neck serve as a constant reminder of the trauma. She wears gloves and covers her neck to try to hide the scars. She must sit in any room facing the door so that she can easily escape if needed. She startles easily. She avoids talking about Somalia as much as possible and gets annoyed, irritable, and angry when friends and family talk about it. She is short tempered and emotionally detached from her family. Her children are struggling in school and social service workers are now making home visits to check on the children.

Depression

Most of the patients with PTSD also suffer from depression. The number of losses encountered by refugees is staggering. Most have lost family members from war or disease and have also lost their country, culture, social network, profession, income, and the ability to use their native language in the country of resettlement. It is quite understandable that depression from loss accompanies PTSD. In our population, they coexist about 80% of the time. Depression alone is a minority diagnosis but does occur in about 20% of patients.

Case study three

Emma is 28-year-old Mexican woman who is married and has two children. She was educated as a scientist and was a scholar in southern Mexico. She and her husband became politically active defending the rights of the indigenous people of southern Mexico. Because of this, her husband was detained and beaten by police. They both received threatening calls telling them that they would be killed if they continued to be active. They escaped to the United States and are applying for political asylum. Her husband continues to have PTSD and depression symptoms, but he is adapting to the new culture and has found gratifying work. Emma has not found work, but has not tried hard. She is less comfortable speaking English than her husband. She is isolated from both the English-speaking (because of language barrier) and Spanish-speaking (because of differences in education and social class) communities. She generally stays at home, even when the children are at school. She becomes especially homesick during the holidays. She looks forward to returning home to Mexico, but cannot because she would likely be killed. She notes that her concentration, interest, and appetite are all diminished. She hopes that things will get better, but cannot imagine how that would happen.

Psychosis

Schizophrenia without PTSD is rather uncommon among refugees but seems to reflect the normal prevalence rate of the general population. However, psychotic symptoms accompanying PTSD is very common. We first noted post-traumatic psychosis among our Cambodian refugees (Kinzie and Boehnlein, 1989). Since that time, multiple writers have stressed the prevalence of psychotic co-morbidity with PTSD (Kozari-Kovacić and Baroveckić, 2005; Sareen *et al.*, 2005; Hardy *et al.*, 2005; Scott *et al.*, 2007; Shevlin *et al.*, 2008; Lindley *et al.*, 2000; Kroll, 2007; Braakman *et al.*, 2008; Bogár and Perczel, 2007; Fan *et al.*, 2008). The majority of these studies have nothing to do with refugees but do indicate that trauma can coexist with, and probably cause, psychotic symptoms in the course of PTSD. It has high enough prevalence for the need to be screened in all refugees undergoing psychiatric evaluation.

Case study four

Faduma is a 26-year-old Somali woman with a history of schizophrenia. Her sister and mother also have psychotic symptoms. Another sister has depression and PTSD. Her father was killed during the war in Somalia and her family threatened. They fled to Kenya. In Kenya, they lived in a refugee camp. Life was difficult with little food and water available. They lived in a small hut and felt unsafe leaving the camp. The family was seen by a psychiatrist about 6 months after coming to the United States. She was noted to have auditory hallucinations of whispers. She also felt the spirits were controlling her. She had nightmares of the violence in Somalia. She was easily taken advantage of by other members of the Somali community. One night some Somali men raped her. She was able to call the police and the men were sent to trial. Around the time of the trial, her symptoms became worse. She started dressing as an American and insisted on speaking in English. She was angry and defiant. She got into frequent fights with her family. She stopped taking antipsychotic medication. Her memories of the rape were intrusive and frequent. She complained of poor sleep. Because of her documental mental health problems, her testimony was seen as not credible. The charges against the men were dropped. She continued to deteriorate to the point of requiring hospitalization.

Cognitive impairment

Many refugees have undergone massive head trauma and suffer from dementing illnesses or forms of encephalitis from infections. These cognitive impairments greatly exacerbate treatment problems and need to be evaluated in the treatment setting.

Case study five

Sadun is a 45-year-old man from Sri Lanka. He was politically active there and was a researcher in one of the major universities. He joined a street protest against the government. The protesters were beaten and Sadun was hit on the head many times with a baton. He developed a subdural hematoma requiring emergency surgery. The scars can be clearly seen on his forehead. Imaging studies revealed severe damage particularly to the frontal cortex. His thoughts and speech were simple and not expected of a university researcher. He was easily preyed upon and had been robbed many times by visitors he thought were friends. He subsequently ended up living in a homeless shelter. His recollection of the beating was vague, but he was fearful of police. On the other hand, he was noted to be too easily trusting and thought relationships were closer than they really were.

Enduring personality change

Although not recognized in DSM-IV, ICD-10 recognizes it and personality change can occur after catastrophic stress and experiences. The key features of these have been found to include hostile or distrustful attitude, somatization, self-injurious behaviour, sexual dysfunction, and enduring guilt. These are extremely resistive to change and persist over a long time (Bauer *et al.*, 1993; Beltran and Silove, 1999; Beltran *et al.*, 2008).

Case study six

Mansoor is a 45-year-old man from Iran. Because of his Bahai religion, he and his family were frequently harassed by the Iranian government. Their property was confiscated and he was imprisoned on several occasions. He was tortured by electric whips and solitary confinement for months at a time. He was likely sexually abused, but refuses to talk about this. After he was released, he and his family escaped to Turkey and then came to the United States. He was seen by a psychiatrist about eight months after coming to the United States. At that time he had intense PSTD symptoms: he was fearful of sleeping, had frequent nightmares about the trauma, and was extremely hypervigilant. These symptoms improved with medications and psychotherapy. However, the patient remains irritable, suspicious, and distrustful. He does not want his wife to leave the house alone because other men may make sexual advances towards her. He believes that his daughters are becoming too Americanized and also may be having sex. He is suspicious of other Bahais because he feels that they did not support him in Iran. He spends most of his time alone watching television and leaves the house to calm down after interacting with family.

Medical problems

Our studies have indicated very high rates of hypertension (about 45%) and diabetes (about 13%) among a mixed group of traumatized refugees (Kinzie *et al.*, 2008). Clearly, ongoing medical problems among refugees are major issues.

Our opinion is that there is such a public health issue that they need to be identified and treated at the earliest evaluation and in ongoing treatment.

___

Case study seven

Arash is a 60-year-old Iranian man who was persecuted in Iran for speaking out against the government. He has PTSD and depression symptoms related to the threats that he received there. Medication for depression and PTSD has helped with sleep and mood symptoms. However, he continues to worry about his children who remain in Iran, but are trying to leave. He is unemployed and faces severe financial hardships. His wife is in poor health. Recently, Arash was diagnosed with hypertension and diabetes mellitus type II. In order to afford medications for diabetes and hypertension and because he was fearful that he was taking too much medication, he stopped taking antidepressants. He presents hopeless and anhedonic. He is tense and irritable. He says that life is not worth living.

___

Course of symptoms

The literature seems to under-recognize the longevity of symptoms and their course of exacerbation and remission. The effect of 9/11, with its traumatic visual images on television, exacerbated the symptoms of even the most stable traumatized refugee patients. There was an increase in depression and PTSD symptoms, especially nightmares (Kinzie *et al.*, 2002). It is now recognized that short-term treatment and evaluation is inappropriate and patients experience ongoing stresses in their lives. Indeed, the diagnosis of PTSD at times seems inappropriate since there is sometimes no 'post', i.e. there are ongoing stresses in some of the neighborhoods the refugees live in, such as gang violence and drug-related illegal activity, which threaten the patients. Other common stresses such as pressures from relatives for money, illnesses, and accidents can completely exacerbate the symptoms.

Other problems

Refugees have many ongoing social problems. The foremost of these is learning the English language or the language of the native country. This can be a profoundly difficult event for people who have little education or who are cognitively disturbed and cannot concentrate. There is pressure from many organizations to get gainful employment rapidly. In the United States this is expected to happen within eight months. At a time of economic recession, this is almost impossible. Patients are often faced with withdrawal of financial funds. Housing is an important issue, as is finding the necessary money for children, medical services, food, and rent. Asylum seekers are an immigrant group, which faces additional problems (Silove *et al.*, 1997). They usually have a pending court date and live in legal limbo, uncertain of whether they will be accepted for refugee status or be sent back to their own country. Their symptoms are greatly exacerbated leading up to and during their court date. There may be a prolonged appeal to a negative court finding, which increases their symptoms as well.

Treatment issues and review

With the multiple psychiatric, medical, and social issues involved in the treatment of refugees, it is a complicated, time-consuming, and professionally driven activity. Clearly, multiple treatment needs are required and comprehensive evaluation and follow-up are needed to ensure there is resolution of some problems and amelioration of the stress on the patient. Unfortunately, there is a lack of good data on treatment outcomes of traumatized refugees. There have been sporadic reports of some counseling techniques or exposure therapy, educational approaches, including one among African refugees (Neuner *et al.*, 2004) and cognitive behaviour and exposure therapy for PTSD in refugees (Paunovic and Öst, 2001). Cognitive behaviour therapy has been used for asylum seekers and for Vietnamese refugees (Bașog̃lu *et al.*, 2004; Hinton *et al.*, 2004). One study examined the use of antidepressants in Bosnian refugees with PTSD (Smajkic *et al.*, 2001). Cognitive behavioural therapy has also been used for refugees and asylum seekers who have traumatic stress symptoms in England (Grey and Young, 2008). None of these reports has addressed the multiple psychosocial medical issues of the patients. There is one good study on mental health and health-related quality of life of tortured refugees using a multidisciplinary treatment (Carlsson *et al.*, 2005). This study had patients in multidimensional treatment, though not including psychotropic medication, for 9 months and included a before and after survey. They found that there was no change in health-related symptoms and their conclusion was that emotional stress seemed to be chronic for the majority of the patients. Our own work with Cambodians who have been in treatment for 10 years showed that a large percentage still had major symptoms (Boehnlein *et al.*, 2004). This dearth of controlled studies is a problem for the field of treatment of traumatized refugees but also underlines the tremendous difficulties in such treatment and its evaluation. As mentioned, refugees come from multiple cultures, speak many languages, and have multiple traumas (some with severe torture) and losses (e.g. loss of family members, home, culture, position in society, and income). Psychiatric treatment may be foreign to them and difficult to accept. In addition, the disorders have a chronic course, as we have documented, with exacerbations and remissions based upon ongoing stresses in the patient's life (Kinzie, 2007). Therefore, it is difficult to do comprehensive studies and it is also difficult to evaluate the outcome of an illness with such a fluctuating course. One of the goals of this chapter is to present an approach to multidimensional treatment to try to address the complicated problems that refugees have in their adjustment to a foreign country.

Intercultural Psychiatric Program clinical approach

This section describes the clinical approach used by the Intercultural Psychiatric Program (IPP) over its 30 years of operation. IPP has incorporated many new refugee groups during this time. The approach has been rather constant throughout.

Psychiatrists

It is a psychiatric-driven programme in which the main treatment and evaluators are University Department of Psychiatry faculty members, all of whom have experience in both cross-cultural psychiatry and in trauma. The psychiatrists have been recruited for their personal qualities of interest in other cultures, warm, gentle, accepting personal styles, and, above all, a clinical competence.

Counsellors

Each psychiatrist is teamed up with a single counsellor for a specific group of patients. For example, Counsellor A works with Vietnamese and will always be assigned to Psychiatrist A. The two of them will them have a group of patients, typically 50 to 100, as their caseload. The counsellors are all members of the ethnic community they serve; that is, the majority of them have been refugees themselves, have come to the United States, received training in our programme, and, in most cases, obtained graduate or postgraduate degrees in psychology or social work. They serve, first of all, as interpreters for the psychiatrists during the psychiatric interviews and treatment sessions. They also serve as case managers between sessions; that is, the patients can call them about various problems, including logistical problems, help with social issues, and medication issues. As the counsellors gain experience, they also do individual counseling and conduct group therapy sessions of a special type (see later).

The setting for IPP originally was part of the psychiatric outpatient department in the Department of Psychiatry. It evolved to have its own physical space with its reception area and records separate from the hospital. All staff members, including administrative staff and secretaries, are recruited because they are sensitive, warm, easy-going people who enjoy working with people of other cultures. Confidentiality is an extremely important part of the training programme. The counsellors and psychiatrists have ongoing training sessions about various issues in mental health, psychiatric diagnosis, treatment, PTSD, and current laws and regulations regarding the treatment of the mentally ill. The programme is a fully approved programme of the mental health division of the state of Oregon and operates like any other mental health clinic, subject to inspection and evaluation by the state and federal agencies, which are associated with Medicare and Medicaid funding. Some grant support from the Office of Refugee Resettlement of the U.S. government and the United Nations Voluntary Fund for Victims of Torture have added financial assistance (Kinzie, 1988).

Diagnostic interview

The diagnostic interview is also the beginning of setting up a relationship with the patient and to form the basis for ongoing treatment. In our setting, the patient has minimal contacts to make for referral. When calling in, they are referred immediately to the counsellor for that ethnic group, i.e. Somali, Bosnian, Kurdish, etc. The counsellor takes a brief history and then sets up a mental health assessment within a week. The psychiatrist interview comes within 2 weeks of this. The counsellor and psychiatrist then are also the treating team. There is no transfer to other treaters and there is a minimum of complications. The setting for the interview needs to be a comfortable and easy to reach place for refugees with the staff totally comfortable with people who may not speak English and have concerns and anxiety about coming to a psychiatric clinic. Being greeted by the counsellor with whom they have spoken on the phone is very helpful and having a critical mass of other refugees from their ethnic group greatly aids in initiation and diagnostic process. The room should be comfortable with three chairs equal distance apart and a warm setting.

The diagnostic interview is a complicated process of which the primary purpose is to establish a relationship and a treatment contract. The exact information is not always as important and much is often missed in the anxiety of the first interview. In our session, the psychiatrist asks the questions and the information is translated verbally and non-verbally as much as possible to the patient and back to the psychiatrist. In our experience, it flows quite easily with the counsellor being the cultural informer to both of the other parties, i.e. I've heard the counsellors say to the patients, 'the psychiatrist needs to know the information, although it may not seem important to you'. Information follows a standard format (Kinzie, 1985; Kinzie and Fleck, 1987). After an exchange of greetings, often information about the patient's culture and their current situation in the country is gathered and follows a traditional medical interview, which often concentrates on physical symptoms. This is often very reassuring to patients as they do not have to immediately go into traumatic information. Most patients come with marked physical symptoms, including sleep disturbance, body pains, GI distress, and headaches. These need to be taken seriously with their duration and location noted. Other symptoms need to be reported at this time, particularly those related to PTSD, such as nightmares, intrusive thoughts, avoidance behaviour, irritability, and hyperarousal, as well as depressive symptoms, such as poor sleep and appetite, low mood, and hopelessness with suicidal thoughts. Psychotic symptoms, such as hallucinations and delusions, should be briefly touched on at this point. Following is the standard format for gathering information.

1 Life in their own country before any traumatic events, including family life, parents, children, education, and occupational level.

2 Life during the traumatic events. As much as possible, allow the patients to describe their traumatic events, including losses of family members, separation, maltreatment, torture, seeing dead bodies, and witnessing/observing horrific events. This may be very difficult for the patient. It is not necessary to go into total detail but the point is to let the patient know that the team can handle hearing it and can understand what the patient went through.

3 The escape process, which is often quite heroic, going through battlefields and finally arriving at a refugee camp.

4 The refugee camp experience is often equally traumatic as they are often subjected to lack of food and water, robberies, gang violence, and even murder.

5 The process of coming to the United States, the adjustment to life in the United States, hopes, fears, and problems.

6 Any physical problems the patient has and any medication the patient is currently taking. These should include medication for hypertension and diabetes.

7 Social problems need to be mentioned—for example, financial, housing, problems raising children, asylum, their specific legal status (e.g. refugee, asylum seeker, citizen, undocumented alien, etc.), need to contact family members, or pressure to go to work when they are unable to.

8 There should be a summary statement by the psychiatrist on what he/she has heard and an explanation of the relationship between the symptoms and the events, which make sense to the patient and his/her culture. A common statement is as follows: 'I understand now that you have backaches, headaches, very poor sleep, irritability, and nightmares. You have had a lot of severely bad things happen to you in the past and now those events have come back to affect your mind and your body. Because you've experienced these bad events, your body now is suffering and you have these multiple symptoms. Does this seem reasonable to you?' We try to get an agreement on some understanding of the relationship to social events and trauma.

9 Then we ask for some kind of contract about treatment of symptoms. For example, the psychiatrist might ask, 'What are the symptoms that we should work on first? You mentioned poor sleep, irritability, nightmares, and sadness. Which are the most important to tackle first?' Often they will say, 'All', but at least we have some specific goals that we are working on.

10 I leave the session after making recommendations for treatment saying, 'There are three things you have to do. You have to take your medicine, you have to keep your appointments, and you cannot kill yourself. Do you agree to do these things?' This is primarily to confirm with them the seriousness and commitment I take to their treatment. Suicide is very rare among our Muslim and Buddhist patients but it confirms that we take their lives seriously and we expect them to continue and cooperate in treatment. This has been a very useful approach for us, as 90% of initial and follow-up patient visits are kept, an astoundingly high percentage for a minority mental health clinic.

The initial interview is not rushed and usually takes about 90 minutes. At the end we usually ask if the patient has any questions or if there are any other things we haven't covered. This gives the patient a chance to elaborate on any other issues. At the end of the session, if the patient has not had a primary care physician who cares for his/her hypertension or it is not documented, we take a blood pressure and, if necessary, initiate treatment for hypertension. We also order a Hemoglobin A_1C diabetes evaluation since that can be done without fasting, which is often difficult for patients.

Treatment of refugees

As mentioned, the treatment of refugees is a complex, complicated task. It is long-term—there is no short-term solution—and is characterized by exacerbations and remissions according to the stresses and comforts in the individual patient's life. The two most important therapeutic ingredients are continuity and constancy.

Continuity implies that the team—the psychiatrist and the counsellor—is with the patient throughout the whole treatment; there is no change in counsellor or psychiatrist and they will be with the patient as long as they need to be. This provides an anchor point of stability in an often chaotic life.

Constancy means that the therapist is the same from session to session. There is no sudden change in tactics, no change in approach, and no challenging, which provides increasing trauma to the patient.

A third ingredient is a warm and sometimes gentle humour, which helps the patient feel comfortable. Many of the patient groups—Bosnians and Somalis in particular—cope with stress with humour and a gentle, often self-effacing, humour can be extremely helpful in reducing the difficult stress.

We emphasize no specific approach. However, exposure therapy, cognitive-behavioural therapy, and eye-movement desensitization and reprocessing all are therapies which, in our experience, are contraindicated for this group; they do not address the multiple problems or specific existential issues, especially of severe trauma, faced by this group. Additionally, these approaches are of limited duration. The patients also see them as a gimmick and a trick for problems, which they know don't have an easy solution, e.g. death of spouses, loss of country, loss of children, language problems, etc. Therapy should be aimed at being as long-term as the patient needs and wants it. A general approach is to be supportive in nature and dynamic in the sense of bringing past experiences to bear on their current symptoms and problems.

We have emphasized some general aspects of treatment that need to be done:

1 Non-specific Approaches for Traumatized Refugees

a) Treatment needs to manage major psychiatric illnesses—depression, PTSD, psychosis, dementia.

b) The well-trained mental health workers, as mentioned before, must have good credibility within the community.

c) There must be integration of physical and mental health.

2 Specific Therapeutic Approaches

a) The interaction with the psychiatrist needs to deal with several issues. The patient often has a need, sometimes not, to tell their trauma story. The therapist needs to have the ability to listen. These stories are extremely difficult to listen to, they are difficult to tell, and they have no solution. There is no solution for some of the existentially, profoundly disturbing events that occur. The ability to listen and to be with the patient is the essential treatment. There is no need or ability to try to fix it or to interrupt or distance oneself from the real pain of the patient. In our experience, this is one of the most difficult things for beginning therapists to do.

b) There is a need for constancy over time with the therapist providing a constant source of stability. These are chronic disorders and there is a need for a long-term relationship as the courses wax and wane. The usual course is for symptoms to regress and then reoccur. The presence of the therapist is to provide continuity and safety. Everyday issues, such as the death of relatives, financial problems, and cultural loss, are ongoing for the patient and the relationship with the therapist fills some of this void. The therapist serves as a confidant, a model, and even an authority to give permission to recognize some problems are very difficult for anyone to handle.

c) The patients have a need to give and the therapist needs to receive. Often, as the patient gets better, they have the ability to give something back to the treatment. Our patients usually don't pay anything directly and receive a great deal of help. When they can give something back, it is extremely useful. The first step is often merely to say 'Thank you'. Often they will give something in their groups, perhaps contributing to a particular meal at a celebration—for example, Ramadan for Muslims or Thet for the Vietnamese. The ability to give back to the staff and for the staff to accept this with graciousness will start to cement a more bilateral relationship.

d) A common problem that the patients deal with is the problem of evil— 'Why did these things that are so bad happen to me?' 'What is the reason for it?' 'Why does evil exist?' These troubling questions have no answer. The goal of the therapist is to recognize the validity of such questions and acknowledge that they are difficult to answer. Beyond that, the therapist also needs to have a belief beyond nihilism that a transformation in humans is possible and that people can in fact get better and can improve their quality of life and their own personal qualities. This belief transfers to the patient; they sense of the existential strength that can come from existential loss (Kinzie, 2001).

3 Medications are extremely helpful in treating refugees. They can reduce symptoms quite rapidly and can give immediate relief. We have evaluated medicines in some detail with our patients and found that they are extremely useful. They are not always taken easily and some of our first studies indicated that there was a great deal of non-compliance with medicine (Kinzie *et al.*, 1988). For example, we found in our early studies that many Cambodian and Mien patients were taking none of the antidepressant medications as they found it was very 'strong'. With education, that percentage has now greatly increased and most patients are compliant (see Lin *et al.* in this volume).

a) Antidepressants have been very useful. The more sedative tricyclic antidepressants have a particular value as they can induce sleep and are effective in severe depression. The risk of overdose is very rare in our Muslim and Buddhist patients. Indeed, our clinic has not had any patients commit suicide from overdosing on our medication (in thirty years, there have only been five documented suicides, all by non-medical means).

b) Particularly useful in treating nightmares, has been clonidine. We have found that clonidine is particularly effective with nightmares and hyperarousal symptoms. We have used it for some time now (Kinzie and Leung, 1989). In an all-night study of Cambodians with PTSD using a polysomnograph, we found that the prevalence of nightmares was greatly diminished with clonidine (Kinzie *et al.*, 1994). More recently, our group (Boehnlein and Kinzie, 2007) has made the case for clonidine and prazosin, both CNS noradrenergic antagonists in PTSD, in reducing nightmares. Our data indicate that most people can reduce nightmares within a week or two with an antidepressant and clonidine or prazosin. We strongly recommend these be used in initiating and continuing treatment for traumatized refugees.

c) The SSRIs, particularly fluoxetine, are useful. Though fluoxetine is not so sedative and not valuable with pain symptoms, it is a safe alternative, especially for old people. It has the advantage over other SSRIs in that it is long-acting and the patient can miss a dose or two without any withdrawal effects.

d) Many patients have psychotic symptoms and we've used a variety of medicines. Risperdal seems to be the best tolerated, although we've had patients gain weight with it and, with the high prevalence of diabetes, it is problematic. Often, when patients have more straightforward schizophrenic symptoms, we have used perphenazine and have had minimal problems with tardive dyskinesia or extrapyramidal symptoms (EPS).

4 Group interaction

a) About half of our patients attend a form of group socialization experiences, now run by our counsellors. These are not expressive or dynamically oriented group therapy sessions but much more socialization and psycho-education. They centre on cultural events and practical problems such as raising children, passing the citizenship test, coping with getting licenses and paying rent, and the intricacies of voting. These have been extremely well attended and have provided ongoing socialization experiences, often forming pseudo-families out of people who are quite isolated (Kinzie *et al.*, 1988).

5 Other approaches

a) Most of our patients are involved in traditional religions, primarily Buddhism or Islam. We have supported those and made contact with some of the local religious leaders. Part of our outreach is to provide education about mental illness and to get their help with encouraging ill people to receive treatment. This has been very useful in aiding our acceptance in the community.

b) Many of the younger patients have trouble with whether to adjust to American culture or stay with traditional culture. We have encouraged a bicultural adjustment; that is, continuing the holidays, celebrations, and religions of the traditional culture as well as adjusting as much as possible to the American life of education and interaction with other Americans. This is easier to do for younger people. More traditional older people find this difficult and find themselves in conflict with their children. This is all the source of some education in the group sessions.

c) The asylum patients, as mentioned before, have a very difficult job in that they are often not able to work and have very little social or financial support as their case is in limbo. We have advocated for them when their case seems to be valid and have worked closely with the local legal immigrant association.

d) We have also aided people in getting citizenship, especially those that have been unable to master English, and have assisted patients in their efforts to find jobs and housing. There is a whole series of social events in which our system can be helpful.

6 Problem areas

a) Medication: Non-compliance with medicine or complaints of side effects was an early-on issue. The group therapies have been very helpful in that other patients have to talk about their use of medicine and it encourages patients. Most patients have found relief very rapidly and have accepted medicine, although this does vary from group to group. We discuss medicine side effects and benefits at each session. It is not uncommon for patients to stop medicine as soon as they feel better, only to have a relapse. Most medicine needs to be taken on a rather continual basis and requires education. Some side effects are so severe (i.e. sexual dysfunction) that they do require a change in medicine.

b) Marital distress: Many traumatized couples who both have experienced horrific events find that the ongoing irritability creates a great deal of distress. We give the patients choices about whether to come together or come separately, usually serially one after another. The latter has been the preferred session for most patients. Among the traditional families from Africa and Eastern Europe, divorce is extremely uncommon although many remain very unhappy. With symptomatic relief, the situation often becomes more tolerable and, on occasion, even enjoyable. We give not only practical suggestions about marital therapy but also information about the strong prohibition against violence in the US culture, a fact that seems to be unknown to some other cultures.

c) Raising children has been another major issue. It is understandable that many refugee children adapt rapidly to American ways—e.g. English language, music, dress—which is quite disparate from the parents. This has caused a great deal of problems. Some children, however, are symptomatic among themselves with hyperactivity, poor school performance, alcohol use, and promiscuity. Our child psychiatry section has handled many of these with some good success, but sometimes it has been very difficult for the families to cope with what seems to be a feeling situation.

d) A very common problem occurs when patients get letters from their home country asking for money. The theory seems to be that America is paved with gold and anyone here should have plenty of money to send home. This has been very stressful since most of our patients are on welfare or have minimal income. We've had to encourage them to sometimes stop the connection or to be very frank that they have no money. We have very supportively stated to patients that they are too poor to send money and their job right now is to take care of their family here.

Evaluation

Evaluation of treatment outcome is extremely difficult and in the primitive steps. Our programme utilizes many rather simple ways to evaluate patients. Certainly one is follow-up of appointments, which has been very good, as I mentioned before (90%). The Global Assessment of Functioning (GAF) by the psychiatrist is another one. Most of our patients still maintain in the lower level, i.e. 60 and lower, and so there is not a high rate of improvement by that. The Sheehan Disability Scale, which is a self-rated analogue scale used to rate a person's distress in the areas of work, social life, and family/home responsibilities, is given at admission and at the 1-year update and provides some very useful data about how the patients view themselves. We also have similar data on depression, nightmares, and irritability. The analogue scale is a useful technique to handle some of the patients' subjective evaluation of their progress. We have pilot data on these measures which are basically a visual analogue scale of a line from 1 to 10 with 10 being the worst or most impairment (Table 10.1).

These preliminary data, though collected from different patients (Sheehan version, intrusive thoughts and irritability) and at different times (six months and one year), nevertheless give an indication that such evaluation is possible. They also show disruption of family and social life positive changes. Depression and irritability also significantly decreased but not as much as those on the Sheehan scale. More work on evaluation clearly needs to be done, including more parameters of patient functioning and symptoms.

Table 10.1 Outcome data on Sheehan Disability Scale and symptom checklist

Measure		Mean
Sheehan Disability Scale (N = 25)		
a) Disruption of family life		7.56
	At Intake	5.00
	At 1 year	p<.002*
b) Disruption of social relationship		8.04
	At intake	5.68
	At 1 year	
	p<.002*	
Depression Rating (N = 18)		
	At intake	7.56
	At 6 months	6.67
	p<.033*	
Irritability Rating (N = 18)		
	At intake	5.33
	At 6 months	4.11
	p<.012*	

*by Friedman non-parametric test

Future needs in research

Clearly, evaluation of outcome is a major need in the field. There are many refugee and torture treatment programmes in the world without a sound empirical basis for their efficacy or effectiveness. The problems of course are huge, involving multiple groups and languages as well as multiple traumas in multiple countries. A multi-dimensional approach of taking symptoms, quality of life, adjustment to the culture, and medical needs and help, all need to be considered. Multiple sources of input, such as from clinicians, patients, and counsellors, need to be considered. We are in the process of doing such an evaluation now but we admit that it is a lengthy and difficult procedure.

References

Başoğlu, M., Ekblad, S., Bäärnhielm, S., and Livanou, M. (2004). Cognitive-behavioral treatment of tortured asylum seekers: A case study. *Anxiety Disorders* **18**: 357–369.

Bauer, M., Priebe, S., Häring, B., and Adamczak, K. (1993). Long-term mental sequelae of political imprisonment in East Germany. *Journal of Nervous and Mental Disease* **181**(4): 257–262.

Beiser, M. and Hou, F. (2001). Language acquisition, unemployment and depressive disorder among Southeast Asian refugees: a 10-year study. *Social Science and Medicine* **53**(10): 1321–1334.

Beltran, R.O. and Silove, D. (1999). Expert opinions about the ICD-10 category of enduring personality change after catastrophic experience. *Comprehensive Psychiatry* **40**(5): 396–403.

Beltran, R.O., Llewellyn, G.M., and Silove, D. (2008). Clinicians' understanding of International Statistical Classification of Diseases and Related Health Problems, 10th Revision diagnostic criteria: F62.0 enduring personality change after catastrophic experience. *Comprehensive Psychiatry* **49**(6): 593–602.

Boehnlein, J.K. and Kinzie, J.D. (2007). Pharmacologic reduction of CNS noradrenergic activity in PTSD: the case for clonidine and prazosin. *Journal of Psychiatric Practice* **13**(2): 72–78.

Boehnlein, J.K., Kinzie, J.D., Sekiya, U., Riley, C., Pou, K., and Rosborough, B. (2004). A ten-year treatment outcome study of traumatized Cambodian refugees. *Journal of Nervous and Mental Disease* **192**(10): 658–663.

Bogár, K. and Perczel, D.F. (2007). Trauma and psychosis. *Psychiatiar Hungarica* **22**(4): 300–310.

Braakman, M.H., Kortmann, F.A., van den Brink, W., and Verkes, R.J. (2008). Posttraumatic stress disorder with secondary psychotic features: Neurobiological findings. *Progress in Brain Research* **167**: 299–302.

Carlson, E.B. and Rosser-Hogan, R. (1993). Mental health status of Cambodian refugees ten years after leaving their homes. *American Journal of Orthopsychiatry* **63**(2): 223–231.

Carlsson, J.M., Mortensen, E.L., and Kastrup, M. (2005). A follow-up study of mental health and health-related quality of life in tortured refugees in multidisciplinary treatment. *Journal of Nervous and Mental Disease* **191**: 651–657.

Drozdek, B. (1997). Follow-up study of concentration camp survivors from Bosnia-Herzegovina: Three years later. *Journal of Nervous and Mental Disease* **185**(11): 690–694.

Fan, X., Henderson, D.C., Nguyen, D.D., et al. (2008). Posttraumatic stress disorder, cognitive function and quality of life in patients with schizophrenia. *Psychiatry Research* **159**(1–2): 140–146.

Fazel, M., Wheeler, J., and Danesh, J. (2005). Prevalence of serious mental disorder in 7000 refugees resettled in western countries: A systematic review. *Lancet* **365**(9467): 1309–1314.

Fenta, H., Hman, I., and Noh, S. (2004). Determinants of depression among Ethiopian immigrants and refugees in Toronto. *Journal of Nervous and Mental Disease* **192**(5): 363–372.

Gerritsen, A.A., Bramsen, I., Deville, W., van Willigen, L.H., Hovens, J.E., and van der Ploeg, H.M. (2006). Physical and mental health of Afghan, Iranian and Somali asylum seekers and refugees living in the Netherlands. *Social Psychiatry and Psychiatric Epidemiology* **41**(1): 18–26.

Grey, N. and Young, K. (2008). Cognitive behaviour therapy with refugees and asylum seekers experiencing traumatic stress symptoms. *Behavioural and Cognitive Psychotherapy* **36**: 3–19.

Hardy, A., Fowler, D., Freeman, D., et al. (2005). Trauma and hallucinatory experiences in psychosis. *Journal of Nervous and Mental Disease* **193**(8): 501–507.

Hauff, E. and Vaglum, P. (1994). Chronic posttraumatic stress disorder in Vietnamese refugees. A prospective community study of prevalence, course, psychopathology, and stressors. *Journal of Nervous and Mental Disease* **182**(2): 85–90.

Hinton, D.E., Pham, T., Tran, M., Safren, S.A., Otto, M.W., and Pollack, M.H. (2004). CBT for Vietnamese refugees with treatment-resistant PTSD and panic attacks: A pilot study. *Journal of Traumatic Stress* **17**(5): 429–433.

Jaranson, J.M., Butcher, J., Halcon, L., et al. (2004). Somali and Oromo refugees: correlates of torture and trauma history. *American Journal of Public Health* **94**(4): 591–598.

Kinzie, J.D. (1985). Cultural Aspects of Psychiatric Treatment with Indochinese Refugees. *American Journal of Social Psychiatry* **5**(1): 47–53.

Kinzie, J.D. (1986). The establishment of outpatient mental health services for Southeast Asian refugees. In C.L. Williams and J. Westermeyer (Eds.), *Refugee Mental Health in Resettlement Countries*, pp. 217–230. Washington DC: Hemisphere Publishing Corporation.

Kinzie, J.D. (1988). Development, staffing, and structure of psychiatric clinics. In J. Westermeyer, C.L. Williams, and A.N. Nguyen (eds), *Mental Health Services for Refugees*, (DHHS Publication NO. [ADM] 91-1824), pp. 146–156. Washington, D.C.: US Government Printing Office.

Kinzie, J.D. (2001). Psychotherapy for massively traumatized refugees: the therapist variable. *American Journal of Psychotherapy* **55**(4): 475–490.

Kinzie, J.D. (2007). PTSD among traumatized refugees. In L.J. Kirmayer, R. Lemelson, and M. Bard (Eds.), *Understanding Trauma: Integrating Biological, Clinical, and Cultural Perspectives*, pp. 194–206, Cambridge University Press.

Kinzie, J.D. and Manson, S.M. (1983). Five-Years' experience with Indochinese refugee patients. *Journal of Operational Psychiatry* **14**(2): 105–111.

Kinzie, J.D. and Fleck, J. (1987). Psychotherapy with severely traumatized refugees. *American Journal of Psychotherapy* **41**(1): 82–94.

Kinzie, J.D. and Boehnlein, J.K. (1989). Post-traumatic psychosis among Cambodian refugees. *Journal of Traumatic Stress* **2**(2): 185–198.

Kinzie, J.D. and Leung, P. (1989). Clonidine in Cambodian patients with Posttraumatic Stress Disorder. *The Journal of Nervous and Mental Disease* **177**(9): 546–550.

Kinzie, J.D., Tran, K.A., Breckenridge, A., and Bloom, J.D. (1980). An Indochinese refugee psychiatric clinic: Culturally accepted treatment approaches. *The American Journal of Psychiatry* **137**(11): 1429–1432.

Kinzie, J.D., Sack, R.L., and Riley, C.M. (1994). The polysomnographic effects of clonidine on sleep disorders in Posttraumatic Stress Disorder: A pilot study with Cambodian patients. *The Journal of Nervous and Mental Disease* **182**(10): 585–587.

Kinzie, J.D., Leung, P., Boehnlein, J.K., and Fleck, J. (1987). Antidepressant blood levels in Southeast Asians: clinical and cultural implications. *The Journal of Nervous and Mental Disease* **175**(8): 480–485.

Kinzie, J.D., Boehnlein, J.K., Riley, C., and Sparr, L. (2002). The effects of September 11 on traumatized refugees: Reactivation of posttraumatic stress disorder. *The Journal of Nervous and Mental Disease* **190**(7): 437–441.

Kinzie, J.D., Fredrickson, R.H., Ben, R., Fleck, J., and Karls, W. (1984). Posttraumatic stress disorder among survivors of Cambodian concentration camps. *The American Journal of Psychiatry* **141**(5): 645–650.

Kinzie, J.D., Boehnlein, J.K., Leung, P.K., *et al.* (1990). The prevalence of posttraumatic stress disorder and its clinical significance among Southeast Asian refugees. *The American Journal of Psychiatry* **147**(7): 913–917.

Kinzie, J.D., Leung, P., Bui, A., *et al.* (1988). Group therapy with Southeast Asian refugees. *Community Mental Health Journal* **24**(2): 157–166.

Kinzie, J.D., Riley, C., McFarland, B., *et al.* (2008). High prevalence rates of diabetes and hypertension among refugee psychiatric patients. *Journal of Nervous and Mental Disease* **196**(2): 108–112.

Kozarić-Kovacić, D. and Barovecki, A. (2005). Prevalence of psychotic comorbidity in combat-related post-traumatic stress disorder. *Military Medicine* **170**(3): 223–226.

Kroll, J.L. (2007). New directions in the conceptualization of psychotic disorders. *Current Opinion in Psychiatry* **20**(6): 573–577.

Lindley, S.E., Carlson, E., and Sheikh, J. (2000). Psychotic symptoms in posttraumatic stress disorder. *CNS Spectrums* **5**(9): 52–57.

Marshall, G.N., Schell, T.L., Elliott, M.N., Berthold, S.M., and Chun, C-A. (2005). Mental health of Cambodian refugees 2 decades after resettlement in the United States. *Journal of the American Medical Association* **294**(5): 571–579.

Neuner, F., Schauer, M., Klaschik, C., Karunakara, U., and Elbert, T. (2004). A comparison of narrative exposure therapy, supportive counseling, and psychoeducation for treating posttraumatic stress disorder in an African refugee settlement. *Journal of Consulting and Clinical Psychology* **72**(4): 579–587.

Paunovic, N. and Öst, L-G. (2001). Cognitive-behavior therapy vs exposure therapy in the treatment of PTSD in refugees. *Behaviour Research and Therapy* **39**: 1183–1197.

Sareen, J., Cox, B.J., Goodwin, R.D., and J.G. Asmundson, G. (2005). Co-occurrence of posttraumatic stress disorder with positive psychotic symptoms in a nationally representative sample. *Journal of Traumatic Stress* **18**(4): 313–322.

Scott, J., Chant, D., Andrews, G., Martin, G., and McGrath, J. (2007). Association between trauma exposure and delusional experiences in a large community-based sample. *The British Journal of Psychiatry* **190**: 339–343.

Shevlin, M., Houston, J.E., Dorahy, M.J., and Adamson, G. (2008). Cumulative traumas and psychosis: an analysis of the national comorbidity survey and the British Psychiatric Morbidity Survey. *Schizophrenia Bulletin* **34**(1): 193–199.

Silove, D., Sinnerbrink, I., Field, A., Manicavasagar, V., and Steel, Z. (1997). Anxiety, depression and PTSD in asylum-seekers: Associations with pre-migration trauma and post-migration stressors. *British Journal of Psychiatry* **170**: 351–357.

Smajkic, A., Weine, S., Djuric-Bijedic, Boskailo E., Lewis, J., and Pavkovic, I. (2001). Sertraline, Paroxetine, and Venlafaxine in refugee posttraumatic stress disorder with depression symptoms. *Journal of Traumatic Stress* **14**(3): 445–452.

UNHCR (2007). *Global Trends.* Retrieved December 15, 2008, from UNHCR – The UN Refugee Agency: http://www.unhcr.org/statistics/STATISTICS/4852366f2.pdf

Chapter 11

Psychopharmacology for refugees and asylum seekers

Keh-Ming Lin, Tonya Fancher, and
Freda Cheung

Since antiquity and throughout the world, forced migration and immigration due to war, natural catastrophes or man-made disasters have been extremely common.[1] The gravity and long-term health consequences of the traumata typically associated with displacement are well recognized. And efforts to provide care have focused on 'tangible' issues such as safety, shelter, and problems due to malnutrition and infectious diseases.[2–5] Less concerted efforts have been made to address appropriate mental healthcare services[6–10] or psychopharmacotherapeutic support[8,11] despite the fact that refugees suffer from extremely high rates of psychiatric problems[12] and are commonly prescribed psychotropics.[13]

In this chapter, the authors review the promise and challenges of psychopharmacotherapy for refugee patients with an emphasis on the importance of accurate diagnosis, systematic assessment of patients' belief systems, involvement of family and other trusted community members, and careful attention to medication adherence. A brief overview of the rapidly expanding literature on pharmacogenetics/pharmacogenomics and its relevance to refugee populations is also included.[14,15] Since traumata, disaster and forced migration know no geographical and national boundaries, and refugees/asylum seekers come from diverse sociocultural and historical backgrounds, it is not the purpose of this chapter to provide specific information to any particular refugee groups. Instead, it focuses on providing general principles, using data from specific groups only for the purpose of highlighting issues. The chapter concludes with brief summary points for care providers working 'in the trenches' and suggestions for future research.

Treatment begins with assessment/diagnosis

Inaccurate diagnosis can lead to unnecessary or harmful treatment. As is true with other branches of medicine, the formulation of a treatment plan starts with a careful assessment of the patient's clinical condition. The patients' divergent socioculturaland personal backgrounds—as is typically the case with refugee patients[16-18]—further complicate such diagnostic challenges. Clinicians unfamiliar with refugee and cross-cultural patients may be confused or frustrated by their symptom presentation, particularly the use of 'idioms of distress' that often result from differences in the conceptualization of suffering and illnesses. As an example, the prominent use of somatic symptoms to express distress among refugee patients may mislead clinicians accustomed to viewing psychiatric problems largely from a psychological angle.[18-23] Refugees' life experiences—typically imbued with memories of torture, betrayal, separation, and multiple losses, and suffused with a profound sense of anger, shame, and alienation—are not easily shared with clinicians. Further, refugee patients may distrust anyone representing authority. Patients may perceive the gulf between them and care providers as unbridgeable, further aggravating the sense of uncertainty in the therapeutic encounter and risking therapeutic nihilism.

Contrary to the bleak picture depicted earlier, the extant literature demonstrates that contemporary psychiatric theories and practices still are remarkably relevant and useful for patients with divergent refugee experiences and cultural backgrounds, provided that clinicians are willing to reach out and be vigilant of their own limitations.[1,10,24,25] Broadly defined syndromal categories, such as depression, psychosis, and post-traumatic stress disorder (PTSD), can be meaningfully applied in refugee populations and psychotropics (antidepressants, antipsychotics, anti-adrenergics), that ameliorate or attenuate their target symptoms, also work well.[26-28] When used appropriately, psychiatric medications indeed represent very powerful armamentaria that can relieve some of the demoralizing symptoms, improve level of functioning and quality of life, as well as facilitate the process of recovery and re-integration.

PTSD represents the most common and disturbing condition for refugee populations. Although rigorously designed studies have not been conducted with refugee populations, clinical observations and experience indicate that similar approaches could be successfully applied with refugee PTSD patients. Pharmacological interventions that appear useful for such patients include selective serotonin reuptake inhibitors (SSRIs, such as, fluoxetine, paroxetine, sertraline, citalopram) and newer generation antidepressants (e.g. venlafaxine, mirtazapine, bupropion, nefazodone). These treatments appear to be more effective in controlling hyper-arousal symptoms (flashbacks, physiological reactivity, and psychological stress associated with traumatic memories) than the avoidance symptoms or emotional numbing.[26,27,29,30]. Other drugs with some evidence of clinical utility include tricyclic antidepressants, monoamine oxidase inhibitors,[31] anti-adrenergics (clonidine, propranolol),[32,33] atypical antipsychotics, anticonvulsants, and mood stabilizers. Benzodiazepines are commonly prescribed; however, the utility of such agents in the treatment of PTSD remains controversial.[26]

Co-morbidity is highly prevalent but often neglected. Co-morbidity may be conceptually divided into three dimensions: (1) the co-occurrence of multiple psychiatric conditions; (2) the co-occurrence of psychiatric and physical problems; and (3) the co-occurrence of psychiatric disorders and addiction problems. Patients suffering from co-morbid conditions are particularly challenging for at least two reasons: (1) treatment may not be effective unless the co-morbid conditions are taken into consideration and adequately addressed, and (2) co-morbidity typically leads to the prescription of multiple medications whose pharmacological properties may interact, resulting in loss of efficacy or adverse effects. Since most clinical trials and funded research programmes exclude patients with such co-morbidities,[34,35] empirical evidence for the optimal care of these patients is grossly inadequate.

Co-morbidities are likely to be even more prominent among refugee patients. Studies have demonstrated that among refugee patients the co-occurrence of PTSD, depression, anxiety disorders, and sleep disorders is the rule rather than exception.[22,36,37] In the typically prolonged process of escape and resettlement, refugees may experience physical assault, infection, starvation, and grossly inadequate health care. Thus they are likely to have multiple, concurrent physical health problems[37–39] that often confound psychiatric diagnosis (i.e. physical conditions mistaken as psychosomatic problems, and vice versa) and complicate treatment decisions. Co-morbid addictive conditions also represent significant issues among refugee patients.[40–42] Reflecting their cultural backgrounds and level of acculturation, different types of addictive behaviours may assume particular prominence. For example, Southeast Asians may have a lower rate of alcohol abuse and dependence as compared to Western populations,[43] but may be more likely to be victims of compulsive gambling.[44–46] Hmong and others of tribal origin might be more susceptible to opioid abuse and addiction.[47,48] When ignored, these co-morbid problems may also work to confuse assessment and undercut the effects of pharmacotherapy.

Divergence in medication beliefs and the importance of a 'negotiated approach'

A large number of influential works by scholars in the fields of social sciences, medicine, and psychiatry have persuasively demonstrated that, in any given society, the gap in the perspectives, beliefs, and approaches between health professionals, patients, and the general public is not only substantial but also is widening.[49–54] Confronted with such discrepancies, health professionals often assume that the culprit is the 'ignorance' of the patients and the general public, indicating the need for improving our public education and outreach efforts. Although these are indeed important efforts, the exclusive focus on the patients is misleading. What is equally important, if not even more so, is that modern biomedicine has distanced and insulated its practitioners from those they aim to serve. In many ways, one could argue that biomedicine has become a culture in itself, increasingly relying on biological reductionism, focusing predominantly on efficiency and 'technological fix', and its assumptions and value systems have become increasingly at odds with the rest of the society. Buttressed with a whole century of remarkable progress in life science and medicine, and enduring through the long process of learning the creed and trade of medicine or related fields, healthcare professionals have been indoctrinated into over-valuing and over estimating the power of their theories and practices. The process of professionalization also diminishes clinicians' sense of the magnitude of uncertainties inherent in clinical care, which has been and will always be part of clinical decisions. Such an inflated sense of self-assurance further encourages healthcare providers to view alternative explanations as bizarre, backward, and perhaps not worthy of attention, consequently further alienating those they strive to serve.

Divergence in cultural and personal life experiences between professionals and patients further widens such gaps. For example, the concept of depression as a disease may be foreign to most refugee patients,[56,57] the wisdom for long-term medication to maintain therapeutic gain or to prevent relapse may elude them,[58] and medication side effects may serve to reinforce their preconceived beliefs that modern 'Western' pharmaceuticals are indeed too 'strong' for them and are likely to do them more harm than good. Although such suspicions might appear ludicrous at first glance, the concerns may not be unfounded, especially as research demonstrates that iatrogenic hazards are rampant, and medical mistakes rank high as a cause of morbidity and mortality among hospitalized patients.

'Instrumental' and 'symbolic' effects of pharmacological agents

The effects of medications are not just mediated through their 'instrumental' (pharmacological, biological) properties. Although often not the focus of clinicians' attention, 'symbolic' effects ('non-pharmacological', including 'placebo responses') account for much of the therapeutic response, as eloquently demonstrated in practically all randomized controlled trials (RCT), where placebo effects typically account for 30–60% of the improvement.

Intervention methods deemed as 'truly' effective usually add an additional 20% over those therapeutic gains that could be achieved even with substances that were pharmacologically inert.[59] Although sparse, the extant literature demonstrates that patients' beliefs and expectations powerfully determine the magnitude of such symbolic effects. Thus, in addition to striving to 'do no harm', clinicians should also strive to maximize the placebo response.

Cultural formulation as a useful clinical tool

Clinicians who are willing to suspend their perspectives and value judgement stand a better chance of achieving a therapeutic alliance and enhanced adherence.[60–62] In addition, participation in such decision-making processes also is inherently empowering to patients, 'paradoxically' enabling them to become more open to new ideas and perspectives presented by the professionals, even if they might initially appeared 'absurd' or confusing to them.

As part of the Diagnostic and Statistical Manual of Mental Disorders, Version IV (DSM-IV), and discussed extensively in review articles,[51,52,63–66] Cultural Formulation (CF) guidelines represent a useful tool for assisting clinicians to achieve the goals discussed earlier. The CF provides a framework for the systematic exploration of cultural information relevant in clinical encounters, covering issues related to cultural identity, cultural explanations of the individual's illness, cultural factors related to psychosocial environment and levels of functioning, cultural elements of the relationship between the individual and the clinician. Evolving from the concept of 'explanatory model' originally proposed by Kleinman,[53] the CF prompts clinicians to ask specific questions on patients' views about the cause, onset, course, severity, and possible outcomes, as well as their understanding regarding treatment options and their expected effectiveness, both 'indigenous' and 'biomedical'. Done properly, the model should yield crucial information regarding patients' idioms of distress, illness categories meaningful to them, their past experiences in help-seeking, and their expectations regarding current encounters with the healthcare system, including their notion about medications being offered. As expected, the model has been applied to the treatment of major depression in non-Western populations, demonstrating better outcome as compared to treatment as usual.[67]

Concurrent use of 'alternative' medicine and traditional healing methods

The CF model should also provide clinicians with valuable information regarding various 'alternative' healthcare practices available to the patients,[54,68,69] including the use of herbs that often are pharmacologically active and have a high potential of interacting with prescribed medications. The use of alternative treatment methods is widespread in all cultural groups, including those deeply influenced by contemporary Western biomedical traditions. Patients tend to keep this information 'underground' because of fear of ridicule or criticism by their clinicians. Consequently, clinicians vastly underestimate the role of 'alternative' or 'indigenous' practices in patient care, regarding them either as nuisance or outright quackery. Instead, perhaps a more useful approach would be to place modern 'Western' biomedicine, including psychiatry, as a part of the wide range of health and healing traditions and practices that might be available to the patient.[70–77] Rather than assuming that ours are the only show in town, we should present our approaches as viable, perhaps in some ways safer and more effective, alternatives among the full array of treatment and coping options. Again, although such a perspective is important and useful for the care of all patients, it becomes even more crucial when working with patients with cross-cultural and/or refugee backgrounds.

Involvement of the family and other significant member(s) of patients' social network

Modern 'Western' biomedicine also is peculiar in its almost exclusive attention to the individual, and in the extent of its neglect of the involvement and influence of the family as well as the social and communal aspect of health and illnesses. Instead of viewing them as potential allies, family and community members are often regarded as intrusive and burdensome, particularly in cross-cultural settings, where health and illnesses are typically seen as familial and even communal, rather than purely personal problems.[8,78,79]

For refugee groups such as Hmong or others of mountainous/isolated origin, where low literacy is common, and exposure to Western cultures and lifestyles is limited, the involvement of family members and community leaders is even more crucial. Medical information typically filters through community leaders, translators, bilingual workers, and family members who function as cultural brokers. These brokers' roles are bi-directional: their function is not just to convey the opinions and recommendations from professionals to their patients, but even more importantly, to provide cultural information and patients' personal and social realities for care providers. It is thus advantageous to regard these cultural brokers as partners rather than 'auxiliaries', a proposition that is often mentioned but not often realized.

Medication adherence

Even without apparent cultural or linguistic barriers, problems with medication adherence (compliance) are pervasive, (commonly exceeding 50%[80–82]) especially for those suffering from chronic conditions (such as diabetes, hypertension, and asthma) or requiring long-term medications. Clinicians often are blissfully unaware of the extent of their patients' failure in treatment adherence, and consequently miss the opportunity to attempt intervention that might be most pivotal in determining their patients' therapeutic outcome.

A number of factors adversely affect adherence, including medication side effects, complexity of the prescription (e.g. single daily dosing versus multiple dosing; multiple drugs), cognitive capacity of the patient, logistic challenges (e.g. lack of transportation), as well as financial strains.[83] However, as important as they are, their influences pale away when compared to disparities between patients' and clinician's beliefs and expectations.[84–89] Such cognitive dissonance is substantial in any clinical encounter, but often much more prominent and troubling with refugee patients. As discussed in the previous section, the CF model represents a rational and effective tool for bridging communication gaps and achieving therapeutic goals.

Inter-individual and cross-ethnic variations in pharmacological responses

Integral with the attention to 'non-pharmacological' issues discussed earlier, it is equally important for clinicians to be aware of the magnitude of inter-individual as well as cross-ethnic variations in drug responses that are biologically based.[90–93] Contrary to general perception, diversity is the norm rather than exception in pharmacological responses, both in terms of how medications are processed (absorbed, distributed, broken-down, eliminated) in the body (pharmacokinetics), and how they affect biological targets (receptors, transporters, production and elimination of neurotransmitters) (pharmacodynamics). As an example, for the majority of the medicines in common use (such as most neuroleptics and antidepressants), variations in drug blood levels after standard dosing commonly approaches 100 folds in any apparently homogeneous populations. The usual dosing strategies, such as those commonly found in the drug information packages, target only those falling into the mid-range of the distribution, ignoring those falling on either side of the curve. Thus, the process of identifying the 'right' medication and defining the right dose range for any particular patient remains largely accomplished by 'trial and error'. Failure in keeping such response variations in mind represents a major reason for treatment failure and excessive adverse effects.[15]

Superimposed on this already considerable individual variations, ethnic and cultural factors further exert significant impact on both the pharmacokinetic and pharmacodynamics processes, sometimes resulting in major differences in risk–benefit ratios and dosing recommendations across ethnic groups.[91,94–96] Mechanisms responsible for these variations, both via genetic and environmental influences, have been largely elucidated; and they explain both inter-individual and cross-ethnic variations. At the genetic level, genes involved in both pharmacokinetic and pharamcodynamic processes have now been known to be highly polymorphic, meaning that multiple forms of the gene typically exist in most populations, leading to huge variations in drug response. As a prominent example, the drug-metabolizing enzymes CYP2D6 have more than 50 distinct variant alleles, many of which are functionally significant, leading to the production of enzymes with divergent activities, effectively dividing patients into the following four groups: poor metabolizers (PMs, those with two defective genes, leading to the complete absence of CYP2D6), slow metabolizers (SMs, those with one defective gene, or with two variant genes that are less effective in producing the enzyme), extensive metabolizers (EMs, those with two functional 'wild-type' genes) and ultra-rapid metabolizers (UMs, those with more than two copies of the gene, leading to 'excessive' production of the enzyme). Since CYP2D6 participates in the metabolism of close to 50% of the drugs currently on the market, these genotypes phenotypes often lead to major differences in the concentration of the drugs in the body and the brain, remarkable divergence in therapeutic responses, and propensity for side effects.[97–100]

As is true with the majority of the genes that have been studied, CYP2D6 genotypes are highly unevenly distributed across ethnic/racial groups. Although the majority of Caucasians (those of European ancestry) are EMs, a substantial proportion of them (5–9%) are PMs. This bimodal distribution of the enzyme activity is mostly the consequence of a specific allele labeled as CY2D6*4, which is rarely found in non-Caucasians. Instead, the majority (up to 70%) of East Asians carry a distinct allele (CYP2D6*10) that produces a less effective form of the enzyme, putting most of them into the SM category. Caused by yet another specific allele (CYP2D6*17) that is commonly seen only in those of Sub-Saharan African origin (20–40%), African Americans and Black Africans also are more likely to be SMs. UMs are highly prevalent among Ethiopians (29%), Arabs (19%), Ethiopian and Sephardic Jews (18 and 13%), and southern Spaniards (5%), but are relatively rare (less than 1%) in other populations.[101–104]

Superimposed on these remarkable genetically based ethnic/racial variations, the function of many of these genes also is highly responsive to environmental cues.

Thus, within the constraints of the genetic disposition, the production of the enzymes often is modulated by their own substrates (substances metabolized by them) or other chemicals, such that the activities of the enzymes are regulated by substances the organism is exposed to. This is not only the case with manufactured drugs, but also with natural substances present in the diet or medicinal herbs, and often is the basis for drug-drug, nutrient-drug, and herb-drug interactions.[105,106] Dietary practices and the utilization of herbs vary widely across cultural groups, and contribute substantively to group variations in drug responses. For examples, a number of earlier studies showed that, in comparison to their Caucasian counterparts, Sudanese and South Indians residing in their original countries were significantly slower in the metabolism of drugs such as antipyrine and clomipramine (thus requiring lower doses for the same effects). But as they immigrated to Western countries and gradually adapted to the diet of the host society, the metabolism of these drugs speeded up, reaching the level of the Caucasians.[107,108] Two decades later, mechanisms responsible for such variations have been largely elucidated. It turns out that most of such nutrient–drug interactions could be explained by alterations in the expression and activities of some of the key drug metabolizing enzymes, especially CYP3A4 and CYP1A2. CYP3A4 is responsible for the metabolism of many antidepressants, benzodiazepines, antibiotics, and antiviral agents,[109,110] whose production could be turned up or down depending on the kind of substances patients have been exposed to. Dramatic examples of such interactions include the effect of grapefruit juice as an inhibitor, and St. John's wort as an inducer, leading to either toxicity or inadequate dosing when they are taken concurrently with drugs metabolized by CYP3A4.[111–116]

Mediated by alterations in the expression of CYP1A2, another major drug metabolizing enzyme,[112,117,118] the stimulating effect of cigarettes and food such as broccoli and char-broiled meat products on drug metabolism serves as another prominent example for such interactions. Although mechanisms responsible for such interactions[119] make a fascinating story by themselves, what matters clinically is that this enzyme also participates in the metabolism of many commonly used antipsychotics and antidepressants, and the alteration of its expression level, caused by exposure to smoking specific diet, could render previously appropriate drug doses inadequate, again requiring adjustment to maintain their therapeutic effects.

Use of herbal preparations and herb-drug interactions

The use of herbs is central to all healing traditions.[120–122] Most 'Western' medicines, commonly regarded as the opposite of herbs, could actually trace their origin back to botanicals from an earlier era. Opioids (heroine, codeine, hydro-cordone), ephedrine, and St. John's wort are but some of the most prominent examples.[123–125] Contrary to general perceptions and biases (especially among health professionals), most herbs, Western or 'indigenous', have their intrinsic effects, and possess biological properties that may be therapeutic or toxic. Since the use of these traditional formularies or concoctions have been passed down for generations and are deeply entrenched in patients' cultural traditions, attempts to 'educate' patients away from their use are not likely to be successful, often leading instead to resistance, either open or hidden, thereby further diminishing clinician–patient trust and communication.

However, this does not mean that clinicians should totally ignore the existence of herbal use in patient care. Herbs themselves could have intrinsic toxic properties, especially when used inappropriately; they may be adulterated in the process of processing or transportation; they may alter the user's physiological functions, leading to effects such as excessive sedation or anticholinergic responses (dry mouth, palpitation, delirium), especially when taken concurrently with prescribed drugs with similar pharmacological properties. Even more importantly, as is true with other natural substances, herbs are metabolized by the same enzymes as those metabolizing prescribed drugs, and thus often have potent effects on the expression of these enzymes, affecting the concentration and potency of the prescribed drugs, or vise versa. Taking CYP3A4 as the most prominent example, recent studies identified St. John's wort as an extremely potent inducer for the enzyme, and conversely, grapefruit juice and some of the other citrus products profoundly inhibit the enzyme's production. Since many drugs, including trazodone, nefazodone, triazolam, antiviral drugs, and drugs often used for the treatment of HIV are metabolized primarily by CYP3A4, the concurrent use of herbs with such properties would dramatically alter the dosing and side effects of the prescribed drugs, at times leading to dire consequences.[126–128]

The picture painted earlier might appear complicated and complicating, but perhaps the following general principles might help clinicians to deal more effectively with issues involving the concurrent use of herbs: (1) be open and receptive to the use of herbs, inquiring about their use and purported effects; (2) consult with local experts or traditional literature when available, regarding potential toxicity and physiological effects of the herbs utilized. Extensive compilation and codification of such information, in the form of pharmacopoeia, are readily available from major medical traditions, such as traditional Chinese medicine, the Indian Ayuverdic medicine, or those influenced by the Mayan–Aztec traditions; (3) when initiating psychopharmacological therapy, be cognizant of possible herb-drug interactions. Titrate with additional

caution ('start low, go slow'); and, finally, (4) unless the herbs taken are potentially toxic or otherwise counterproductive, advise patients of the potential of
herb-drug interactions, and the importance of avoiding sudden changes (starting, stopping, or altering composition or 'dose') in the use of herbal prepara-
tions in order to minimize the possibility of altering metabolism and action of
the prescribed drugs.

Conclusions and future directions

In this paper, the authors aim at providing clinicians with a framework
that should be useful in conceptualizing their approaches when working with
refugee patients. In such a context, it maybe useful to keep in mind that almost
all of the issues clinicians are confronted with while working with these patients
also are those they need to pay attention to in their routine practices. Clinicians
need to be cognizant of the extent of inter-individual and cross-group variations in treatment responses, with genetic, environmental, personal (life experiences), and sociocultural factors all contributing to such variations. It also is
crucial to be mindful of the divergence between their own and patients' versions of pathoetiology, pathophysiology, and treatment outcomes, and to
regard clinical care as joint, collaborative ventures, with the goals of not only
optimizing medications' instrumental (i.e. pharmacological) effects, but even
more importantly, to maximize medication adherence as well as the symbolic
dimension of the therapeutic effects (i.e. 'placebo response'). For obvious reasons, these challenges become even more salient and crucial in clinical encounters involving those with refugee and/or cross-cultural backgrounds. To be
successful, clinicians need to cultivate the fortitude for tolerating a higher level
of uncertainty inherent in all clinical transactions, to be on the look out for
surprises, and to view ethnic and cultural variations in drug responses as challenges rather than nuisance. Clinicians who are open to these challenges will be
amply rewarded with improved communication, collaboration, and better
treatment responses as well as patient/family satisfaction and gratitude.

General principles aside, many important, practical issues await further
clarification. Ideally, such research efforts should be systematic rather
than piecemeal in nature and should include both qualitative and quantita-
tive methodologies, leading to hypothesis generation as well as hypothesis
testing. Beginning from case reports, descriptions of clinical experiences and
insights, as well as studies based on administrative/claim data, these efforts
should progress to open trials and RCTs, in order to clarify issues such as the
maximization of adherence, nature, and prevalence of the use of herbal prepa-
rations, genetic and environmental determinants of medication responses for
specific refugee groups, and the utility of therapeutic drug monitoring and

pharmacogenetic/pharmacogenomic approaches in the care of such patients. Insights derived from such efforts would lead to new and more effective therapeutic approaches, whose effectiveness should be further examined at the programme level (practice research), along with professional education and information dissemination.[35,129] Cognizant of the fact that, unfortunately, new refugee groups are constantly emerging, and people of refugee and displacement experiences represent a sizable section of all populations, the field needs to ensure that there is continuity in the accumulation of knowledge base, such that experiences and insight gained from works with earlier refugee groups benefit subsequent waves of refugees, so as to minimized the 're-invention of the wheel'. Such goals can only be achieved with the existence of stable and durable infrastructures supporting systematic research efforts in an ongoing manner.

Acknowledgments

The authors thank Ms. Mai See Yang, MS, for her assistance in the preparation of this manuscript.

References

1 Holzman, W, Bornemann, T., (Eds.) (1990). *Mental Health of Immigrants and Refugees.* Austin, Texas: Hogg Foundation for Mental health, University of Texas.

2 Kandula, N., Kersey, M., and Lurie, N. (2004). Assuring the health of immigrants: what the leading health indicators tell us. *Annual Review of Public Health* 25: 357–376.

3 Carlock, D. (2007). Finding information on immigrant and refugee health. *Journal of Transcultural Nursing* 18(4): 373.

4 Ingleby, D. (2005). *Forced Migration and Mental Health: Rethinking the Care of Refugees and Displaced Persons.* New York: Springer.

5 Center for Disease Control and Prevention (CDCP) (2010). Immigrant and Refugee. Retrieved from health. http://www.cdc.gov/immigrantrefugeehealth/index.html.

6 Smith, M., Cartaya, O., Mendoza, R., Lesser, I., and Lin, K. (1998). Conceptual models and psychopharmacological treatment of torture victims. In J. Jaranson and M. Popkin, (Eds.), *Caring for Victims of Torture*, pp. 149–169, Washington, DC: American Psychiatric Press.

7 Lin, K. (1986). Psychopathology and social disruption in refugees. In C. Williams and J. Westermeyer, (Eds.), *Refugees and Mental Health*, pp. 61–73, Washington, DC: Hemisphere Publishing Corporation.

8 Lin, K. and Shen, W. (1991). Pharmacotherapy for southeast Asian psychiatric patients. *Journal of Nervous & Mental Disease* 179(6): 346.

9 Owan, T. (1985). Southeast Asian Mental Health: Treatment, Prevention, Services, Training and Research. Rockville, MD: National Institute of Mental Health.

10 Kinzie, J. (2006). Immigrants and refugees: The psychiatric perspective. *Transcultural Psychiatry* 43(4): 577.

11 Smith, M., Cartaya, O., Mendoza, R., Lesser, I., and Lin, K. M. (1998). Conceptual models and psychopharmacological treatment of torture victims. In J.M. Jaranson and M.K. Popkin (Eds.), *Caring for Victims of Torture*. Washington, D. C., American Psychiatric Press, pp. 149–169.

12 Chung, R.C. and Kagawa-Singer, M. (1993). Predictors of psychological distress among Southeast Asian refugees. *Social Science & Medicine* **36**(5): 631–639.

13 Kinzie, J., Tran, K., Breckenridge, A., and Bloom, J. (1980). An Indochinese refugee psychiatric clinic: Culturally accepted treatment approaches. *American Journal Psychiatry* **137**(11): 1429–1432.

14 Lin, K., Perlis, R., and Wan, Y. (2008). Pharmacogenomic strategy for individualizing antidepressant therapy. *Dialogues in Clinical Neuroscience* **10**(4): 401.

15 Lin, K.M., Chen, C.H., and Chen, C.Y. (2008). Ethnopsychopharmacology. *International Review of Psychiatry* **20**(5): 452–459.

16 Uba, L. (1992). Cultural barriers to health care for Southeast Asian refugees. *Public Health Reports* **107**(5): 544–548.

17 Berthold, S.M., Wong, E.C., Schell, T.L., *et al.* (2007). U.S. Cambodian refugees' use of complementary and alternative medicine for mental health problems. *Psychiatric Services* **58**(9): 1212–1218.

18 Chung, R. and Lin. K. (1994). Helpseeking behavior among Southeast Asian refugees. *Journal of Community Psychology* **22**: 109–120.

19 Gerritsen, A., Bramsen, I., Devillé, W., van Willigen, L., Hovens, J., and van der Ploeg, H. (2004). Health and health care utilisation among asylum seekers and refugees in the Netherlands: Design of a study. *BMC Public Health* **4**(1): 7.

20 Hinton, D. and Hinton, S. (2002). Panic disorder, somatization, and the new cross-cultural psychiatry: The seven bodies of a medical anthropology of panic. *Culture, Medicine and Psychiatry* **26**(2): 155–178.

21 Castillo, R., Waitzkin, H., Ramirez, Y., and Escobar, J. (1995). Somatization in primary care, with a focus on immigrants and refugees. *Archives of Family Medicine* **4**(7): 637.

22 Moore, J.L. and Boehnlein, J. (1991). Posttraumatic stress disorder, depression, and somatic symptoms in U.S. Mien patients. *Journal of Nervous & Mental Disease* **179**: 728–733.

23 Westermeyer, J., Bouafuely, M., Neider, J., and Callies, A. (1989). Somatization among refugees: An epidmiologic study. *Psychosomatics* **30**: 34–43.

24 Mollica, R., Wyshak, G., De Marneffe, D., Khuon, F., and Lavelle, J. (1987). Indochinese Versions of the Hopkins Symptom Checklist-25: A Screening Instrument for the Psychiatric Care of Refugees. American Psychiatric Association, 497–500.

25 Kinzie, J., Fredrickson, R., Ben, R., Fleck, J., and Karls, W. (1984). Posttraumatic stress disorder among survivors of Cambodian concentration campus. *American Journal of Psychiatry* **141**(5): 645–650.

26 Friedman, M. (2002). Future pharmacotherapy for post-traumatic stress disorder: prevention and treatment. *Psychiatric Clinics of North America* **25**(2): 427–441.

27 Stein, D., Ipser, J., and McAnda, N. (2009). Pharmacotherapy of posttraumatic stress disorder: A review of meta-analyses and treatment guidelines. *CNS spectrums* **14**(1 Suppl 1): 25.

28 Friedman, M. (1988). Toward Rational Pharmacotherapy for Posttraumatic Stress Disorder: An Interim Report. American Psychiatric Association, 281–285.

29 Sullivan, G. and Neria Y. (2009). Pharmacotherapy of PTSD: Current status and controversies. *Psychiatric Annals* **39**(6): 342.

30 Smajkic, A., Weine, S., Duric-Bijedic, Z., Boskailo, E., Lewis, J., and Pavkovic, I. (2001). Sertralilne, paroxetine and venlafaxine in refugee post traumatic stress disorder with depression symptoms. *Medicinski Arhiv* **55**: 35–38.

31 DeMartino, R., Mollica, R., and Wilk, V. (1995). Monoamine oxidase inhibitors in posttraumatic stress disorder: Promise and problems in Indochinese survivors of trauma. *Journal of Nervous and Mental Disease* **183**(8): 510.

32 Kinzie, J. and Leung, P. (1989). Clonidine in Cambodian patients with posttraumatic stress disorder. *Journal of Nervous and Mental Disorders* **177**(9): 546–550.

33 Kinzie, J., Sack, R., and Riley, C. (1994). The polysomnographic effects of clondine on sleep disorders in posttraumatic stress disorder: A pilot study with Cambodian patients. *The Journal of Nervous and Mental Disease* **182**(10): 585.

34 Lebowitz, B. and Rudorfer, M. (1998). Treatment research at the millennium: From efficacy to effectiveness. *Journal of Clinical Psychopharmacology* **18**(1): 1.

35 National Institute of Health (NIMH) (1999). Bridging Science and Service: A Report. Rockville, MD: National Institute of Health.

36 Lin, K. (1986). Psychopathology and social disruption in refugees. *Refugee Mental Health in Resettlement Countries* 61–73.

37 Hollifield, M., Warner, T., Lian, N., *et al.* (2002). Measuring trauma and health status in refugees a critical review. *Journal of American Medical Association* **288**(5): 611–621.

38 Ta, K., Westermeyer, J., and Neider, J. (1996). Physical disorders among Southeast Asian refugee outpatients with psychiatric disorders. *Psychiatric Services* **47**(9): 975.

39 Kinzie, J.D., Denney, D., Riley, C., Boehnlein, J., McFarland, B., and Leung, P. (2008). High prevalence rates of diabetes and hypertension among refugee psychiatric patients. *Journal of Nervous and Mental Disease.* **196**(2): 108.

40 Marshall, G., Schell, T., Elliott, M., Berthold, S., and Chun, C. (2005). Mental Health of Cambodian Refugees 2 Decades after Resettlement in the United States. American Medical Association, 571–579.

41 Chang, J., Rhee, S., and Berthold, S. (2008). Child abuse and neglect in Cambodian refugee families: Characteristics and implications for practice. *Child Welfare* **87**(1): 20.

42 Kozarić-Kovačić, D., Ljubin, T., and Grappe, M. (2000). Comorbidity of posttraumatic stress disorder and alcohol dependence in displaced persons. *Croatian Medical Journal* **41**(2): 173–178.

43 D'Amico, E., Schell, T., Marshall, G., and Hambarsoomians, K. (2007). Problem drinking among Cambodian refugees in the United States: How big of a problem is it? *Journal of Studies on Alcohol and Drugs* **68**(1):11.

44 Marshall, G., Elliott, M., and Schell, T. (2009). Prevalence and correlates of lifetime disordered gambling in Cambodian refugees residing in Long Beach, CA. *Journal of Immigrant and Minority Health* **11**(1): 35–40.

45 Petry, N., Armentano, C., Kuoch, T., Norinth, T., and Smith, L. (2003). Gambling participation and problems among South East Asian refugees to the United States. *Psychiatric Services* **54**(8): 1142.

46 Niederland, W. (1984). Compulsive gambling and the 'survivor syndrome'. *American Journal of Psychiatry* **141**(8): 1013.

47 Westermeyer, J., Lyfoung, T., and Neider, J. (1989). An epidemic of opium dependence among Asian refugees in Minnesota: Characteristics and causes. *Addiction* **84**(7): 785–789.

48 Westermeyer, J., Lyfoung, T., Westermeyer, M., and Neider, J. (1991). Opium addiction among Indochinese refugees in the United States: Characteristics of addicts and their opium use. *The American Journal of Drug and Alcohol Abuse* **17**(3): 267–277.

49 Mezzich, J., Kirmayer, L., Kleinman, A., and Fabrega, Jr H. (1999). The place of culture in DSM-IV. *Journal of Nervous & Mental Disease* **187**(8): 457.

50 Lewis-Fernandez, R. (2009). The cultural formulation. *Transcult Psychiatry* **46**: 379–382.

51 Lewis-Fernández, R. and Diaz, N. (2002). The cultural formulation: A method for assessing cultural factors affecting the clinical encounter. *Psychiatric Quarterly* **73**(4): 271–295.

52 Mezzich, J.E. (1995). Cultural formulation and comprehensive diagnosis. Clinical and research perspectives. *Psychiatric Clinics of North America* **18**: 649–657.

53 Kleinman, A. (1978). Clinical Relevance of Anthropological and Cross-Cultural Research: Concepts and Strategies. American Psychiatric Association, 427–431.

54 Kleinman, A. (1980). *Patients and Healers in the Context of Culture. An Exploration of the Borderland Between Anthropology, Medicine and Psychiatry.* Berkeley: University of California Press.

55 Fadiman, A. (1998). *The Spirit Catches You and You Fall Down: A Hmong Child, her American Doctors, and the Collision of Two Cultures.* New York: Farrar, Straus and Giroux.

56 Daley, T. (2005). Beliefs about treatment of mental health problems among Cambodian American children and parents. *Social Science and Medicine* **61**(11): 2384–2395.

57 Kleinman, A. (2004). Culture and depression. *New England Journal of Medicine* **351**: 951–953.

58 Kinzie, J. and Fleck, J. (1987). Psychotherapy with severely traumatized refugees. *American Journal of Psychotherapy* **41**(1): 82–94.

59 Smith, M., Lin, K., and Mendoza, R. (1993). Non-biological issues affecting psychopharmacotherapy: Cultural considerations. *Psychopharmacology and Psychobiology of Ethnicity.* Washington, DC: American Psychiartic Press, pp. 37–58.

60 Weiss, M., Doongaji, D., Siddhartha, S., *et al.* (1992). The Explanatory Model Interview Catalogue (EMIC). Contribution to cross-cultural research methods from a study of leprosy and mental health. *The British Journal of Psychiatry* **160**(6): 819–830.

61 Cruz, M. and Pincus, H. (2002). Research on the influence that communication in psychiatric encounters has on treatment. *Psychiatric Services* **53**(10): 1253.

62 Eisenthal, S., Emery, R., Lazare, A., and Udin, H. (1979). 'Adherence' and the negotiated approach to patienthood. *Archives of General Psychiatry* **36**(4): 393.

63 Lim, R. (2006). *Clinical Manual of Cultural Psychiatry.* Washington, DC: American Psychiatric Pub, Inc.

64 Kirmayer, L., Groleau, D., Guzder, J., Blake, C., and Jarvis, E. (2003). Cultural consultation: a model of mental health service for multicultural societies. *Canadian Journal of Psychiatry* **48**(3): 145–153.

65 Kirmayer, L., Thombs, B., Jurcik, T., Jarvis, G, and Guzder, J. (2008). Use of an expanded version of the DSM-IV outline for cultural formulation on a cultural consultation service. *Psychiatric Services* **59**(6): 683.

66 Lu, F.G. (2006). DSM-IV outline for cultural formulation: Bringing culture into the clinical encounter. *Focus* **4**(1): 9–10.

67 Yeung, A., Chang, D., Gresham, Jr R., Nierenberg, A., and Fava, M. (2004). Illness beliefs of depressed Chinese American patients in primary care. *Journal of Nervous and Mental Disease* **192**(4): 324.

68 Lewis-Fernandez, R. and Kleinman, A. (1995). Cultural psychiatry: theoretical, clinical, and research issues. *The Psychiatric Clinics of North America* **18**(3): 433–448.

69 Lin, K., Demonteverde, L., and Nuccio, I. (1990). Religion, healing and mental health among Filipino–Americans. *International Journal of Mental Health* **19**(3): 40–44.

70 Pickwell, S. (1999). Multilevel healing pursuits of Cambodian refugees. *Journal of Immigrant Health* **1**(3): 165–179.

71 Kirmayer, L. and Minas, H. (2000). The future of cultural psychiatry: An international perspective. *Canadian Journal of Psychiatry* **45**(5): 438–446.

72 Levin, N. and Levin, D. (1982). A folk medical practice mimicking child abuse. *Hospital Practice (Office ed.)* **17**(7): 17.

73 Phan, T. (2000). Investigating the use of services for Vietnamese with mental illness. *Journal of Community Health* **25**(5): 411–425.

74 Feldman, K. (1984). Pseudoabusive burns in Asian refugees. *Archives of Pediatrics and Adolescent Medicine* **138**(8): 768–769.

75 Tseng, W. and McDermott, Jr J. (1981). Minor psychiatric disorder. *Culture, Mind, and Therapy: Introduction to Cultural Psychiatry*. New York: Brunner/Mazel.

76 Leslie, C. (1976). *Asian Medical Systems*. Berkeley: University of California Press.

77 Hinton, L. and Kleinman, A. (1995). An agenda for research. In R. Desjarlais, L. Eisenberg, B. Good, and A. Kleinman, (Eds.), *World Mental Health: Problems and Priorities in Low Income Countries*. New York: Oxford University Press.

78 Gordon, H., Paterniti, D., and Wray, N. (2004). Race and patient refusal of invasive cardiac procedures. *Journal of General Internal Medicine* **19**(9): 962–966.

79 Lefley, H. (1998). Families, culture, and mental illness: constructing new realities. *Psychiatry* **61**(4): 335.

80 Julius, R., Novitsky, Jr M., and Dubin, W. (2009). Medication adherence: a review of the literature and implications for clinical practice. *Journal of Psychiatric Practice* **15**(1): 34.

81 Mitchell, A. (2007). Adherence behaviour with psychotropic medication is a form of self-medication. *Medical Hypotheses* **68**(1): 12–21.

82 WHO. (2003). Adherence to long term therapies: evidence for action. http://www.who.int/chronic_conditions/adherencereport/en/.

83 Sackett, D.L., Haynes, R.B., Gibson, E.S., Hackett, B.C., Taylor, D.W., and Roberts, R.S. (1975). Randomised clinical trials of strategies for improving medication compliance in primary hypertension. *Lancet* **7918**: 1205–1207.

84 Sue, S. (1977). Community mental health services to minority groups: some optimism, some pessimism. *American Psychologist* **32**: 616–624.

85 Sue, S., Fujino, D.C., Hu, L.T., Takeuchi, D.T., and Zane, N.W. (1991). Community mental health services for ethnic minority groups: A test of the cultural responsiveness hypothesis. *Journal of Consulting and Clinical Psychology* **59**(4): 533–540.

86 Zane, N.W.S., Enomoto, K., and Chun, C. (1994). Treatment outcomes of Asian and White American clients in outpatient therapy. *Journal of Community Psychology* **22**: 177–191.

87 Kinzie, J.D., Leung, P., Boehnlein, J.K., and Fleck, J. (1987). Antidepressant blood levels in Southeast Asians. Clinical and cultural implications. *Journal of Nervous and Mental Disorders* **175**(8): 480–485.

88 Kroll, J., Habenicht, M., Mackenzie, T., *et al.* (1989). Depression and posttraumatic stress disorder in Southeast Asian refugees. *American Journal of Psychiatry* **146**(12): 1592–1597.

89 Kroll, J., Linde, P., Habenicht, M., *et al.* (1990). Medication compliance, antidepressant blood levels, and side effects in Southeast Asian patients. Journal of Clinical Psychopharmacology **10**(4): 279–283.

90 Kalow, W., Ozdemir, V., Tang, B., Tothfalusi, L., and Endrenyi, L. (1999). The science of pharmacological variability: an essay. *Clinical Pharmacology and Therapeutics* **66**(5): 445–447.

91 Chen, C., Chen, C., and Lin, K. (2008). Ethnopsychopharmacology. International Review of Psychiatry (Abingdon, England) **20**(5): 452.

92 Darmansjah, I. and Muchtar, A. (1992). Dose-response variation among different populations. *Clinical Pharmacology and Therapeutics* **52**(5): 449–452.

93 Lin, K., Poland, R., and Anderson, D. (1995). Psychopharmacology, ethnicity and culture. *Transcultural Psychiatry Research Review* **32**: 1–40.

94 Lin, K., Poland, R., and Nakasaki, G. (1993). *Psychopharmacology and Psychobiology of Ethnicity.* Washington DC: American Psychiatric Publications Inc.

95 Lin, K. and Smith, M. (2000). Psychopharmacotherapy in the context of culture & ethnicity. In P. Ruiz (Ed.), *Ethnicity and Psychopharmacology.* Vol. 13, pp. 1–36, Washington, DC: American Psychiatric Association.

96 Temple, R. and Stockbridge, N. (2007). BiDil for heart failure in black patients: The US Food and Drug Administration perspective. *Annals of Internal Medicine* **146**(1): 57.

97 Ingelman-Sundberg, M. (2004). Pharmacogenetics of cytochrome P450 and its applications in drug therapy: the past, present and future. *Trends in Pharmacological Sciences* **25**(4): 193–200.

98 Mendoza, R., Wan, Y., Poland, R., Smith, M., and Lin, K.M. (2001). CYP2D6 polymorphism in a Mexican American population. *Clinical Pharmacology and Therapeutics* **70**(6): 552–560.

99 Wan, Y., Poland, R., Han, G., Konishi, T., Zheng, Y.P., and Lin, K.M. (2001). Analysis of the CYP2D6 gene polymorphism and enzyme activity in African–Americans in southern California. *Pharmacogenetics and Genomics* **11**(6): 489.

100 Luo, H. and Wan, Y. (2006). Polymorphisms of genes encoding phase I enzymes in Mexican Americans – an ethnic comparison study. *Current Pharmacogenomics* **4**(4): 345–353.

101 Lundqvist, E., Johansson, I., and Ingelman-Sundberg, M. (1999). Genetic mechanisms for duplication and multiduplication of the human CYP2D6 gene and methods for detection of duplicated CYP2D6 genes. *Gene* **226**(2): 327–338.

102 Luo, H., Aloumanis, V., Lin, K., Gurwitz, D., and Wan, Y. (2004). Polymorphisms of CYP2C19 and CYP2D6 in Israeli ethnic groups. *American Journal of PharmacoGenomics* **4**(6): 395.

103 Akullu, E., Persson, I., Bertilsson, L., Johansson, I., Rodrigues, F., and Ingelman-Sundberg, M. (1996). Frequent distribution of ultrarapid metabolizers of debrisoquine in an Ethiopian population carrying duplicated and multiduplicated functional CYP2D6 alleles. *Journal of Pharmacology and Experimental Therapeutics* **278**(1): 441–446.

104 Dahl, M., Yue, Q., Roh, H., *et al.* (1995). Genetic analysis of the CYP2D locus in relation to debrisoquine hydroxylation capacity in Korean, Japanese and Chinese subjects. *Pharmacogenetics* **5**(3): 159.

105 Anderson, K. and Kappas, A. (1991). Dietary regulation of cytochrome P450. *Annual Review of Nutrition* **11**(1): 141–167.

106 Sorensen, J. (2002). Herb–drug, food–drug, nutrient–drug, and drug–drug interactions: mechanisms involved and their medical implications. *The Journal of Alternative and Complementary Medicine* **8**(3): 293–308.

107 Branch, R., Salih, S., and Homeida, M. (1978). Racial differences in drug metabolizing ability: a study with antipyrine in the Sudan. *Clinical Pharmacology and Therapeutics* **24**(3): 283.

108 Lewis, P., Rack, P., Vaddadi, K., and Allen, J. (1980). Ethnic differences in drug response. *Postgraduate Medical Journal* **56**: 46.

109 Spina, E., Santoro, V., and D'Arrigo, C. (2008). Clinically relevant pharmacokinetic drug interactions with second-generation antidepressants: an update. *Clinical Therapeutics* **30**(7): 1206–1227.

110 Zanger, U., Turpeinen, M., Klein, K., and Schwab, M. (2008). Functional pharmacogenetics/genomics of human cytochromes P450 involved in drug biotransformation. *Analytical and Bioanalytical Chemistry* **392**(6): 1093–1108.

111 Elewski, B. and Tavakkol, A. (2005). Safety and tolerability of oral antifungal agents in the treatment of fungal nail disease: a proven reality. *Therapeutics and Clinical Risk Management* **1**(4): 299.

112 Simard, C., O'Hara, G., Prévost, J., Guilbaud, R., Massé, R., and Turgeon, J. (2001). Study of the drug–drug interaction between simvastatin and cisapride in man. *European Journal of Clinical Pharmacology* **57**(3): 229–234.

113 Synold, T., Dussault, I., and Forman, B. (2001). The orphan nuclear receptor SXR coordinately regulates drug metabolism and efflux. *Nature Medicine* **7**(5): 584–590.

114 Pal, D. and Mitra, A. (2006). MDR- and CYP3A4-mediated drug–herbal interactions. *Life Sciences* **78**(18): 2131–2145.

115 Blumberg, B. and Evans, R. (1998). Orphan nuclear receptors – new ligands and new possibilities. *Genes and Development* 3149–3155.

116 Fuhr, U. (2000). Induction of drug metabolising enzymes: pharmacokinetic and toxicological consequences in humans. *Clinical Pharmacokinetics* **38**(6): 493.

117 Kroon, L. (2007). Drug interactions with smoking. *American Journal of Health-System Pharmacy* **64**(18): 1917.

118 Faber, M., Jetter, A., and Fuhr, U. (2005). Assessment of CYP1A2 activity in clinical practice: why, how, and when? *Basic and Clinical Pharmacology and Toxicology* **97**(3): 125–134.

119 Nebert, D., Roe, A., Dieter, M., Solis, W., Yang, Y., and Dalton, T. (2000). Role of the aromatic hydrocarbon receptor and [Ah] gene battery in the oxidative stress response, cell cycle control, and apoptosis. *Biochemical Pharmacology* **59**(1): 65–85.

120 Steiner, R. (1986). *Folk Medicine in the Art and the Science*. York, PA: Maple Press Company.

121 WHO. (1999). *WHO Monographs on Selected Medicinal Plants*. Geneva: WHO Press.

122 Spinella, M. (2001). *The Pharmacology of Herbal Medicine*. Cambridge, MA: The MIT Press.

123 Eisenberg, D., Davis, R., Ettner, S., *et al.* (1998). Trends in Alternative Medicine Use in the United States, 1990–1997 Results of a Follow-Up National Survey. *JAMA*, **280**(18): 1569–1575.

124 Ernst, E., De Smet, P., Shaw, D., and Murray, V. (1998). Traditional remedies and the 'test of time'. *European Journal of Clinical Pharmacology* **54**(2): 99–100.

125 Yager, J., Siegfreid, S., and DiMatteo, T. (1999). Use of Alternative Remedies by Psychiatric Patients: Illustrative Vignettes and a Discussion of the Issues. *American Psychiatric Association*, 1432–1438.

126 Wang, Z., Gorski, J., Hamman, M., Huang, S., Lesko, L., and Hall, S. (2001). The effects of St John's wort (Hypericum perforatum) on human cytochrome P450 activity. *Clinical Pharmacology and Therapeutics* **70**(4): 317–326.

127 Ishihara, K., Kushida, H., Yuzurihara, M., *et al.* (2000). Interaction of drugs and Chinese herbs: pharmacokinetic changes of tolbutamide and diazepam caused by extract of Angelica dahurica. *The Journal of Pharmacy and Pharmacology* **52**(8): 1023.

128 Guo, L., Taniguchi, M., Xiao, Y., Baba, K., Ohta, T., and Yamazoe, Y. (2000). Inhibitory effect of natural furanocoumarins on human microsomal cytochrome P450 3A activity. *The Japanese Journal of Pharmacology* **82**(2): 122–129.

129 NIH (2009). National Center for Complementary and Alternative Medicine (NCCAM).

Chapter 12

Psychotherapy and refugees

Russell F. Lim and Alan K. Koike

Introduction

Case study one

ML is a 50-year-old Hmong woman, who states that she 'thinks too much'. She came to the United States in 1982, after five years in a refugee camp in Thailand. She was born in Laos and fled to the jungles of Laos with her family in 1975 after the United States military pulled out of Southeast Asia. She witnessed both of her parents and a brother killed in the jungle by communist Lao soldiers. She complains of headaches, weakness, and whole body pain. She is reluctant to engage in psychotherapy and states 'I will cry if I think about the past. I do not want to talk about it'.

Estimates of the number of refugees worldwide vary from 14.9 million refugees, and 22 million internally displaced persons in 2002, as reported by the United States Committee for Refugees (NCPTSD, 2008), to 11.4 million refugees worldwide by the end of 2007 as stated by United Nations High Commissioner on Refugees (UNHC, 2008). Studies have found high rates of exposure to violence and other pre-migration traumas in refugee populations (Marshall *et al.*, 2005) such as starvation (67%), torture (37%), rape, feeling near death (37–62%), and witnessing the killing of friends and family members (35%) (NCPTSD, 2008). In addition, refugees often experience post-migration stressors such as loss, acculturation problems, racism, and poverty. The subsequent effects of such traumas include high rates of mental illness, especially post-traumatic stress disorder (PTSD) (4–86%) and major depressive disorder (MDD) (5–31%) (Marshall *et al.*, 2005; NCPTSD, 2008).

The American Psychiatric Association (APA) Practice Guidelines for the Treatment of Patients with Acute Stress Disorder and post-traumatic stress disorder (APA, 2004) recommends cognitive behavioral therapy (CBT) as an effective treatment for acute and chronic PTSD. Eye movement desensitization and reprocessing (EMDR) are also considered effective. Stress inoculation, imagery rehearsal, and prolonged exposure techniques may also be indicated for treatment of PTSD, particularly for symptoms such as anxiety and avoidance.

Psychodynamic psychotherapy may be useful in addressing developmental and interpersonal issues as they are related to PTSD (APA, 2004). Unfortunately, little research has been done on the use of these therapies in refugee populations.

The prospect of doing psychotherapy with refugees and survivors of torture often seems like a daunting task, with little empirical evidence to guide the therapist. Refugees often present with severe symptoms from multiple horrific traumas. The concept of complex PTSD has often been associated with refugees and includes the view of oneself as helpless and damaged, difficulties with trust and relationships, alteration in affect regulation, dissociation, and somatization (Herman, 1997). Added challenges to psychotherapy include cultural and linguistic barriers, the instability of their current living situations, and poverty. Therapists attempting psychotherapy with the refugee population must not make the assumption that Western-based models of psychotherapy will be appropriate without modifications, since the clients often will not share the same beliefs, values, and customs as the therapists. In this chapter, we will review selected literature on psychotherapy in various refugee populations so that therapists may have some guidance on how best to modify their approaches to provide culturally appropriate and effective psychotherapy to their refugee clients.

Useful frameworks for assessment and treatment

Blackwell (2005) wrote about an approach to counseling that begins with an assessment of the refugee, and continues through the political, cultural, interpersonal, and intra-psychic levels, and also involves the therapist going through these same four levels for themselves.

Refugees

We will begin our discussion of refugees with a question: Who becomes a refugee? These unfortunate individuals are usually the losers of a political conflict, and have no home to return to since they are *persona non grata* in their homeland. As mentioned previously, they experience many losses and traumas, and often have PTSD and MDD. Therefore, the reason for their flight from their home is a part and parcel of their identity, and even though therapists may be reluctant to ask the client to talk about his or her political history, it is an essential part of the old and new identity of the refugee. Clinicians should also feel free to seek cultural consultation, or gain more background information about the patient's culture and history to augment the assessment interview.

From a structural point of view, the use of a migration history, as described by Lee (1990), can be helpful in organizing a refugee's history. Eliciting a

Table 12.1 Migration history

Pre-migration history
Country of origin, family, education, socioeconomic status, community and family support, political issues, war, trauma
Experience of migration
Migrant versus refugee—Why did they leave? Who was left behind? Who paid for their trip? Means of escape, trauma
Degree of loss
Loss of family members, relatives, and friends
Material losses: business, careers, properties
Loss of cultural milieu, community, religious, and spiritual support
Traumatic experience
Physical—Torture, rape, starvation, imprisonment
Psychological—Rage, depression, guilt, grief, post-traumatic stress disorder.
Work and financial history
Original line of work, current occupation, socioeconomic status
Support systems
Community support, religion, family
Medical history
Beliefs in herbal medicine, somatic complaints
The family's concept of illness
What do family members think the problem is? Its cause? What do they do for help? What result is expected?
Level of acculturation
First or second generation
Impact on development
Level of adjustment, assess developmental tasks

Source: Adapted from Lee, 1990.

migration history is often crucial (see Table 12.1) to understanding the client's experience, as well as developing rapport. Elements of the migration history that should be obtained include the refugee's life before migration, reason for migration, time spent in transit, and losses and trauma associated with migration, as well as traumatic events before, during, and after migration, also known as the pre-migration, transition, and post-migration periods.

Most of the research on refugee mental health has focused on past traumas and their sequelae. However, Goodkind (2005) argues that high levels of distress among refugees are often caused by daily stressors they face in exile situations. These include their marginal position and relative powerlessness in their new surroundings, poverty, loss of community and social support, and loss of status and meaningful social roles. These factors need to be considered when doing therapy with refugees.

Therapists need to ask how the client sees their role in their home country in the past, and in the present, in the context of the political conflict in their homeland. Have they been political activists? Does this cause the patient shame by having put their family members at risk? Were they betrayed by their own people? Will they continue to be activists in exile? How do they feel about their new home and government? The legacy of colonialism can be positive, in which case they may idealize the colonist nation, or negative, if the colonizer has been oppressive, and the client and their families can be disillusioned to find themselves a member of the underclass.

At the cultural level, the refugee's cultural transition is never finished. The client has to leave their old and familiar culture, and join another new and unfamiliar one. Cultural imperialism, or forcing individuals not from a culture to behave as if they are from that culture is similar to a category fallacy, a term Arthur Kleinman (1977) created to describe how patients from different backgrounds are forced to fit into the host culture's diagnostic schema. Having some knowledge about the patient's culture is helpful, but not sufficient, as cultures are not static, and conflicts are common, and values are learned from other cultures; in addition, there are sub-cultures, and the client maintains relationships with other cultures. Old cultures are idealized, and held onto as a place of safety. Gender and age roles change from the Old World into the new, creating more conflicts between the generations in a refugee family.

At the interpersonal level, refugees can feel cut off from their support systems, and the communities that formerly gave them strength. Refugees have many losses and forced separations, which can lead to incomplete grieving, possibly due to the inability to perform a necessary burial ritual, and experience much guilt for having left loved ones behind, and in the current political situation in their homeland, their safety would be jeopardized by communication with them. Another common feeling is regret, for things not done or said. Refugees are transformed by torture, as they no longer see the world as a safe place. Their relationships are affected by conflicts of loyalty, and the consequences of actions or inactions. Women and children especially feel torn between two cultures due to changes in their roles secondary to the loss of the father or inability to speak the host countries' language. In this context, the therapist can become a safe witness and confidant.

At the intra-psychic level, refugees may have lost their humanity and their individuality. A common reaction is psychic numbing, followed by fragmentation. They have a need to remember, and a wish to forget. The past is so horrible, that it must be released in small portions to come to terms with it, without overwhelming the patient and resulting in the loss of the present. A common reaction is regression and withdrawal. The patient fluctuates between victim and survivor, the first unable to do simple things, the second is capable and resilient, and in truth they will always be both, just as they have to live in two cultures. Survivor guilt is common, and in some cases warranted as compromises and confessions may have been made. Anger and rage are also common, as the ability to regulate one's emotions has been broken down. However, recognizing feelings of revenge and violence remind the patient of the persecutor, and being like the abuser is very threatening to the patient. The experience of shame and failure is a common reaction as they were not able to protect themselves against the trauma, which contradicts their necessary belief of control over their ability to maintain their own safety.

Therapists

As for the therapist, they will have to undergo some important self assessment, starting with their basic attributes. Where is the therapist from, and what country are they doing their work in? The patient will have their own ideas about the therapist's politics, and the therapist has their own ideas about their politics and their host country, as well, since political neutrality is impossible. The therapist needs to ask the patient about their political history, since they are the expert in this area.

Therapists tend to be unaware of their own cultures, not being aware that there are 'universal ideas' that they took to be 'universal'. As it is impossible to be both a therapist and an anthropologist, the therapist needs to be aware of the role of culture in their own lives. The therapist must be able to work in the middle of the spectrum between true cultural sensitivity to imperialism and universality, and to take on the challenge of truly understanding another's experience in their's and in the therapist's context. Thus, the Western ideal of therapeutic neutrality is almost impossible, as therapists all have a gender, a cultural identity, a set of moral beliefs, and a preference for a mode of therapy, and an agency that the therapist works for, with its own culture and mission.

On an interpersonal level, many therapists are unprepared for the intensity of the encounter between the patient and the therapist. The client may show extreme neediness or idealization, in the context of relating stories and feelings of horror and suffering. Clients may direct rage towards therapists that could not be directed towards their persecutors, or they may be meet with resentment towards their level of achievement. Therapists may feel helpless to meet all of the clients' needs. There may be conflicts with the agency and its goals for patients. Piwowarczyk (2005) argues that the therapist needs to be aware of the spiritual aspects of their work with refugees. Working with victims of torture, in particular, forces the therapist to face their own existential beliefs about the concepts of good and evil. By bearing witness to man's cruelty to his fellow man, the therapist empowers the torture victim and begins the healing process. Piwowarczyk argues that for some trauma survivors, spiritual understanding is the only path to recovery.

Intra-psychically, therapists must be aware of counter-transference towards the patient and possible boundary violations. They may also feel that they are beyond racism, but must remain vigilant for any possible stereotypes, preconceptions, and prejudices. Being aware of one's own defenses is the key to recognizing and avoiding tricky situations in the therapeutic relationship. Therapists also need to care for themselves while doing trauma psychotherapy and need to watch out for burn out and vicarious traumatization (see Chapter 19 in this volume).

Kinzie (2001) also stated that there are four therapist variables that will enhance the therapist's success with refugees that have experienced trauma: the ability to listen, to stay, to receive, and to believe. Refugees have a need to tell their stories, and effective therapists listen and are present without interrupting, distancing with a question, over-identifying, or giving premature support. The therapist needs to be a constant object that stays with the refugee during difficult times of symptom re-activation. Refugees often need to give gifts to show their gratitude for the therapist's help, and the therapist should feel comfortable accepting small gifts of food or other small items graciously and genuinely, and not refuse out of the Western taboo of not receiving gifts from clients. Finally, the therapist has to believe not only that the evil of which the client speaks is possible, but they must also believe that healing is still possible.

Treatment strategies

There have been many treatment strategies discussed in the literature, from multi-level psychotherapy, CBT, EMDR, narrative therapy, testimony therapy, dance therapy, group therapy, and trans-cultural models, among others. We will review some salient examples to help guide the therapist seeing refugees in choosing a psychotherapy modality.

As mentioned previously, therapists need to be culturally sensitive, to understand the patient's worldview and sociopolitical background, to assess their pre-migration history, the patient's identification with their culture of origin, and to demonstrate cultural empathy which is *not* equivalent to Western empathy. This requires that the therapist must complete a self-assessment and increase their awareness of the effect of their ethnicity to the client. Therapists must be able to tolerate hearing stories of great sadness and savage cruelty. Indeed, therapists need to be aware that not all Western methods will work on refugees, such as reconstruction, or re-experiencing the trauma.

Kinzie and Fleck (1987) described eight essential components to successful psychotherapeutic interactions with refugees, and they include: 1) creating a non-threatening environment; 2) having an awareness of avoidance as a defense against PTSD; 3) expecting a flood of emotions as numbing is worked through; 4) having a long-term relationship with the client; 5) focusing on sleep disorders and mood symptoms; 6) watching for present-day triggers for re-experiencing trauma; 7) using community supports to help patients with day-to-day stresses; and not being afraid to use religious, cultural, or spiritual support; and 8) realizing that sometimes the existential approach is the best, and the therapist should simply be there and available for the client.

The multilevel model of psychotherapy was described by Bemak, Chung, and Pederson (2003), and consists of four phases: 1) mental health education; 2) individual, group, and/or family psychotherapy; 3) cultural empowerment; and 4) indigenous healing. Level one involves educating clients about mainstream mental health practices, establishing the therapeutic relationship, discussing the cultural beliefs and values of the client, setting the frame, time boundaries, and expectations of the use of medications.

The second level is applying Western techniques, such as individual, group, and family therapy that are individualized for that patient's cultural background. The therapy can be more directive and active than normally seen with Westernized patients. CBT and dream work are examples of psychotherapy that are compatible with Buddhist and Latino cultures. For children, they suggest storytelling and projective drawing. Since many refugees come from collectivist cultures, their recommendation is to use family therapy and group therapy. Group therapy relies on three of Yalom's therapeutic factors: universality, altruism, and corrective emotional experiences (2005). The therapist must also use culturally relative diagnoses, using concepts and ideas familiar to the patient, such as culture bound syndromes, when appropriate.

Level three involves creating a sense of cultural and environmental mastery. Therapists can adopt a social advocacy role in family reunification, welfare benefits, social services, financial support, and housing. They can also help to teach clients to deal with racism. The fourth level involves the integration of Western methods with indigenous ones. The therapist can engage the comunity, including monks, priests, community leaders, such as elders, shamans, or indigenous healers. These healers use a variety of methods, including physical treatments, such as cupping, coining, and acupuncture, magic healing methods, such as animal sacrifice and other rituals, and medications, such as herbs, soups, oils, or teas, and counseling.

Hinton and Otto (2006) described using a culturally modified, somatically focused cognitive–behavioral therapy (CBT) approach with traumatized Cambodian refugees. They noted that the DSM IV-TR (Diagnostic and

Statistical Manual, Fourth Edition, Text Revision) (APA, 2000) criteria for PTSD may not represent the symptoms seen in response to trauma across cultures. They emphasized the need to focus on somatic symptoms when treating traumatized refugees, and suggested that careful attention be paid to anger and survival guilt. They discouraged the use of abstract questions, or questions about flashbacks, and believed that patients often will not talk about their trauma experiences. The authors believe that trauma-related memories are connected to a wide range of physical sensations. In the initial evaluation, the clinician should pay attention to somatic complaints and determine how the sensations are induced. In treatment, the clinician should identify the sequences that generate symptoms, teach methods of somatic relaxation, have the patient give a narrative to the somatic flashback, elicit and modify somatic symptoms, explore culturally relevant metaphors for symptoms, perform exposure to somatic sensations, and re-associate positive affect and memory to somatic sensations. The authors compared the combination of sertraline and CBT to sertraline alone for ten Cambodian refugee women with PTSD and found the combined treatment with CBT resulted in significant reduction in PTSD and associated symptoms (Otto, 2003). This same research group then adapted this CBT technique with Vietnamese refugees (Hinton *et al.*, 2006). They describe a culturally sensitive treatment for PTSD with headache and dizziness-focused panic attacks.

Schulz, Huber, and Resick (2006) commented on the cultural issues that influence mental health service delivery for refugees. They reported that the War Trauma Recovery Project, Inc. of St. Louis, Missouri, used cognitive processing therapy (CPT) in the treatment of Bosnian refugees with PTSD. Although most clinicians in the United States provide psychotherapy in English, most refugees come to the United States not speaking English. In this project, they preferred to use an interpreting method in which the interpreter would translate several phrases at a time using the third person. They do not find it helpful for the interpreter to play the role of cultural broker. In their work with Bosnian refugees, the authors found that bereavement was almost universal. Many clients experienced physical symptoms, in addition to severe emotional distress when discussing war traumas. They noticed a different emotional expression among Bosnian clients compared to other refugee groups. Many Bosnians reported a 'choking sensation' during PTSD experiencing events. They responded well to behavioral interventions, such as relaxation techniques and the improvement of self-care such as better nutrition. The authors modified CPT to include behavior strategies that targeted emotion tolerance and anxiety reduction such as relaxation breathing and other relaxation techniques at the beginning of therapy. They then addressed environmental factors, analyzing and challenging schemas. Finally, they had clients face the trauma experiences through exposure work. Although CPT has a 12-session protocol, this group averaged 17 sessions lasting from one to two hours. The authors felt that Bosnian refugees responded well to cognitive therapy. Exposure therapy was also felt to be an important component of their treatment, but it was almost always delayed until the latter part of treatment. The creation of an environment of trust and safety is essential to the success of the therapy. They felt that the approach had to be tailored to each individual client and could not be manualized. The article did not describe the training of the therapists, so it is unclear how well they understood the cultural nuances of the therapy, but they did adapt it to the Bosnian patients by lengthening the course of psychotherapy.

Ilic (2004) described the successful use of EMDR in a case example of a 47-year-old Croatian man, who was a refugee in Serbia. According to the author, the Centre for Rehabilitation of Torture Victims in Belgrade has used EMDR in treating over 160 clients with PTSD. Ilic points out that success depended on client motivation, with secondary gain and acceptance of the victim's role being the main obstacles to improvement.

Bower and his colleagues (2004) also described a case of successful treatment with EMDR at the Florida Center for Survivors of Torture. This case was of a 44-year-old Bosnian woman living in the United States, who suffered severe depression, PTSD, and general anxiety symptoms. As part of her torture, the woman was raped multiple times by soldiers, and during one episode, the soldiers tattooed their names all over her body. This particular client received case management; laser surgery for tattoo removal, antidepressant medication, traditional talk therapy, and CBT, but it was not until she had EMDR therapy that she reported a significant reduction in PTSD symptoms. The authors stated that it was a combination of antidepressant medications, traditional talk, and EMDR therapies that provided a holistic approach that resulted in the reduction of her PTSD and depressive symptoms.

Clinicians at the International Rehabilitation a Research Centre for Torture Victims in Copenhagen were among the first to describe psychotherapy in their work with South American refugees from Chile, Argentina, and Uruguay. This model emphasized the need to explore memories of torture. Patients were encouraged to reveal as much detail as possible about their traumatic experiences. In doing so, patients began to understand the 'impossible choices' they faced as victims of torture, and how the guilt and responsibility for the trauma must fall on their torturers. The psychotherapy was intensive, one and a half hour long sessions, often twice a week. Ortmann and his colleagues (1987) reported that 90% of 38 patients treated at the centre had substantially improved or recovered after treatment ranging from a few weeks to eighteen months.

Onyut and colleagues (2005) reported on the use of Narrative Exposure Therapy (NET) in the treatment in six Somali children suffering from PTSD. The children were aged 12–17 years, and located in a refugee settlement in Uganda. They were treated with 4 to 6 individual sessions by expert clinicians. NET was developed for the treatment of PTSD as a result of organized violence. It is a short-term approach based on CBT exposure therapy, which is specifically designed for survivors of war and torture. Clients are repeatedly asked to talk about the worst traumatic event in detail and re-experience the emotions associated with the event. This causes habituation of the emotion response to the traumatic memory, and reconstructs a consistent autobiographic narrative. This study described two cases of NET in depth and presented data from a pilot study assessing PTSD symptoms using the CIDI (Composite International Diagnostic Interview) Sections K and E at pre-treatment, post-treatment, and 9-month follow-up. The study found a reduction in symptoms post-treatment and at 9-month follow-up.

Although there are no controlled studies of testimony therapy, there are two papers that state that it is beneficial in certain cases, as it is the public acknowledgement that the trauma was a group experience. Cienfuegos and Morelli (1983) developed the use of testimony psychotherapy in Chile. Within the context of intensive psychotherapy, the clients recounted their torture experiences and their sessions were audio taped for transcription. The survivor and therapist produced a written testimony that could be further analyzed and used as an indictment against the torturers. Testimony psychotherapy is a brief individual method of psychotherapy for torture survivors. The therapy is both a private and public means to personal recovery through bearing witness to historical and social consequences of political violence. The technique is based on the belief that collective traumatization is as important as individual traumatization. It works through the narration of a person's experience of collective traumatization in a new context in which their memories can be used to develop new understandings of history. The authors describe the use of testimony psychotherapy in 39 clients and found the technique to be successful for the majority of torture survivors.

Weine and his colleagues (1998) reported on the use of testimony psychotherapy in 20 traumatized adult refugees from Bosnia-Herzegovia, and they also believed that there was value in emphasizing the collective traumatization of the group. Twenty Bosnian refugees in Chicago who had witnessed genocide received an average of six sessions, each lasting approximately 90 minutes. All sessions were taped, transcribed, and a final document was given to the survivor at the final session. A second copy was held in an oral history archives for the project. Practitioners of testimony psychotherapy feel that it allows survivors some symptom relief from PTSD. Bosnians also experienced trauma as a collective as well as individual experience. For them, what the insurgents targeted was not only just their individual lives but also their collective way of life. The testimony helped them find meaning, communicate, and teach what it means to survive political violence and to be Bosnian. The study reported a reduction in the rate of PTSD diagnosis; PTSD symptom severity; a decrease in re-experiencing, avoidance, hyper-arousal, and depressive symptoms; and an increase in GAF scale scores. Weine emphasizes that testimony psychotherapy is relational and that the therapy is integrative and allows the survivor to put seemingly unrelated fragments into a coherent story. It is a ritual in the oral tradition, and it creates a social context that is important to survivors.

Rechtman (1997) presented a case of transcultural psychotherapy with a Cambodian refugee with schizoaffective disorder in Paris. In 1990, a Southeast Asian psychiatric programme was founded in Paris to serve Southeast Asian refugees. Ten Cambodian refugees were treated with intensive psychodynamic psychotherapy by the author. The author emphasized not only the role of retrieving traumatic memories and reducing anxiety symptoms, and how exposure therapy is helpful, but also that it must be done carefully. The therapist must also consider cultural concepts of emotion, sadness, and trauma from non-Western cultures. He must also be aware of how culturally different clients express their suffering in their own terms. During his therapy session, he used an interpreter, as he was not fluent in Southeast Asian languages. Rechtman emphasized the need to think beyond just idioms of distress, and discussed the topic of cultural bereavement that mimics PTSD, but is not considered a disease, but a somewhat normal response to the catastrophic loss of social structure and culture. He does not try to obtain a trauma story, as that would be harmful to the patient. There is no attempt at abreaction, which Rechtman views as dangerous. He focuses on the symptoms, and the trauma is brought to consciousness. Rechtman felt that it was important to work in the survivor's native language, hence the use of the interpreter. Finally, he felt that the therapist had to have knowledge of the client's cultural background, and that this knowledge is essential, but not adequate to fully understand the client's experience.

Mollica and Lavell (1988) argued that the intensive psychotherapies are not useful in Southeast Asian refugees because they are foreign to the cultures and run the risk of severely retraumatizing clients. Like Rechtman, they have not found the analysis of the trauma story to be therapeutic, but does acknowledge that it is important for the therapist to know the client's trauma history.

They advocated for brief contact model with frequent visits and an emphasis on support and concrete assistance with such things as housing and employment.

Kinzie and his colleagues (1988) described their experience in starting a group therapy programme with Southeast Asian refugees at an Indochinese refugee psychiatric clinic at the Oregon Health Sciences University. They argued that refugees are often isolated. They share diagnoses and social problems, and can benefit from interacting with other refugees who share a common past and language. The groups involved four ethnic groups: Vietnamese, Cambodian, Lao, and Mien. The groups varied from 7 to 22 individuals. The Mien group was split into separate groups by gender so that the women would not be inhibited by the presence of men. Social activities brought out group cohesion and support, and promoted cultural identity. Loss was a frequent theme of the groups as were generational and cultural conflicts and psychosomatic symptoms. Attempts to introduce elements of formal psychotherapy to some of the groups had mixed results. The authors concluded that the groups could not replace individual sessions with the psychiatrist.

A novel approach utilizing dance as a mode of therapy with children from war-torn countries is described by Harris (2007). He argued that accessing a community's cultural resources through creative artistic expression promotes resiliency in the face of trauma. He further argued that the psychophysiology of trauma involves reliving traumatic experiences 'at the body level'. Dance movement therapy (DMT) is effective at overcoming cultural differences and helps torture victims learn skills to deal with their traumatic memories. Three basic principles of DMT include: 1) movement reflects personality; 2) the relationship established between the therapist and patient through movement supports healing and behavioral change; and 3) significant changes occur on the movement level that can affect physical and emotional functioning. Harris gives two examples of the use of DMT with refugee children. In the first example, recognizing the importance of dance in Dinka culture, Harris approached resettled Sudanese youth in Philadelphia, Pennsylvania, and met with about 40 of them for 18, two-hour sessions over the course of an academic year in order for the youth to teach him their traditional dances. He argued that the ritualized dance provided a therapeutic container for the youth's anxieties and emotions that was free from the shame associated with Western mental health interventions and the use of dance reinforced traditional coping mechanisms among this population. The second example was the use of three time-limited DMT groups, consisting of young adult women, adult Muslim men, and child soldiers in each of three towns in the Kailahun district of Sierra Leone. In tandem with teams of local trauma counselors, Harris met with clients in the first two groups for nine weekly sessions. The DMT involved a series of structured exercises in addition to improvisatory movement experiences. The groups enabled participants to reduce hyper-arousal, depression, and anxiety, manage difficult emotions, and express suppressed rage and anger.

Supervision

Usually one-on-one, supervision presents an opportunity to go in-depth on the therapist's work with clients, a fairly safe place to talk about personal reactions, and may mimic the therapeutic work with the client. However, the perspective is limited to be from one person, and only one to hold the powerful feelings, as well as there is no peer support present. Group supervision is recommended for its multiple perspectives, containment of feelings, and support for the supervisees.

Conclusions

Psychotherapy for refugees is crucial to their recovery from trauma, and its sequelae of PTSD and MDD. There are many examples of effective psychotherapy that have been successfully modified for use in different cultural groups. The characteristics that they shared were an attempt to avoid focusing on the traumatic events in order to avoid re-traumatization, but instead to focus on the symptoms and their meaning to the client. Only one author suggested that intense exposure to the worst traumatic memories (NET) was beneficial in Somali children from Uganda. Most included an education component, where patients were taught new skills to manage their symptoms. They also had a training component for the therapist to become knowledgeable in the patient's culture and experience. The most effective methods included CPT, CBT, group, dance, and individual therapy, suggesting that the healing principles were universal once the patient's experience, cultural values, beliefs, and customs were incorporated into existing therapeutic modalities that were then modified and informed by the perspective of the client, further suggesting that a manualized approach was not helpful with diverse populations of refugees. More research is needed to quantify the success of other modalities yet to be reported in the literature. A culturally sensitive clinician should be able to conduct effective psychotherapy with refugees following the principles reviewed in this chapter, including knowing the client's political history, cultural beliefs, values, and customs, interpersonal relationships, and their intra-psychic struggles, as well as the therapist's own history, values, relationships, and intra-psychic struggles. The therapist can then create a multilevelled approach using any of the techniques mentioned in this chapter, while doing mental health education, cultural empowerment, and indigenous healing.

References

American Psychiatric Association. (2000). *Diagnostic and Statistical Manual, Fourth Edition, Text Revision*, Washington, DC: APPI.

American Psychiatric Association. (2004). *Practice Guidelines: Treatment of Patients with Acute Stress Disorder and Posttraumatic Stress Disorder*. Washington, DC: APPI.

Bemak, F., Chung, R.C.Y., and Pedersen, P.B. (2003). *Counseling Refugees: A Psychosocial Approach to Innovative Multicultural Interventions*. Westport, CN: Greenwood Press.

Blackwell, D. (2003). *Counseling and Psychotherapy with Refugees*. Philadelphia, PA: Jessica Kingsley Publishers.

Bower, R.D., Pahl, L., and Bernstein, M.A. (2004). Case presentation of a tattoo-mutilated, Bosnian torture survivor. *Torture* **14**(1): 16–24.

Cienfuegos, A. and Monelli, C. (1983). The testimony of political repression as a therapeutic instrument. *American Orthopsychiatry* **53**: 43–51.

Goodkind, J.R. (2005). Effectiveness of a community-based advocacy and learning program for Hmong refugees. *American Journal of Community Psychology* **36**: 3/4, 387–408.

Harris, D.A. (2007). Dance/movement therapy approaches to fostering resilience and recovery among African adolescent torture survivors. *Torture* **17**(2): 134–155.

Herman, J.L. (1997). *Trauma and Recovery: The Aftermath of Violence – from Domestic Abuse to Political Terror*. New York: Free Press.

Hinton, D.E., Safren, S.A., Pollack, M.H., and Tran, M. (2006). Cognitive-behavior therapy for Vietnamese refugees with PTSD and comorbid panic attacks. *Cognitive and Behavioral Practice* **13**: 271–281.

Hinton, D.E. and Otto, M.W. (2006). Symptom presentation and symptom meaning among traumatized Cambodian refugees: Relevance to a somatically focused cognitive-behavior therapy. *Cognitive and Behavioral Practice* **13**: 249–260.

Ilic, Z. (2004). EMDR in the treatment of posttraumatic stress disorder with prisoners of war. In Z. Spiric, G. Knezevic, V. Joric, and G. Opacic (Eds.) *Torture in War: Consequences and Rehabilitation of Victims-Yugoslav Experience*, pp. 281–291, Belgrade: International Aid Network.

Kinzie, J.D. (2001). Psychotherapy for massively traumatized refugees: the therapist variable. *American Journal of Psychotherapy* **55**(4): 475–490.

Kinzie, J.D. and Fleck, J. (1987). Psychotherapy with severely traumatized refugees. *American Journal of Psychotherapy* **41**: 82–94.

Kinzie, J.D., Leung, P., Bui, A., *et al.* (1988). Group therapy with Southeast Asian refugees *Community Ment Health J* **24**(2): 157–166.

Kleinman, A.M. (1977). Depresssion, somatization, and the new cross-cultural psychiatry. *Social Science and Medicine* **11**: 3–10.

Lee, E. (1990). Assessment and treatment of Chinese–American immigrant families. In G.W. Saba, B.M. Karrer, and K.V. Hardy, (Eds.), *Minorities and Family Therapy*, pp. 99–122, New York: Haworth Press.

Marshall, G.N., Schell, T.L., Elliot, M.N., Berthold, S. M., and Chun, C. (2005). Mental health of Cambodian refugees two decades after resettlement in the United States. *Journal of American Medical Association* **294**(5): 571–579.

Mollica, R. and Lavell, J. (1998). Southeast Asian refugees. In L. Comas-Diaz and
E. Griffiths, (Eds.), *Clinical Guidelines in Cross-Cultural Mental Health*, New York:
Wiley.

National Center for PTSD. (2008). Fact Sheet: PTSD in Refugees. Available at: http://www.
ncptsd.va.gov/ncmain/ncdocs/fact_shts/fs-refugees.html. (Accessed October 24, 2008).

Onyut, P.L., Neuner, F., Schauer, E., Ertl, V., Odenwald, M., and Schauer, M. (2005).
Narrative exposure therapy as a treatment for child war survivors with posttraumatic
stress disorder: Two case reports and a pilot study in an African refugee settlement.
BMC Psychiatry 5: 7.

Ortmann, J., Genefke, I., Jakobsen, L., and Lunde, I. (1987). Rehabilitation of torture
victims: an interdisciplinary treatment model. *American Journal of Social Psychiatry*
3: 161–167.

Otto M.W., Hinton, D.E., Korbly N.B., Chea, A., Ba, P., and Gershuny, B.S. (2003).
Treatment of pharmacotherapy–refractory posttraumatic stress disorder among
Cambodian refugees: A pilot study of combination treatment with cognitive–behavior
therapy vs. sertraline alone. *Behaviour Research and Therapy* 41(11): 1271–1276.

Piwowarczyk, L. (2005). Engaging the sacred in treatment. *Torture* 15(1): 1–8.

Rechtman, P. (1997). Transcultural psychotherapy with Cambodian refugees in Paris.
Transcultural Psychiatry 34(3): 359–375.

Schulz, P.M., Huber, L.C., and Resick, P.A. (2006). Practical adaptations of cognitive
processing therapy with Bosnian refugees: implications for adapting practice to a
multicultural clientele. *Cognitive and Behavioral Practice* 13: 310–321.

United Nations High Commissioner on Refugees. (2008). 2007 Global Trends: Refugees,
Asylum-Seekers, Returnees, Internally Displaced and Stateless Persons.
Available at: http://www.unhcr.org/statistics/STATISTICS/4852366f2.pdf.
(Accessed November 23, 2008).

Weine, S.M., Kulenovic, A.D., Pavkovic, I., and Gibbons, R. (1998). Testimony
psychotherapy in Bosnian refugees: A pilot study. *American Journal of Psychology*
155(12): 1720–1726.

Yalom, I. and Leszcz, M. (2005). *The Theory and Practice of Group Psychotherapy,
Fifth Edition*. New York: Basic Books.

Chapter 13

Post-traumatic stress disorder

Nick Grey, Damon Lab, and Kerry Young

Introduction

This chapter describes the nature of post-traumatic stress disorder (PTSD) and considers how it may apply to people who are refugees and asylum seekers. The main empirical treatments for PTSD in general populations are outlined, and the evidence in refugee and asylum seeker populations summarized. The chapter goes on to provide some guidance regarding clinical practice, such as identifying PTSD, what initial interventions should be provided and by whom, and when to refer on to more specialized services. An established phasic model of intervention is used as the framework for such clinical decision making.

What is PTSD?

It has long been evident that experiencing a traumatic event can cause psychological problems. However, PTSD is a relatively recent addition to psychiatric classification. A key question is 'what makes an event traumatic?' Earlier classifications required the stressor to be 'outside the range of usual human experience' and that it 'would be markedly distressing to anyone' (APA, 1987). However PTSD is also caused by events that are actually very common, such as road traffic accidents, or physical and sexual assaults.

Current formal diagnostic criteria are now more specific. A traumatic event is one in which the individual 'experienced, witnessed, or was confronted with an event or events that involved actual or threatened death or serious injury, or a threat to the physical integrity of self or others' and that the person's 'response involved intense fear, helplessness, or horror' (APA, 1994). In addition, to meet DSM-IV criteria for PTSD an individual also needs to experience at least one 're-experiencing' symptom, three 'avoidance or numbing' symptoms, and two 'hyperarousal' symptoms. Re-experiencing symptoms include intrusive memories, nightmares, flashbacks, and emotional or physiological reactivity to reminders. Avoidance and numbing symptoms include avoidance of thoughts, feelings, or conversations related to the trauma, avoidance of places, people, or activities that act as reminders, psychogenic amnesia, diminished interest or participation in activities, feelings of detachment or estrangement, a restricted range of affect ('feeling numb'), and a foreshortened sense of future. Hyperarousal symptoms include difficulty in falling or staying asleep, irritability, difficulty concentrating, hypervigilance, and an exaggerated startle response ('feeling jumpy'). This spectrum of symptoms must have lasted longer than a month, and interfere significantly with the person's functioning.

In children there are some adaptations to these criteria. The response at the time of trauma may be expressed by disorganized or agitated behaviour rather than intense fear, helplessness, or horror. Re-experiencing criteria in young children include trauma-specific re-enactment and/or repetitive play in which themes or aspects of the trauma are expressed, and frightening dreams without recognizable content.

Similar criteria are also given by the World Health Organization in the International Classification of Diseases and Related Health Problems (ICD: WHO, 1992). Of note is that PTSD is classified as an anxiety disorder in DSM whereas in ICD it is classified under reactions to severe stress and adjustment disorders. Furthermore, factor analyses of traumatic stress symptoms have indicated that a four-factor structure (re-experiencing, avoidance, numbing, and hyperarousal) is a better fit to the available data than a three-factor structure (with avoidance and numbing combined together as in DSM-IV) (Foa, Riggs, and Gershuny, 1995).

Multiple and prolonged traumatic events, such as torture, may lead to more complex traumatic stress presentations, which result in a profound impact on the client not captured by PTSD. ICD-10 attempts to cover these presentations with the diagnosis Enduring Personality Change Following Catastrophic Experience (EPC; WHO, 1992). The criteria include a permanently hostile or distrustful attitude to the world, social withdrawal, a constant feeling of empti- ness or hopelessness, an enduring feeling of being 'on edge', including hyper- vigilance and irritability, and a permanent feeling of being changed or different from others. Herman (1992) refers to 'complex trauma', which, in addition to symptoms of PTSD, also includes phenomena such as difficulties in affect regulation, self-harm, and disruptions in identity. The utility of terms such as complex trauma or EPC is currently unclear.

The diagnosis of PTSD in refugee and asylum seeker populations

The utility of psychiatric diagnoses, rooted mainly in a Western-based medical model across non-Western cultures, is often debated and this has been particularly true for PTSD (Kagee and Naidoo, 2004). Most refugees and asylum seekers have escaped situations that would clearly meet the above criteria for being 'traumatic'. PTSD has come under the spotlight in terms of how useful it is as a diagnosis to capture the mental health problems refugees experience following exposure to traumatic events.

First, the tendency for the media and even some professionals to assume all refugees fleeing conflict are 'traumatized' and the consequent overemphasis on PTSD has been noted (e.g. Summerfield, 2001). Related to this is the criticism that receiving a mental illness diagnosis such as PTSD can medicalize the plight of those fleeing conflict, unfairly shifting the emphasis away from seeing torture and war as human rights issues and locating the problem within the 'sick' individual. However, these discourses are separate from the question of whether the constellation of symptoms that constitute a diagnosis of PTSD can be consistently observed in populations of refugees who have experienced trauma across the globe.

Literature in the transcultural psychiatry field raises awareness that the spiritual, social, and moral context of an individual mediates expression of psychological distress, meaning responses to trauma will not be uniform across cultures. Specific presentations following trauma involving religious meaning and particular physical symptoms, for example, have been found in samples from Bhutan (Van Ommeren et al., 2001), Mozambique (Igreja, Kleijn, and Richters, 2006), Cambodia (Hinton et al., 2005; Hinton et al., 2006), and Burundi (Yeomans, Herbet, and Forman, 2008). However there is good evidence for the stability of the symptom structure of PTSD cross culturally (Sack, Seeley, and Clarke, 1997; Palmieri, Marshall, and Schell, 2007; Rasmussen, Smith, and Keller, 2007), and PTSD is therefore seen by most as a useful concept for understanding reactions to trauma across cultures (deJong, 2004).

Prevalence of PTSD in refugee and asylum seeker populations

Prevalence rates of PTSD in refugee populations vary depending on country of origin, sample size, duration displaced, assessment method, and language of interviewer. Fazel, Wheeler, and Danesh (2005) conducted a systematic review of studies looking at general refugee populations (i.e. excluding studies using clinic-based samples) living in developed countries. Seventeen surveys of adult refugee populations met their research criteria and the average prevalence rate for PTSD across these studies was 9% (CI 8–10%). Five studies looking at child refugees found a slightly higher rate of 11% (CI 7–17%).

Prevalence rates of PTSD in individuals living in refugee camps in neighbouring countries reveals higher rates of morbidity. Mollica and colleagues (1999) found that 39% of Bosnians living in a refugee camp in Croatia met criteria for PTSD. A lower estimate of 12% was found in a study of Guatemalan refugees living in camps located in the next-door state of Chiapas in Mexico (Sabin *et al.*, 2003). The participants in this survey had been settled in Mexico for much longer than in the previous study, which may explain the significant difference in rates (as well as possibly supporting the evidence for the importance of social factors in the maintenance of PTSD for refugees). Within clinical populations, a study of Afghanis attending a psychiatric clinic in a refugee camp in Peshawar in neighbouring Pakistan found that nearly 80% met criteria for PTSD (Naeem *et al.*, 2005).

Rates of PTSD in samples taken from clinic populations of refugees living in the West are also considerably higher than those found in general refugee populations. Weine *et al.* (1995) found 65% of Bosnian refugees in a US clinic met the criteria for a diagnosis of PSTD. In a sample of Cambodian refugees attending a psychiatric clinic in the United States, Hinton and colleagues (2006) found that 56% of subjects were symptomatic for the disorder. In the United Kingdom, McColl and Johnson (2006) conducted a survey of London community psychiatric services and found that 42% of the refugee patients on their caseloads had a likely diagnosis of PTSD. High morbidity rates have also been found in clinic samples of child refugees, with Kinzie and colleagues (2006) finding that 63% of war trauma exposed Latin American children at a specialist clinic in the United States met criteria for PTSD.

Risk factors for the development of PTSD

Factors in exile such as social isolation and unemployment are stronger predictors of depressive morbidity than trauma factors (van Velsen, Gorst-Unsworth, and Turner, 1996; Gorst-Unsworth and Goldenberg, 1998; Hermansson, Timpka, and Thyberg, 2002; Miller *et al.*, 2002). Identified risk factors for development of PTSD and depression include a loss of social network, fear of repatriation, and family separation (Steel *et al.*, 2006). These hold clear policy implications. However, individual experience also helps account for the development of psychological problems. The higher the level of trauma exposure, the higher the psychological morbidity (Mollica *et al.*, 1998). In particular, if an individual has been tortured they are more likely to experience PTSD (Holtz, 1998; Silove *et al.*, 2002). Intrusive PTSD symptoms are associated with impact/physical torture and isolation, whereas avoidant symptoms are associated with sexual torture (van Velsen, Gorst-Unsworth, and Turner,, 1996). The latter may be mediated by high levels of shame. Intra-individual factors that protect against developing psychological problems include religious faith (Shrestha *et al.*, 1998), political commitment, and, in those who have been tortured, a preparedness for this outcome (Basoglu *et al.*, 1997).

In summary, although refugees and asylum seekers who have experienced trauma may present with a variety of symptoms dependent on their particular culture, spiritual beliefs, and illness models, there is good evidence that symptoms of PTSD are prevalent in this group, particularly in those seeking help for emotional distress.

Effective treatments for PTSD

Pharmacological treatments

The use of SSRIs for PTSD is indicated from systematic reviews (Stein, Ipser, and Seedat, 2006). They should be given in similar dosages as used for depression and response is gradual. Improvement is usually partial and there are no data guiding the length of treatment (Nagy and Marshall, 2002). Due to high co-morbidity of PTSD with depression, antidepressants are very often prescribed in clinical practice. For a review of pharmacotherapy of PTSD and trauma-related disorders see Dent and Bremner (2009).

Psychological treatments

A number of strategies have been used (also see Lim and Koike in this volume, Chapter 12). Exposure-based treatments are the most effective for PTSD and are recommended over pharmacological treatments in routine practice (NCCMH, 2005; Foa et al., 2008). These involve discussing the details of the traumatic event, usually many times, and often listening to the audiotapes of such sessions, or writing a narrative of the experience. There are a number of different versions of such cognitive behavioural therapies (CBT). The best established protocols, for both adults and children, in both research settings and in dissemination studies, are for Prolonged Exposure (PE: Foa et al., 2005, 2007), Cognitive Processing Therapy (CPT; Resick and Schnicke, 1993), and Cognitive Therapy for PTSD (CT; Ehlers and Clark, 2000; Ehlers et al., 2005, 2010).

Eye Movement Desensitization and Reprocessing (EMDR; Shapiro, 1995) is a structured treatment that consists of visualizing a moment of the traumatic event while being aware of related thoughts and feelings at the same time as attending to a distracting stimulus (usually saccadic eye movements). Evidence for the effectiveness of EMDR in the treatment of PTSD is extensive and comparable to that of exposure-based treatments (Bisson et al., 2007).

Evidence in refugee and asylum seeker populations

There are few randomized treatment outcome studies with refugee populations. Those that exist provide evidence for the effectiveness of (broadly) cognitive behavioural therapies and all contain some elements of exposure (see Table 13.1).

There is little evidence for the lasting efficacy of medication for PTSD in refugees and asylum seekers (Smajkic *et al.*, 2001).

Guidelines for clinical practice

Regardless of the specific techniques used there are a number of general guidelines to consider when working with traumatized refugees and asylum seekers.

Assessment

Establishing some trust and rapport is important in any assessment. This applies particularly to those who have experienced interpersonal traumas such as rape or torture, in which trust in others may have been significantly damaged. Feelings of shame associated with sexual abuse or other humiliating treatment or having perpetrated acts of violence need to be dealt with sensitively. It is important to establish the client's level of knowledge and provide information about the nature of the service to which they have been referred, the role of mental health professionals, and rules about confidentiality.

The client's main pre-occupations, possible goals, and standard background information and history should be elicited. Although obtaining a trauma history is necessary to make a diagnosis of PTSD, at first assessment it is probably better to ask only for a brief history of trauma in their country of origin, together with an account of their flight. In addition, details of specific psychological difficulties should be gathered as usual.

Recounting traumatic events is usually distressing (for the clinician too) and individuals may experience flashbacks in the room during the interview process. In some cases clinicians may need to remind clients where they are and that they are safe now in order to 'ground' them. When assessing traumatic stress symptoms, special attention should be paid to which aspects, of what may be an extensive trauma history, are being re-experienced by the client, in the form of intrusions, flashbacks, or nightmares. Care should be taken to distinguish intrusive memories of what actually happened at the time of the traumatic event from post-traumatic ruminative thoughts and images of the consequences and sequelae. Intrusive memories are also seen in disorders such as depression, and following bereavement.

Although PTSD symptoms might be spontaneously reported in the course of the assessment, structured interviews are the most reliable and valid way of establishing whether someone meets the diagnostic criteria for PTSD. A common interview is the Structured Clinical Interview for DSM (SCID; First *et al.*, 1996). However, probably the nearest thing that there is to a

Table 13.1 Comparing psychological treatments for PTSD in refugees and asylum seekers

Treatment	Main trauma-focused intervention	Evidence in general PTSD populations	Evidence in refugee and asylum seeker populations	Further issues
Testimony	Repeated transcriptions of traumatic events.	Little available	Some available (Weine et al., 1998).	Political origins documenting human rights abuses in Chile (Cienfuegos and Monelli, 1983).
CBT (includes PE, CPT, CT)	Exposure/reliving of traumatic events through imaginal exposure and/or writing.	Excellent, recommended treatment	Good evidence. Exposure therapy, Paunovic and Ost (2001). CBT, Otto et al. (2003) CPT, Schulz et al. (2006). Many case descriptions for other CBT.	Relatively more focus on identifying and altering meanings in addition to discussion of traumatic material.
NET	Detailed transcribed description of traumatic events in context of life story.	Some emerging	Very good. Neuner et al. (2004). Schauer et al. (2005) Using lay counsellors with limited training in refugee camp (Neuner et al., 2008). Preliminary evidence for children (Onyut et al., 2005).	Use of narratives for political means explicit. Developed originally to be used in refugee camps. See Mueller (2009) for role of NET in CBT.
EMDR	Keeping image of key events in consciousness.	Very good, recommended treatment	Little available. Service audit from Lab et al. (2008). Preliminary evidence for children (Oras et al., 2004).	Therapy less verbal therefore it minimizes language issues

CBT Cognitive Behaviour Therapy; PE Prolonged Exposure; CPT Cognitive Processing Therapy; CT Cognitive Therapy; NET Narrative Exposure Therapy; EMDR Eye Movement Desensitization and Reprocessing.

'gold standard' for PTSD assessment is the Clinician Administered PTSD Scale (CAPS: Blake *et al.*, 1990), which is used extensively in current PTSD research.

If language constraints permit, self-report questionnaires are very useful instruments to efficiently obtain a lot of information both at assessment and during the course of treatment. There are a number of well-established general symptom measures with good psychometric properties. The most widely used is the Impact of Event Scale (Horowitz, Wilner, and Alvarez, 1979). The better, revised version comprises 22 items asking about each of the symptom clusters of intrusions, avoidance, and hyperarousal (IES-R; Weiss and Marmar, 1997). A good alternative scale is the 17 item Post-traumatic Diagnostic Scale (Foa *et al.*, 1997), which more carefully follows the DSM-IV criteria for PTSD. Other trauma-specific scales are also available, such as the Harvard Trauma Questionnaire (HTQ: Mollica *et al.*, 1992), which has been widely used in refugee populations. Although these measures have been shown to be acceptable in eliciting PTSD symptoms in refugee populations (IES: Söndergaard, Ekblad, and Theorell, 2003; PDS: Norris and Aroian, 2008; HTQ: Hollifield *et al.*, 2002) normative data for non-Western samples is sparse; so care should be taken in applying the various clinical cut-offs suggested.

These scales cannot provide a diagnosis of PTSD. Rather they provide additional information that can corroborate and lend weight to a clinical assessment. Furthermore it is sensible to enquire further about the answers provided on the self-report questionnaires. An individual may indicate that they regularly have 'intrusive memories' but this would not necessarily distinguish between flashbacks of the event or later rumination. If the person has experienced multiple traumatic events it is important to know with respect to which event or events the questionnaire has been completed.

Intervention: a phased approach

The National Institute for Health and Clinical Excellence (NICE) in the United Kingdom recommends a phased approach (NCCMH, 2005), which broadly follows the framework set out by Herman (1992). Treatment may move back and forth between phases as events occur. The treatment path will vary according to the client's precise presentation. Due to multiple problems and the use of interpreters, treatment is more likely to need approximately 18–25 sessions or more, rather than the common 12–16 sessions of CBT for PTSD (Grey and Young, 2008).

Making a diagnosis of PTSD for someone who has been experiencing flashbacks, nightmares, and other distressing symptoms can, in itself, be therapeutic. Some traumatized individuals feel as if they are 'going mad', particularly in relation to the intrusive thoughts and images of past events they re-experience.

Table 13.2 Phased intervention

Phase/goals	How achieved	Which professionals involved	Considerations
Establishing safety	Ongoing assessment and formulation; normalization. Meet primary needs; housing, asylum status, social contact. Medical assessment; physiotherapy, medical interventions. Psychiatric assessment; antidepressant medication.	Multidisciplinary: social workers, psychiatrists, clinical psychologists, physiotherapists, occupational therapists.	May be repeated; need to return to this phase during a treatment episode.
'Remembrance'	Trauma focused therapy: PE, CT, NET, CPT, EMDR, testimony	Trained trauma therapists. Although NET has also been used with lay counsellors following training (Neuner et al., in press).	This is the 'classic' PTSD therapy.
Reconnection	Family reunion, valued and enjoyable activities, political commitment.	Formal therapeutic input, but also broader social networks such as community organizations, religious leaders, political groups.	Includes work on loss of trust, and spiritual and religious dimensions.

Explaining that such symptoms are 'a normal reaction to an abnormal event' will usually help sufferers to feel less frightened. Written information in the client's preferred language should be provided whenever possible. Such 'normalization' is a key intervention that all professionals working with people with PTSD should provide. These principles are also described by Lim and Koike in this volume (see Chapter 12).

Phase 1: Establishing safety

Broadly speaking, assessment and normalization form part of establishing safety. Clients may be so preoccupied with their asylum status, accommodation, finances, family separation, physical complaints, occupational or social functioning that they can think or talk about little else. If this is the case, then it may be that specific therapy for traumatic stress symptoms should be delayed until these issues are less preoccupying or, indeed, resolved. However, general counselling or activating other networks can still be supportive. Common onward referrals might include psychiatric assessment for medication, medical assessment of torture injuries or chronic pain, contact with housing authorities, benefits agencies, or legal advisors. A lack of trust in others may make clients reluctant to pursue these avenues and may come to be an agreed goal for treatment (Grey and Young, 2008).

It is important, where possible, to utilize existing methods of coping and heighten the client's own resilience. Finding appropriate social support structures such as community organizations or a local temple/church can also be of great benefit. Drawing on religious beliefs might be extremely important for some individuals. In India, Sachs and colleagues (2008) found that only one of 749 Tibetan refugees met the criteria for PTSD despite high rates of trauma exposure (including torture), which they partly attributed to religious practice. Thus, explanations and context become extremely significant.

There are no definitive rules as to when an individual will be ready for trauma-focused therapy. Lack of refugee status is not a reason for not providing specific therapy. If a person has not received refugee status and is expecting to be deported in the very imminent future, therapy aimed specifically at traumatic stress symptoms may not be possible. However, others may be awaiting status and not perceive immediate threat of removal and be better able to address their traumatic stress symptoms at this stage. Moving on to the next stage needs to be negotiated between client and therapist keeping in mind that there can be significant (and understandable) avoidance of confronting painful memories by both parties that may need to be overcome. Patients should never be coerced into dealing with their trauma but should be helped to make an informed decision following psycho-education about the method and hope for positive outcome.

Phase 2: Trauma-focused therapy

The general principles and techniques of trauma-focused approaches remain the same for working with refugees as for other populations. Where the client has been involved in only a few traumatic events, or has experienced many, but re-experiences only a few, then reliving of each event can be attempted. Often, however, refugees have been involved in a series of traumas and will present with re-experiencing symptoms related to many, and it may not be possible to undertake reliving of all troubling events. In these circumstances the same basic approach is adopted by a variety of therapies (EMDR, NET, and other established CBT protocols). First the whole story of the traumatic experiences is described before then focusing on specific parts of the narrative that are most emotional, the 'worst moments'. When using EMDR for more complex/multiple traumatic experiences, possible adaptations include more time for preparation work to provide the client with sufficient strategies for grounding at the end of a session.

Specific cognitive themes to address may include mental defeat and permanent change (Ehlers, Maercker, and Boos, 2000). Additionally, clients may also struggle to understand how others come to commit atrocities and may challenge beliefs about human nature, making the integration of these experiences more difficult. Possible psycho-sociological explanations can be discussed and related to the client's experience (Grey and Young, 2008; Young, 2009). The importance of social factors, wider systemic models, and social identity theory models are also clearly applicable, perhaps particularly when considering the development of state organized violence and inter-ethnic conflict (Silove, 1999).

Phase 3: Social reintegration

We emphasize the need for broader social interventions for people, which include links with community organizations and other suitable groups, and helping to obtain suitable housing and refugee status. The individual therapy interventions that we discuss in this chapter are not at the expense of these broader issues but merely recognize that, even with good provision of social care, individuals can still experience significant psychological distress. We encourage enquiring about traditional approaches to such distress that may be used within a cultural group, and for the person to use any such approaches that seem appropriate, such as particular grief rituals. We also encourage people to talk with other members of their family and community, including community elders or religious leaders, to establish what others believe too.

Working with interpreters

It is not always necessary to use an interpreter if either client or therapist is able to speak the other's language, albeit not completely fluently, if a slower pace is adopted. However, it is often wise to employ an interpreter so that the client can express important concepts or meanings that are crucial for therapy. The most important aspect of providing good therapy in this context is that a three-way trusting relationship can be developed between the client, interpreter, and therapist (Haenel, 1997; Tribe and Raval, 2002). This may require changes of interpreter if necessary. Therapist and interpreter characteristics such as age, gender, and ethnicity may be important. The latter can be particularly sensitive as some refugees may not want members of their own community interpreting for reasons of perceived confidentiality and shame.

There is evidence that trauma-focused therapy through an interpreter can be effective (Schulz et al., 2006; d'Ardenne et al., 2007). Specific adaptations to the reliving process in trauma-focused therapy may be necessary (see d'Ardenne and Farmer, 2009). First, the interpreter must understand the rationale of the treatment, to expect high levels of distress in clients, and to not act in a way that might prevent this despite any understandable desire to 'help' the client. Second, it can be helpful if the interpreter is able to translate simultaneously by sitting close to the therapist and whisper the translation into their ear so as not to interfere with the processing. Third, the importance of exact translation should be emphasized so that meaning is not lost. Fourth, debriefing with the interpreter at the end of a session is important.

Future developments

It is clear that further research examining the effectiveness of established treatments for PTSD in refugee populations needs to be carried out. The timing of therapy should also be investigated; particularly the question of when is it still advisable to engage in trauma-focused work if the patient is under threat of deportation to the country where they were traumatized. Lastly, continued research into cultural differences in responses to trauma, and expression of symptoms, is still needed for these factors to be best taken into account by treating clinicians.

References

American Psychiatric Association. (1987). *Diagnostic and Statistical Manual of Mental Disorders* (3rd edition revised). Washington DC: Author.

American Psychiatric Association. (1994). *Diagnostic and Statistical Manual of Mental Disorders* (4th edition). Washington DC: Author.

d'Ardenne, P., Ruaro, L., Cestari, L., Wakhoury, W., and Priebe, S. (2007). Does interpreter-mediated CBT with traumatized refugee people work? A comparison of patient outcomes in East London. *Behavioural and Cognitive Psychotherapy* 35: 293–301.

d'Ardenne, P. and Farmer, E. (2009). Using interpreters in trauma therapy. In N. Grey (Ed.) *A Casebook of Cognitive Therapy for Traumatic Stress Reactions*, Hove: Routledge.

Basoglu, M., Mineka, S., Paker, M., Aker, T., Livanou, M., and Gok, S. (1997). Psychological preparedness for trauma as a protective factor in survivors of torture. *Psychological Medicine* **27**: 1421–1433.

Bichescu, D., Neuner, F., Schauer, M., and Elbert, T. (2007). Narrative exposure therapy of political imprisonment-related chronic trauma spectrum disorders: A randomized controlled trial. *Behaviour Research and Therapy* **45**: 2212–2220.

Bisson, J.I., Ehlers, A., Matthews, R., Pilling, S., Richards, D., and Turner, S. (2007). Psychological treatments for chronic post-traumatic stress disorder. Systematic review and meta-analysis. *British Journal of Psychiatry* **190**: 97–104.

Blake, D., Weathers, F., Nagy, L., *et al.* (1990). Clinician Administered PTSD Scale (CAPS). National Center for PTSD, Behavioural Sciences Division, Boston.

Cienfuegos, A.J. and Monelli, C. (1983). The testimony of political repression as a therapeutic instrument. *American Journal of Orthopsychiatry* **53**: 41–53.

de Jong, J. (2004). Public mental health and culture: disasters as a challenge to western mental health care models, the self, and PTSD. In J. Wilson and B. Drozdek (eds.), *Broken Spirits: the treatment of traumatized asylum seekers, refugees, war and torture victims.* New York: Routledge.

Dent, M.F. and Bremner, J.D. (2009). Pharmacotherapy for posttraumatic stress disorder and other trauma-related disorders. In M.M. Antony and M.B. Stein (Eds.), *Oxford Handbook of Anxiety and Related Disorders.* Oxford: OUP.

Ehlers, A. and Clark, D.M. (2000). A cognitive model of post-traumatic stress disorder. *Behaviour Research and Therapy* **38**: 319–345.

Ehlers, A., Clark, D.M., Hackmann, A., McManus, F., and Fennell, M. (2005). Cognitive therapy for posttraumatic stress disorder: Development and evaluation. *Behaviour Research and Therapy* **43**: 413–431.

Ehlers, A., Clark, D.M., Hackmann, A., McManus, F., Fennell, M., and Grey, N. (2010). *Cognitive Therapy for PTSD: A Therapist's Guide.* Oxford: Oxford University Press. In preparation.

Ehlers, A., Maercker, A., and Boos, A. (2000). PTSD following political imprisonment: the role of mental defeat, alienation, and perceived permanent change. *Journal of Abnormal Psychology* **109**: 45–55.

Fazel, M., Wheeler, J., and Danesh, J. (2005). Prevalence of serious mental disorder in 7000 refugees resettled in western countries: a systematic review. *The Lancet* **365** (9467): 1309–1314.

First, M.B., Spitzer, R.L., Gibbon, M., and Williams, J.B. (1996). *Structured Clinical Interview for DSM-IV axis I disorders, clinician version.* Washington DC: American Psychiatric Press.

Foa, E.B., Cashman, L., Jaycox, L., and Perry, K. (1997). The validation of a self-report measure of posttraumatic stress disorder: the posttraumatic diagnostic scale. *Psychological Assessment* **9**: 445–451.

Foa, E.B., Keane, T.M., Friedman, M.J., and Cohen, J.A. (Eds.). (2008). *Effective Treatments for Posttraumatic Stress Disorder: Practice Guidelines from the International Society for Traumatic Stress Studies (2nd Edition).* New York: Guilford.

Foa, E.B., Riggs, D.S., and Gershuny, B.S. (1995). Arousal, numbing, and intrusion: symptom structure of PTSD following assault. *American Journal of Psychiatry* **152**: 116–120.

Foa, E.B., Hembree, E.A., Cahill, S.P., *et al.* (2005). Randomized trial of prolonged exposure for post-traumatic stress disorder with and without cognitive restructuring: Outcome at academic and community clinics. *Journal of Consulting and Clinical Psychology* **73**: 953–964.

Foa, E.B., Hembree, E.A., and Rothbaum, B.O. (2007). *Prolonged Exposure Therapy for PTSD: Emotional Processing of Traumatic Experiences: Therapist Guide.* New York: Oxford University Press.

Gorst-Unsworth, C. and Goldenberg, E. (1998). Psychological sequelae of torture and organized violence suffered by refugees from Iraq: Trauma-related factors compared with social factors in exile. *British Journal of Psychiatry* **172**: 90–94.

Grey, N. and Young, K. (2008). Cognitive behaviour therapy with refugees and asylum seekers experiencing traumatic stress symptoms. *Behavioural and Cognitive Psychotherapy* **36**: 3–19.

Haenel, F. (1997). Aspects and problems associated with the use of interpreters in psychotherapy of victims of torture. *Torture* **7**: 68–71.

Herman, J.L. (1992). *Trauma and Recovery.* London: Pandora Books.

Hermansson, A, Timpka, T., and Thyberg, M. (2002). The mental health of war-wounded refuges: an 8 year follow-up. *Journal of Nervous and Mental Disease* **190**: 374–380.

Hinton, D.E, Chhean, D., Pich. V., Um, K., Fama, J.M., and Pollack, M.H. (2005). Neck-focused panic attacks among Cambodian refugees: A logistic and linear regression analysis. *Transcultural Psychiatry* **42**(1): 46–77.

Hinton, D.E., Chhean, D., Pich, V., Pollack, M.H., Orr, S.P., and Pitman, R.K. (2006). Assessment of posttraumatic stress disorder in Cambodian refugees using the Clinician-Administered PTSD Scale: Psychometric properties and symptom severity. *Journal of Traumatic Stress* **19**(3): 405–409.

Hollifield, M., Warner, T.D., Lian, N., Krakow, B., Jenkins, J.H., and Kesler, J. (2002). Measuring trauma and health status in refugees: A critical review. *Journal of American Medical Association* **288**: 611–621.

Holtz, T.H. (1998). Refugee trauma versus torture trauma: A retrospective controlled cohort study of Tibetan refugees. *Journal of Nervous and Mental Disease* **186**: 24–34.

Horowitz, M.J., Wilner, N.J., and Alvarez, W. (1979). The impact of event scale: A measure of subjective stress. *Psychosomatic Medicine* **41**: 209–218.

Igreja, V., Kleijn, W., and Richters, A. (2006). When the war was over, little changed: women's posttraumatic suffering after the war in Mozambique. *Journal of Nervous and Mental Disorder* **194**(7): 502–509.

Kagee, A. and Naidoo, A.V. (2004). Reconceptualizing the sequelae of political torture: limitations of a psychiatric paradigm. *Transcultural Psychiatry* **41**: 46–61.

Kinzie, J.D., Cheng, K., Tsai, J., and Riley, C. (2006). Traumatized refugee children: The case for individualized diagnosis and treatment. *Journal of Nervous and Mental Disease* **194**(7): 534–537.

Lab, D., Santos, I., and de Zulueta, F. (2008) Treating post-traumatic stress disorder in the 'real world': Evaluation of a specialist trauma service and adaptations to standard treatment approaches. *Psychiatric Bulletin* **32**(1): 8–12.

McColl, H. and Johnson S. (2006). Characteristics and needs of asylum seekers and refugees in contact with London community mental health teams: A descriptive investigation. *Social Psychiatry & Psychiatric Epidemiology* **41**(10): 789–795.

Miller, K.E., Weine, S.M., Ramic, A., *et al.* (2002). The relative contribution of war experiences and exile-related stressors to levels of psychological distress among Bosnian refugees. *Journal of Traumatic Stress* **15**: 377–387.

Mollica, R.F., Caspi-Yavin, Y., Bollini, P., Truong, T., Tor, S., and Lavelle, J. (1992). The Harvard Trauma Questionnaire: Validating a cross-cultural instrument for measuring torture, trauma and post-traumatic stress disorder in refugees. *Journal of Nervous and Mental Disease* **180**: 111–116.

Mollica, R.F., Donelan, K., Tor, S., *et al.* (1993). The effect of trauma and con-finement on functional health and mental health status of Cambodians living in Thailand–Cambodia border camps. *Journal of the American Medical Association* **280**: 581–586.

Mollica, R., McInnes, K., Poole, C., and Svang, T. (1998). Dose–effect relationships of trauma to symptoms of depression and posttraumatic stress disorder among Cambodian survivors of mass violence. *British Journal of Psychiatry* **173**: 482–488.

Mollica, R.F., McInnes, K., Sarajlic, N., Lavelle, J., Sarajlic, I., and Massagli, M.P. (1999). Disability Associated with psychiatric comorbidity and health status in Bosnian refugees living in Croatia. *Journal of American Medical Association* **282**(5): 433–439.

Mueller, M. (2009). The role of Narrative Exposure Therapy in cognitive therapy for refugees and asylum seekers. In N. Grey (Ed.), *A Casebook of Cognitive Therapy for Traumatic Stress Reactions.* Hove: Routledge.

Naeem, F., Mufti, K., Ayub, M., *et al.* (2005). Psychiatric morbidity among Afghan refugees in Peshawar, Pakistan. *Journal of Ayub Medical College, Apr–Jun.*

Nagy, L. and Marshall, R. (2002). PTSD psychopharmacology basics for non-physicians and beginning psychiatrists. *PTSD Clinical Quarterly* **11**: 33–39.

National Collaborating Centre for Mental Health. (2005). *Clinical Guideline 26. Post-Traumatic Stress Disorder (PTSD): The Management of PTSD in Adults and Children in Primary and Secondary Care.* London: National Institute for Clinical Excellence.

Neuner, F., Onyut, P., Ertl. V., Schauer, E., Odenwald, M., and Elbert, T. (2008) Treatment of posttraumatic stress disorder by trained lay counsellors in an African refugee settlement – a randomized controlled trial. *Journal of Clinical and Consulting Psychology* **76**: 686–694.

Neuner, F., Schauer, M., Klaschik, C., Karunakara, U., and Elbert, T. (2004). A comparison of narrative exposure treatment, supportive counselling, and psycho-education for treating posttraumatic stress disorder in an African refugee settlement. *Journal of Consulting and Clinical Psychology* **72**: 579–587.

Norris, A.E. and Aroian, K.J. (2008). Avoidance symptoms and assessment of posttraumatic stress disorder in Arab immigrant women. *Journal of Traumatic Stress* **21**: 471–478.

Onyut, L.P., Neuner, F., Schauer, E., *et al.* (2005). Narrative exposure therapy as treatment for war survivors with posttraumatic stress disorder: two case reports and a pilot study in an African refugee settlement. *BMC Psychiatry* **5**: 7.

Oras, R., de Ezpeleta, S.C., and Ahmad, A. (2004). Treatment of traumatized refugee children with Eye Movement Desensitization and Reprocessing in a psychodynamic context. *Nordic Journal of Psychiatry* **58**(3): 199–203.

Otto, M.W., Hinton, D., Korbly, N.B., *et al.* (2003). Treatment of pharmacotherapy–refractory posttraumatic stress disorder among Cambodian refugees: a pilot study of combination treatment with cognitive–behavior therapy vs sertraline alone. *Behaviour Research and Therapy* **41**: 1271–1276.

Palmieri, P.A., Marshall, G.N., and Schell, T.L. (2007). Confirmatory factor analysis of posttraumatic stress symptoms in Cambodian refugees. *Journal of Trauma Stress* **20**(2): 207–216.

Paunovic, N. and Ost, L.-G. (2001). Cognitive–behaviour therapy vs. exposure therapy in the treatment of PTSD in refugees. *Behaviour Research and Therapy* **39**: 1183–1197.

Rasmussen, A., Smith. H., and Keller, A.S. (2007). Factor structure of PTSD symptoms among West and Central African refugees. *Journal of Traumatic Stress* **20**(3): 271–280.

Resick, P.A. and Schnicke, M.K. (1993). *Cognitive Processing Therapy for Rape Victims: A Treatment Manual.* Newbury Park, CA: Sage.

Sabin, M., Lopes Cardozo, B., Nackerud, L., Kaiser, R., and Varese, L. (2003). Factors associated with poor mental health among Guatemalan refugees living in Mexico 20 years after civil conflict. *Journal of American Medical Association* **290**(5): 667–670.

Sachs, E., Rosenfeld, B., Lhewa, D., Rasmussen, A., and Keller, A. (2008). Entering exile: Trauma, mental health, and coping among Tibetan refugees arriving in Dharamsala, India. *Journal of Traumatic Stress* **21**(2): 199–208.

Sack, W.H, Seeley, J.R., and Clarke, G.N. (1997). Does PTSD transcend cultural barriers? A study from the Khmer Adolescent Refugee Project. *Journal of the American Academy of Child and Adolescent Psychiatry* **6**(1): 49–54.

Schauer, M., Neuner, F., and Elbert, T. (2005). *Narrative Exposure Therapy: A Short-Term Intervention for Traumatic Stress Disorders after War, Terror, or Torture.* Gottingen: Hogrefe.

Schulz, P.M., Resick, P.A., Huber, L.C., and Griffin, M.G. (2006). The effectiveness of cognitive processing therapy for PTSD with refugees in a community setting. *Cognitive and Behavioral Practice* **13**: 322–331.

Shapiro, F. (1995). *Eye Movement Desensitization and Reprocessing: basic principles, protocols and procedures.* New York: Guilford Press.

Shrestha, N-M., Sharma, B., Van Ommeran, M., *et al.* (1998). Impact of torture on refugees displaced within the developing world: Symptomatology among Bhutanese refugees in Nepal. *Journal of the American Medical Association* **280**: 443–448.

Silove, D. (1999). The psychosocial effects of torture, mass human rights violations, and refugee trauma: Towards an integrated conceptual framework. *Journal of Nervous and Mental Disease* **187**: 200–207.

Silove, D., Steel, Z., McGorry, P., Miles, V., and Drobny, J. (2002). The impact of torture on post-traumatic stress symptoms in war-affected Tamil refugees and immigrants. *Comprehensive Psychiatry* **43**: 49–55.

Smajkic, A., Weine, S., Djuric-Bijedic, Z., Boskailo, E., Lewis, J., and Pavkovic, I. (2001). Sertraline, paroxetine and venlafaxine in refugee posttraumatic stress disorder with depressive symptoms. *Journal of Traumatic Stress* **14**: 445–452.

Söndergaard, H.P., Ekblad, S., and Theorell, T. (2003). Screening for post-traumatic stress disorder among refugees in Stockholm. *Nordic Journal of Psychiatry* **57**(3):185–189.

Steel, Z., Silove, D., Brooks, R., Momartin, S., Alzuhairi, B., and Susljik, I. (2006). Impact of immigration detention and temporary protection on the mental health of refugees. *British Journal of Psychiatry* **188**: 58–64.

Stein, D.J., Ipser, J.C., and Seedat, S. (2006). Pharmacotherapy for posttraumatic stress disorder. *Cochrane Database of Systematic Reviews* DOI: 10.1002/ 14651858.CD002795. pub2.

Summerfield, D. (2001). Asylum seekers, refugees and mental health services in the UK. *Psychiatric Bulletin* **25**: 161–163.

Tribe, R. and Raval, H. (Eds.). (2002). *Working with Interpreters in Mental Health*. Hove: Brunner–Routledge.

Turner, S.W., Bowie, C., Dunn, G., Shapo, L., and Yule, W. (2003). Mental health of Kosovan Albanian refugees in the UK. *British Journal of Psychiatry* **182**: 444–448.

van Ommeren, M., Sharma B., Komproe, I.H. *et al.* (2001). Trauma and loss as determinants of medically unexplained epidemic illness in a Bhutanese refugee camp. *Psychological Medicine* **31**: 1259–1267.

van Velsen, C., Gorst-Unsworth, C., and Turner, S. (1996). Survivors of torture and organized violence: demography and diagnosis. *Journal of Traumatic Stress* **9**: 181–193.

Weine, S.M., Becker, D.F., McGlashan, T.H., et al. (1995). Psychiatric consequences of 'ethnic cleansing': Clinical assessments and trauma testimonies of newly resettled Bosnian refugees. *American Journal of Psychiatry* **152**: 536–542.

Weine, S.M., Kulenovic, A.D., Pavkovic, I., and Gibbons, R. (1998). Testimony psychotherapy in Bosnian refugees: a pilot study. *American Journal of Psychiatry* **155**: 1720–1726.

Weiss, D.S. and Marmar, C.R. (1997). The impact of event scale – revised. In J.P. Wilson and T.M. Keane (Eds.), *Assessing Psychological Trauma and PTSD: A Handbook for Practitioners*. New York: Guilford Press.

World Health Organization. (1992). *International Statistical Classification of Diseases and Related Health Problems* (10th rev.). Geneva: WHO.

Young, K.A.D. (2009). Cognitive therapy for survivors of torture. In N. Grey (Ed.), *A Casebook of Cognitive Therapy for Traumatic Stress Reactions*. Hove: Routledge.

Yeomans, P.D., Herbert, J.D., and Forman, E.M. (2008). Symptom comparison across multiple solicitation methods among Burundians with traumatic event histories. *Journal of Traumatic Stress* **21**(2): 231–234.

Chapter 14

Suicide in refugees and asylum seekers

Lakshmi Vijayakumar and
A.T. Jotheeswaran

I have been to the doctor because I am very stressed. I feel I am going crazy, I don't
want to go back to my country as a crazy person, dying is better. Before I get crazy,
before I get sick, before I get hospitalized, I prefer to kill myself.

(Ashford, 2003)

Suicide by itself is a global public health problem. Each year, approximately
1 million individuals die by suicide, 10–20 million attempt suicide, and
50–120 million are profoundly affected by suicide or attempt of close relative
or associate (Hendin *et al.*, 2009). The majority of suicides (85%) in the world
occur in low- and middle-income countries. Suicide is now among the top five
causes of death of young adults of both sexes (Table 14.1). The estimated
burden of suicide in the different regions of the world reveal that the burden is
substantial in developing countries (Fig. 14.1).

Various theories and models are applied to understand the cause and effect
of suicide. The models that are applied to study suicide include the public
health model, psychiatric biological medical model, psychological model,
injury control model, sociological model, interpersonal model, stress diathesis
model, and socioeconomic model. A close study of all these models demonstrates one clear idea that there is no single overriding reason for suicide. Apart
from this it must be emphasized that suicide is a human behaviour and, like all
other human behaviours, has multiple causes. To add to this is an important
point, that suicide risk does vary over time through the life of an individual.

Though suicide is an intrinsically individual and personal act, it cannot be
isolated from the concerned individual's sociocultural context. When viewed
through this glass, refugees and those seeking asylum are found to be more
vulnerable to the risk of suicide.

Summerfield, D. (2000) says nearly 1% of people are refugees or displaced
persons resulting from 40% current violent conflicts. Worldwide there are

Table 14.1 The burden of suicide

Region	Numbers of death	DALYs (%)
Africa	50000	0.3
America	69000	1.1
E Mediter.	36000	0.8
Europe	151000	2.0
SE Asia	252000	1.6
W Pacific	286000	2.0
World	844000	1.3

W.H.O.

10 million asylum seekers and refugees. Majority of them reside in low-income countries, sometimes in refugee camps. Only 25% of refugees and asylum seekers are in Europe (McColl *et al.*, 2008).

Seeking asylum or being a refugee radically transforms their lives often by circumstances beyond their control. Majority of them have experienced genocide, imprisonment, violence, trauma, war bereavement, and other harsh circumstances, which make life intolerable and death preferable. The process of seeking asylum can involve hazardous journeys, separations, inhuman conditions, constant fear of being apprehended, and death. Common post migration difficulties are: discrimination, detention, dispersal, destitution, denial of right to work, denial of healthcare, and delayed decision on asylum application.

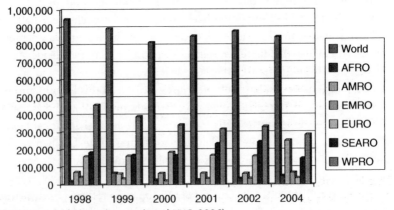

Fig. 14.1 Suicide in various regions (WHO 2006).

It is sometimes referred to as a grief process that comprises seven losses: family and friends, language, culture, homeland, status, contact with the group, and exposure to physical risk (Carta *et al.*, 2005). All these factors distance the individual from the community.

To understand the link between refugee status and suicide, Durkheim's (1897/1952) social integration theory is useful. Social integration refers to the quantity and quality of ties that bind individuals to others, to their community, and the wider society. Durkeim suggested that social integration can be either excessive or insufficient and that in both cases, suicide rates are increased. According to social integration theory, suicide rates tend to be high among groups that have low levels of domestic integration. Refugees and asylum seekers are in that category and consequently are likely to have higher suicide rates.

Following the Henry and Short (1954) theory of suicide, it can be expected that in situations where blame for one's frustrations and suffering can be directed externally, suicide is less likely to happen. Levi (1992), a survivor of Auschwitz concentration camp, pointed out that focusing on the day-to-day survival decreased the likelihood of suicide.

Similar life-saving behaviours and attitudes were described by Kepinski (1970) in his study of survivors of Nazi concentration camps. The three factors which could make a difference between life and death were finding an 'angel' (i.e. a friend) in the hell of the camp, maintaining the will to live through psychosomatic unity, and 'camp autism', which allowed one to focus on internal experience and strongly held personal values and hopes, thereby allowing for psychological isolation from the inhuman conditions. In a similar vein, Solzhenitsyn (1974) and Lipper (1951) noted that the feeling of 'universal innocence' and the realization that the individual's ill fate was shared with so many others suppressed the thoughts of suicide among Gulag prisoners. Mandelstam (1970) and Lipper (1951) observed that the Gulag prisoners' will to survive and their hope of meeting the people they loved helped them to overcome the ordeal and to stay alive (Krysinska and Lester, 2008).

These divergent views underscore the complexity and interaction of various factors for suicide in refugees and asylum seekers.

There is overwhelming evidence that seeking asylum is both directly and indirectly a stressful and disturbing experience and such experience is closely related to suicide and self harming (Procter, 2004).

Method

There is paucity of studies about suicide in refugees and asylum seekers. Lack of reliable data and limited access to official archives and documents has resulted in reliance on anecdotal reports. Suicidal behaviour in refugees is often not reported as it is considered politically sensitive. This is more so in low- and middle-income countries, where majority of the displaced persons reside in refugee camps with poor infrastructure.

Access to records or permission to study suicidal behaviour in refugees is mostly denied. Mental health professionals and human rights activists have been instrumental in generating public concern, which has resulted in policy initiatives in Western countries like Germany, USA, UK, Australia, etc. Unfortunately, low- and middle-income countries, where majority of the refugees in the world reside, lag far behind in research, services, policy, and programmes for refugees.

In this chapter, we present a review conducted to understand the prevalence of suicidal behaviour and predisposing factors for suicidal behaviour among refugees. We ran the literature search using Ovid search in Medline, EMBASE, PsycINFO and SIEC using keywords 'Refugee (asylum seekers) and Suicide'; we exacted 59 articles related to suicide from 864 papers published on refugees. Further there were only seven papers which reported prevalence of suicidal behaviour among refugees.

For convenience the term 'refugees' in this chapter also includes asylum seekers.

Prevalence

Research evidence reports higher incidence of suicide rates among refugees compared to general populations (Mcspadden, 1987). For example studies on Ethiopion immigrants reported suicide rates as five to six times higher in refugee population than in the national population (Arieli and Aycheh, 1993; Arieli *et al.*, 1994, 1996).

The overall prevalence of suicidal behaviour among refugees ranges from 3.4% to 34%. Most of the studies reported suicidal thoughts and ideation. Only two investigated attempted suicide. There is considerable variation between studies in measuring suicidal behavioural. (Table 14.2)

Risk and protective factors

The risk and protective factors associated with suicide in general population are applicable to the refugee population also, albeit with variations mediated by their circumstances.

Sociodemographic factors

It is unclear whether the suicides are different for the different sexes. Dudley (2003) reported that men's and women's rate of suicide behaviour in Australian

Table 14.2 Studies on suicide among refugees

Study	Country	Age group	Participants country of origin	Sample size	Measures	Suicidal behaviour %
Slodnjak V. Kos et al., 2002	Slovenia	14–15 yrs	Bosnia and Herzegovina	N = 460	CDI, IES, WTQ, Teachers report	24.14%
Ferrada-Noli, et al., 1998a	Sweden	Adult	69% Middle East and Africa, 31% Yugoslavia, East Europe, and Latin America	N = 149	DSM-IV, PTSD, CPRS, Suicidal behaviour questionnaire	40% Attempted suicide
Bhuia et al., 2006	London	Adult 18–>35	Somalis	N = 143	MINI-Neuropsychiatry Interview	9.1% Suicidal risk
M. Tousignant et al.,1999	Canada	Adolescents (13–19 yrs)	El Salvador, Cambodia, Laos, Iran, Vietnam, South Asia, Central America	N = 203	DISC-2.25,CGAS	3.4 % Suicide attempt
Rahman et al., 2003	Pakistan	Adult Mean 28.2, SD (7.3)	Afghanistan	N = 297	SRQ-20	34% Suicidal thought
Rashid, 1998	Pakistan	Adult	Kashmir	N = 534	ICD -10 Clinical examination	26.9% Suicidal thought
van Ommeren et al., 2008	Germany	Mean 43.2, (SD 14.9)	Bosnian 29%, Serbian 27%, Kosovo 29%, Iraq 5%, Turkey 8%	N = 100	M.I.N.I, PDS, EUROHIS	Suicidal thought 27.7% Returnees and 43.2% Stayers

Immigration Detention Centres were probably 41 and 26 times the national average, and that male rates were 1.8 times the rate of males in prisons.

Koppenaal *et al.* (2003) analyzed the cause of death among asylum seekers in Netherlands for the period 1998–1999. In the two year study period, 156 asylum seekers died, of which 49 were due to unnatural causes. Compared to the Dutch standard population, the age and gender stratified standard mortality rate (SMR) was 1.23 (1.01–1.23) and 0.85 (0.59–1.11) for male and female asylum seekers. More specifically SMR for male suicides was 2.8 (1.5–4.1).

Staehr and Munk-Andersen (2006) studied suicide and suicidal behaviour among asylum seekers in Denmark during the period 2001–2003 and found that the number of suicide attempts by asylum seekers was 3.4 times higher than Danish residents. Further the rate of suicide increased in the subsequent 2 years. Suicidal behaviour was most frequent between 30 and 39 years.

Refugee women face many dangers while fleeing or in places of settlement including physical and sexual violence, abduction, forced prostitution, and forced sale of children. For many female refugees, the violent situations that cause them to flee their home countries are only the beginning. When women and girls are separated from male family members during flight or are widowed during war, they are especially susceptible to physical abuse and rape. Women and girls have been victimized by pirates, border guards, military units, and male refugees.

Many refugee women are widowed or become separated from their husbands during flight, leaving them with the sole responsibility of their dependent children. This responsibility, added to the isolation and stress experienced as a refugee, increases the risk of mental illness for many women (United Nations High Commissioner for Refugees, 1991).

A cross sectional survey of 297 Afghan mothers with children residing in two refugee camps in North West Frontier Province of Pakistan revealed that 36% of women in the sample (n = 106) screened positive for common mental disorder. Ninety six (91%) of those screened positive had suicidal thoughts in the previous month and nine (8.1%) rated suicidal feelings as their top most concern (Rahman and Hafeez, 2003).

Depression and mental disorder in mothers are known to be associated with emotional, behavioural, and conduct problems in children, thus creating a vicious cycle of despair, despondency, and anti-social behaviour. High levels of suicidal feelings in the primary caregiver may lead to different or more severe psychopathology in the offspring. High rates of hopelessness and suicidal feelings among refugee mothers may have important public health and social implications.

About a third of the refugee women attending PHC facilities in Pakistan screened positive for a mental disorder and, on self-report, had suicidal feelings in the previous 6 months. In a poor and, to a large extent, culturally similar district of neighbouring Punjab province, using the same instrument, it was found that less than 3% of women of 670 surveyed admitted suicidal thoughts (A. Rahman, personal communication).

Glen *et al.* (2007) interviewed 1293 internally displaced female household heads in Nyala district in South Darfur, Sudan, and found that over the previous year 5% reported suicide ideation, 2% reported suicidal attempt, and 2% of households had a member who died by suicide in the previous years.

Karam *et al.* (2007) reviewed published community-based studies that assessed suicidality in the Arab world (which included the following countries: Bahrain, Egypt, Iraq, Jordan, Kuwait, Lebanon, Morocco, Oman, Palestine, Saudi Arabia, Sudan, and United Arab Emirates). The lifetime prevalence of suicide attempt ranged from 0.72% to 6.3%. Compared to female university students, females who were displaced or refugees were significantly more likely to report suicide ideation within the past few weeks.

An epidemiological survey of 203 adolescents from refugee families aged 13–19 years from 35 countries did not find an increase in suicide attempts in the adolescents. Attempted suicide rate of 3% was similar to the rate found in Montreal High School students (Tousignant *et al.*, 1999).

It was expected that Bosnian refugee adolescents who fled from war zones to Slovenia would have increased suicidal ideation. Two years after the beginning of the war in Bosnia, 256 refugee students aged 14–15 years were compared with a sample of 195. Compared to the Slovene peers, the Bosnian refugees show significantly lower rates of suicidal ideation (Slodnjak *et al.*, 2000). Case report of five cases of psychiatric disturbances in unaccompanied children who were refused political asylum showed suicidal thoughts and loss of perception of time (Christensen and Lindskov, 2000).

Psychological factors

Suicidal ideation and psychological problems are inseparable. In fact psychological problems are an over riding factor in a majority of suicide deaths. Research from around the world reveals that 60–95% of people who die by suicide have one or more psychological disorders. The common diagnoses are depression, alcoholism and schizophrenia, post-traumatic stress disorder (PTSD), and other disorders (Vijayakumar *et al.*, 2006).

The majority of asylum seekers and refugees have no mental illness (Watters, 2001; Summerfield, 2003). They use their own resources and coping strategies to deal with the considerable difficulties encountered in their country of origin, during migration, in their new host country, and in the asylum process.

However, studies in high-income countries show that levels of psychopathology and mental illness, in particular anxiety and depression, are higher in refugee and asylum seeker groups than in the general population (Burnett, 2001). Another review found that refugees resettled in Western countries were about 10 times more likely to have PTSD than age-matched general populations in those countries (Fazel *et al.*, 2005). Other studies suggest that there may be more somatic presentation of psychological problems among asylum seekers and refugees (Tribe, 2002; van Ommeren *et al.*, 2002).

Though it is universally accepted and acknowledged that there is a direct and close relation between suicide and psychological disorders there are very few studies which have assessed the association between suicidal behaviour of refugees and psychological disorders.

Ferrada-Noli *et al.*'s (1998a) study of 65 refugees with diagnosis of PTSD found that 40% had made suicidal attempt, 29% had detailed suicidal plan, and 31% had recurrent suicidal thoughts. Suicidal behaviour was significantly greater in refugees with principal PTSD diagnosis than among the others. PTSD patients with comorbid depression reported higher frequency of suicidal thoughts and PTSD non-depressive patients' increased frequency of suicide attempt.

Fazel *et al.* (2005) did a systematic review of the prevalence of serious mental disorder in 6743 refugees resettled in Western countries and found a prevalence rate of 9% for PTSD in adults and 5% for major depression. The prevalence of PTSD in children and adolescents (below 18 years) was found to be 11%. In the studies that provided information on comorbidity, 71% of those diagnosed with major depression had a diagnosis of PTSD and 44% of those diagnosed with PTSD also had a diagnosis of major depression. Depression with comorbidity increases the risk of suicide.

Increasing number of researchers suggest that post migration factors play an important role both in the development and perpetuation of mental disorders such as anxiety disorders, somatisation disorders, and depression (Kivling-Boden and Sundbom, 2002; Knipscheer and Kleber, 2006). Research also has showed that chronic stress and hopelessness increase the risk of suicide.

Alcoholism and substance abuse are closely linked to suicidal behaviour. However, data on these factors in refugees are sparse. Bhui *et al.* (2006) found a higher prevalence of mental disorders in Somali refugees who use khat.

Berk (1998) found a higher rate of alcoholism and suicide among teenagers after the cessation of armed conflict in Bosnia. They had survived the most imminent threat and then succumbed to the long-term stress. Some of these problems were due to demobilization from the army of those teenagers who had been in the military. They were now left with no defined role after having had an important one, which had given them considerable power.

A meta-analysis of studies comparing the mental health of refugees with that of control groups from the host countries found that refugees (including asylum seekers and internally displaced people) had an overall increase in psychopathology (Porter and Haslam, 2005). However, this increase was not an inevitable consequence of acute wartime stress. Refugees who were older, better educated, female, and of rural residence and higher socioeconomic status predisplacement had worse mental health outcomes. Morbidity was significantly associated with post migration factors such as a lack of permanent accommodation and restricted opportunity to work (McColl *et al.*, 2008).

The increased prevalence of psychopathology among the refugees can be an explanation for increased suicidality in the refugees but the pathways and mediators are unclear.

Further psychological assessments in refugees can be complicated by issues of language, culture, etc. Issues of validity occur within transcultural epidemiology, and describing the extent of psychopathology in asylum seekers and refugees can be problematic (van Ommeren *et al.*, 2002).

Sociocultural factors

Loss, trauma, violence, physical abuse, torture, and economic hardships have been linked to suicidal behaviour. Nearly all refugees experience losses and many have suffered multiple traumatic experiences. Post displacement difficulties also cause significant distress. Problems with process of acculturation in a new society have been linked to higher prevalence of mental health problems (Bhugra, 2005).

A case report of a 23-year-old Vietnamese refugee who attempted suicide by self-inflicted abdominal stab describes the teasing of his fellow workers that he was a communist spy, rejection of his romantic advances by an American, and the variety of stressors and lack of services for the refugees (Jack *et al.*, 1984).

Mcspadden (1987) reported high levels of depression and suicide among 59 Ethiopian single male refugees. Interestingly the intensity of the pang of the refugee is directly related to the distance between his or her origin country and host country. The farther the refugee is moved culturally from the country of origin the higher is the alienation, which in turn, triggers suicide thought.

Westman *et al.* (2003) studied the influence of place of birth and socioeconomic factors on attempted suicide in a defined population of 4.5 million people. Refugees from Poland and Iran had a higher hazard ratio of attempted suicide than Swedish control. Women born in Latin America, Asia, and Eastern Europe had a higher rate than Swedish women. The hazard ratio of attempted suicide among women from Iran, Asia, Latin America, and Southern and Eastern Europe considerably exceeded those of men from the same country of origin. Although the risk of attempted suicide declined sharply with increased income in men, it remained high in women. Foreign-born psychiatric patients' risk of committing suicide was the double the risk compared to Swedish psychiatric patients (Johansson *et al.*, 1996).

Bayard-Burfield *et al.* (1999) studied suicide attempts in Swedes and foreign-born people from a defined catchment area during 1991–1994, a time of social change when the number of refugees from Bosnia increased. Foreign-born women aged 35–45 and 45–54 had rates of attempted suicide, which were 1.7 and 2.3% higher than those in Swedish women. Single females had the highest rate of suicide. The country of origin and the culture of the refugee play a significant role in suicidal behaviour.

Method of suicide and time of risk

The suicide method adopted by the refugees or asylum seekers seem to have a very close relationship with two important factors—one being the origin country and the other the type of torture the refugee had undergone.

Relationships were found to exist between the main stressors and the refugees' preference for suicide method. Particularly among PTSD patients with a history of torture, an association was found between the torture method that the victims had been exposed to, and the suicide method used in ideation or attempts. Blunt force applied to the head and body was associated with jumping from height, water torture, with drowning, and sharp force torture with methods involving self-inflicted stabbing or cutting (Ferrada-Noli, 1998b).

In the mid-1980s, intentional overdosage with isoniazd were reported in young South East Asian refugee women. They were aged 14–23, had come to the US within 1 year, and were receiving isoniazid preventive therapy for tuberculosis without disease (Nolan *et al.*, 1988). Blanchard *et al.* (1986) have also reported isoniazid overdose in Cambodian refugees.

These studies reiterate that easy availability of the method to commit suicide increases the risk of suicide.

There is an increased risk of suicide among refugees during the early period of displacement and also long duration of stay in refugee camps or detention centres. Staehr and Munk-Anderson (2006) found that the long waiting time (average 20.8 months) faced by asylum seekers combined with rejection of asylum cases trigger a rapid suicide ideation. It was also found that 44% of suicidal attempts occur within 6 months of arrival (Table 14.3).

Table 14.3 Probable factors for suicide in refugees and asylum seekers

Sociodemographic factors	Psychological disorders	Pre-migration difficulties	Post displacement difficulties	Personal factors
Female gender	PTSD		Longer stay in detention centres	Lack of religious belief
Far East and South East Asia	Depression	Exposure to trauma violence, abuse, loss, etc.	Deportation	
	Anxiety and Somatoform disorder		Reduced economic resources	Low resilience Reduced
Older adolescents Educated	Comorbidity		Cultural barriers	problem solving ability
Prior higher socioeconomic status			Exclusion	
Single			Stigma	

Protective factors, which are likely to reduce suicidal behaviour in refugees, have not been adequately researched. Religiosity is a protective factor but Ferrada-Noli (1995) stated that religiosity was not found to be a significant deterrent of suicidal behaviour. Jahangir *et al.* (1998) stated that depressed Afghan refugees with a higher degree of religiosity are less vulnerable to suicidal attempts or plans.

No single factor is a necessary component in the etiology of suicidal thoughts and behaviours. Suicidal behaviour results due to a complex interaction of the various domains of risk and protective factors.

Using the overlap model of suicide risks of Blumenthal and Kupfer (1990), the different domains of risk are presented in the following Venn diagram and the person at the highest risk of suicide is in the shaded area where all the circles intersect (Fig. 14.2).

Prevention

Prevention and intervention programmes to reduce suicidal behaviour in refugees and asylum seekers have not been reported in a single study.

Suicide prevention strategies that show promise in the general population may not be generalizable to the refugee population because of the different context within which these interventions have been implemented. Some of the risk factors are the same but some are different, and this has implication in suicide prevention efforts.

A social and public health approach acknowledges that suicide is preventable, and promotes a framework for developing an integrated system of interventions across multiple levels including the individual, family, the community, and the healthcare system (Vijayakumar *et al.*, 2005), and this approach can be applied to reduce suicidal behaviour in refugees. Priority should be given to

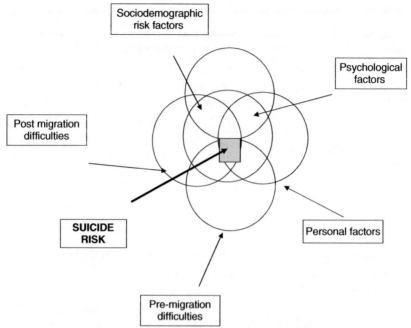

Fig. 14.2 Model of suicide risk in refugees and asylum seekers.

developing a culturally and contextually appropriate tool for assessment of suicide ideation and behaviour in refugees and asylum seekers.

The position statement of the Royal College of Psychiatrists suggests the following three main areas of action to promote health and to prevent the development of mental and physical illnesses in refugee and asylum seeking population.

1 Public policy that minimizes the impact of social risk factors for physical and mental illness.

2 Equitable access to a full range of health, social care, and legal services.

3 That public bodies organize to fulfil their duties under national and international law. (R. C. P., 2007)

The above policies and programmes, if implemented, are likely to reduce suicides in the refugees. In addition certain specific programmes may have additional value

1 Counselling and provision of emotional support both at the time of arrival and more importantly at the time of relocation or repatriation.

2 Early education on the language and culture of the host country.

3 Early provision for economic activity.

4 Ensuring communication and connections to the family, friends, NGOs, and ethnic groups.

5 Media efforts to portray the refugees in a positive framework.

Conclusions

Refugees experience greater trauma and psychological problems and as a consequence have increased suicidal behaviour. Suicidal behaviour among refugees has received very little investigation and deriving hypotheses to understand causal factors are difficult due to limited research and publication in the area. Hence there is an urgent need for further research, which will help in formulating appropriate, relevant, and cost-effective suicide prevention programmes for refugees.

A conservative estimate of suicidal behaviour prevalence of 10% implies that there are at least a million refugees and asylum seekers who are at risk of suicide. Despite the enormity of the problem it has received scant attention from mental health professionals and policy makers. There is an urgent need to acknowledge the magnitude of the problem, and this requires easy access to accurate and transparent data. The process must occur at all levels of service. At the individual level refugees must be provided a compassionate and caring environment to express their suicidal thoughts/plans without fear of marginalization and stigmatization. Mental health professionals, health and media personnel, policy makers, and NGOs must be sensitized to the needs of the refugees and the context of their circumstances. Finally, programmes and interventions should culminate in a society where refugees and asylum seekers are perceived as valued and respected members of the community. Suicide prevention in refugees and asylum seekers should be considered as social and ethical objectives rather than a traditional exercise in health sector.

References

Arieli, A. and Aycheh, S. (1993). Psychopathological aspects of the Ethiopian immigrants to Israel. *Isreal Journal of Medical Science* **29**: 411–418.

Arieli, A., Gilat, I., and Aycheh, S. (1994). Suicide by Ethiopian immigrants in Israel. *Harefuah* **123**: 45–70.

Arieli, A., Gilat, I., and Aycheh, S. (1996). Suicide among Ethiopian Jews: A survey conducted by means of a psychological autopsy. *Journal of Nervous and Mental Disorders* **184**: 317–319.

Ashford, K. (2003). Seeking trust in asylum. *The Adelaide Review* Nov (2–3). Adelaide News. www.Adelaiderview.com/au/archives.

Bayard-Burfield, L., Sundquist, J., Johansson, S.E., and Traskman-Bendz, L. (1999). Attempted suicide among Swedish-born people and foreign-born migrants. *Archives of Suicide Research* **2**(3): 171–181.

Berk, J.H. (1998). Trauma and resilience during war: A look at the children and humanitarian aid workers of Bosnia. *Psychoanalytic Review* **85**(4): 640–658.

Bhugra, D. (2005). Cultural identities and cultural congruency: A new model for evaluating mental distress in immigrants. *Acta Psychiatrica Scandinavica* **111**(2): 84–93.

Bhui, K., Craig, T., Mohamud, S., *et al*. (2006). Mental disorders among Somali refugees: Developing culturally appropriate measures and assessing sociocultural risk factors. *Social Psychiatry and Psychiatric Epidemiology* **41**(5): 400–408.

Blanchard, P.D., Yao, J.D., McAlpine, D.E., and Hurt, R.D. (1986). Isoniazid overdose in the Cambodian population of Olmsted County, Minnesota. *Journal of American Medical Association* **256**: 3131–3133.

Blumenthal, S.J. and Kupfer, D.J. (1990). *Suicide Over the Life Cycle – Risk Factors, Assessment, and treatment of Suicidal Patients (Ed.)*. Washington DC: American Psychiatric Press Inc.

Burnett, A. and Peel, M. (2001). Health needs of asylum-seekers and refugees. *British Medical Journal* **322**: 544–546.

Carta, M.G., Bernal, M., Haro-Abad, J.M., *et al*. (2005). Migration and mental health in Europe (The state of the mental health in Europe working group: Appendix I). *Clinical Practice and Epidemiology in Mental Health* **1**: 13.

Christensen, A.M. and Lindskov, T. (2000). When time stops … Psychiatric reactions to deportation orders of unaccompanied children and teenagers seeking asylum. *Ugeskr Laeger* **162**(16): 2338–2339.

Dudley, M. (2003). Contradictory Australian national policies on self harm and suicide: the case of asylum seekers in mandatory detention. *Australasian Psychiatry* **11** (Suppl.): 102–108.

Durkheim E. (1897/1952). *Suicide, a Study in Sociology*. Translated by J.A. Spaulding and G. Simpson, London: Routledge and Kegan Paul.

Fazel, M., Wheeler, J. and Danesh, J. (2005). Prevalence of serious mental disorder in 7000 refugees resettled in western countries: a systematic review. *Lancet* **365**: 1309–1314.

Ferrada-Noli, M., Asberg, M., Ormstad, K., Lundin, T., and Sundbom, E. (1998a). Suicidal behaviour after severe trauma. Part one: PTSD diagnosis, psychiatric comorbidity, and assessments of suicidal behaviour. *Journal of Traumatic Stress* **11**: 103–112.

Ferrada-Noli, M., Asberg, M., and Ormstad K. (1998b). Suicidal behavior after severe trauma. Part 2: The association between methods of torture and of suicidal ideation in posttraumatic stress disorder. *Journal of Traumatic Stress* **11**(1): 113–124.

Ferrada-Noli, M., Asberg, M., Ormstad, K., and Nordstrom, P. (1995). Definite and undetermined forensic diagnoses of suicide among immigrants in Sweden. *Acta Psychiatrica Scandinavica* **91**: 130–135.

Glen, K., Rabih, T., and Lynn, L. (2007). Basic health, women's health, and mental health among internally displaced persons in Nyala province, South Darfur, Sudan. *American Journal of Public Health* **2**(97): 353–361.

Hendin, H., Phillips, M.R., Vijayakumar, L. Pirkis, J., Wang, H., and Yip, P. (2009). Epidemiology in Asia. Suicide and Suicide Prevention (Ed.), pp. 1–5, World Heath Organisation.

Henry, A. and Short, J. (1954). *Suicide and Homicide*. New York: Free Press.

Jack, R.A., Nicassio, P.M., and West, W.S. (1984). Acute paranoid disorder in a Southeast Asian refugee. *Journal of Nervous and Mental Disease* **172**(8): 495–497.

Jahangir, F., Rehman, H., Jan, T. (1998). Degree of religiosity and vulnerability to suicidal attempt/plans in depressive patients among Afghan refugees. *International Journal for the Psychology of Religion* **8**(4): 265–269.

Johansson, L.M., Johansson, S.-E., Sundquist, J., and Bergman, B. (1996). Suicide among psychiatric in-patients in Stockholm, Sweden. *Archives of Suicide Research* **2**(3): 171–181.

Karam, E.G, Hajjar, R.V., Salamoun, M. M. (2007). Suicidality in the Arab World. *Arab Journal of Psychiatry* **18**(2): 99–107.

Kepinski, A. (1970). Tzw KZ-syndrom: Proba syntezy (in Polish). The KZ-Syndrome: A summary. *Prazeglad Lekarski* **1**: 18–23.

Kivling-Boden, G. and Sundbom, E. (2002). The relationship between post-traumatic symptoms and life in exile in a clinical group of refugees from the former Yugoslavia. *Acta Psychiatrica Scandinavica* **111**(5): 351–357.

Knipscheer, J.W. and Kleber, R.J. (2006). The relative contribution of posttraumatic and acculturative stress to subjective mental health among Bosnian refugees. *Journal of Clinical Psychology* **62**(3): 339–335.

Koppenaal, H., Bos, C.A., and Broer, J. (2003). High mortality due to infectious diseases and unnatural causes of death among asylum seekers in the Netherlands, 1998–1999. *Ned Tijdschr Geneeskd* **9**(147): 391–395.

Krysinska, K. and Lester, D. (2008). Suicide in the Soviet Gulag camps. *Archives of Suicide Research* **12**: 170–179.

Levi, P. (1992). Shame. In J. Miller (Ed.), *On Suicide*, pp. 181–188, Pub. San Francisco Chronicle, San Francisco.

Lipper, E. (1951). *Eleven Years in Soviet Prison Camps*. Chicago: Regnery.

Mandelstam, N. (1970). *Hope Against Hope. A Memoir*. New York: Artheneum.

McColl, H., McKenzie, K., and Bhui K. (2008). Mental health care of asylum-seekers and refugees. *Advances in Psychiatric Treatment* **14**: 452–459.

Mcspadden, L.A. (1987). Ethiopian refugee resettlement in the Western United States: social context and psychological well-being. *International Migration Review* **21**: 796–819.

Nolan, C.M., Elarth, A.M., and Barr, H.W. (1988). Intentional isoniazid overdosage in young Southeast Asian refugee women. *Chest* **93**(4): 803–806.

Porter, M. and Haslam, N. (2005). Predisplacement and postdisplacement factors associated with mental health of refugees and internally displaced persons: a meta-analysis. *Journal of American Medical Association* **294**: 602–612.

Procter, N. (2004). Emergency mental health nursing for refugees and asylum seekers. *Australian Nursing Journal* **12**: 21–23.

Rashid, K.H. (1998). Post-traumatic stress disorder in Kashmiri refugees. *Journal of the College of Physicians and Surgeons Pakistan* **8**(1): 29–32.

Rahman, A. and Hafeez, A. (2003). Suicidal feelings run high among mothers in refugee camps: a cross-sectional survey. *Acta Psychiatrica Scandinavia* **108**: 392–393.

Royal College of Psychiatrists. (2007). *Improving Services for Refugees and Asylum Seekers: Position Statement*. Royal College of Psychiatrists (http://www.rcpsych.ac.uk/docs/ Refugee%20asylum%20seeker%20consensus%20final.doc).

Slodnjak, V., Kos, A., and Yule, W. (2000). Depression and parasuicide in refugee and Slovene adolescents. *Crisis* **21**: 190.

Solzhenitsyn, A. (1974). *The Gulag Archipelago* (Vol.2). Glasgow: Collins/Fontana.

Staehr, M.A. and Munk-Andersen, E. (2006). Suicide and suicidal behavior among asylum seekers in Denmark during the period 2001–2003. A retrospective study. *Ugeskr Laeger* **168**(17): 1650–1653.

Summerfield, D. (2000). War and mental health: a brief overview. *BioMed Journal* **321**: 3323–3325.

Summerfield, D. (2003). Mental health of refugees. *British Journal of Psychiatry* **183**: 459–460.

Tousignant, M., Habimana, E., Biron, C., Malo, C., Sidoli-LeBlanc, E., and Bendris, N. (1999). The Quebec adolescent refugee project: Psychopathology and family variables in a sample from 35 nations. *Journal of the American Academy of Child and Adolescent Psychiatry* **38**(11): 1426–1432.

Tribe, R. (2002). Mental health of refugees and asylum-seekers. *Advances in Psychiatric Treatment* **8**(4): 240–246.

United Nations High Commissioner for Refugees (2006). Edition UNHCR 2006, Geneva.

Van Ommeren, M., Sharma, B., Sharma, G.K., Komproe, I., Cardena, E. and de Jong, J.T. (2002). The relationship between somatic and PTSD symptoms among Bhutanese refugee torture survivors: examination of comorbidity with anxiety and depression. *Journal of Traumatic Stress.* **11**(1): 113–124.

Vijayakumar, L. (2006). Suicide & mental disorders – a maze? *Indian Journal of Medical Research* **124**: 271–374.

Vijayakumar, L, John S., Pirkis J., and Whiteford, H. (2005). Suicide in developing countries: Risk Factors. *Crisis* **26**(3): 112–119.

Von Lersner, U., Wiens, U., Elbert, T., and Neuner, F. (2008). Mental health of returnees: Refugees in Germany prior to their state-sponsored repatriation. *BMC International Health and Human Rights* **8**: doi 1472-698X8/8.

Watters, C. (2001). Emerging paradigms in the mental health care of refugees. *Social Science and Medicine* **52**: 1709–1718.

Westman, J., Hasselstrom, J., Johansson, S.E., and Sundquist, J. (2003). The influences of place of birth and socioeconomic factors on attempted suicide in a defined population of 4.5 million people. *Archives of General Psychiatry* **60**: 409–414.

WHO (2006). 'Building Awareness – Reducing Risk' – Mental Illness and Suicide – Suicide: A Growing Global Burden. www.geocities.com/uwispa/Suicide_A_Growing_Global_Burden.pdf

World Health Organisation (2006). Safer access to pesticide – community intervention. *NLM Classification WA* **240**: 1–4.

Chapter 15

Loss and cultural bereavement

Wojtek Wojcik and Dinesh Bhugra

'You shall leave everything you love most: this is the arrow that the bow of exile shoots first. You are to know the bitter taste of other's bread, how salt[y] it is, and know how hard a path it is for one who goes ascending and descending others' stairs'.

(Dante Alighieri, 1321)

Introduction

This chapter explores another component of the asylum seeker or refugee's experience, namely that of the loss of what is left behind when one leaves not out of choice but of forced necessity. To help shed light and explore this topic, the concept of cultural bereavement is discussed; a traditional model of grief and bereavement is applied to loss in forced migration. This is at first glance the corollary of cultural assimilation, in that someone bereft will struggle to assimilate and fit in, whilst one who has made an apparently easy transition and is well supported will be less likely to grieve. In fact, an appreciation of both is important and meaningful to understanding the experience of a person. Dante Alighieri (quoted above) harboured chronic feelings of loss and resentment following his exile from Florence, despite living elsewhere in Italy and being feted in his new host city. Few share his ability to articulate their feelings so clearly; the greater the importance of the empathic clinician in exploring such difficulties with patients.

Applying the familiar framework of grief to this unfamiliar ground fosters an understanding which may be critical to the therapeutic encounter. As with bereavement, the effect of exile can run deep and be an underlying factor in presenting psychopathology, which, if the process of bereavement is ignored, can lead to the patient's difficulties being misunderstood. The lost object (to use the term from psychoanalytic theory), rather than someone recently deceased, can be the totality of home with the social roots, references to early memories, and shared values that this entails. It may become relevant immediately following migration or much later, in someone who initially was relieved to have escaped and assimilated very well.

The overall aim of this chapter is to raise awareness of and provide a few questions with which the experience of exile and loss can be further explored, to benefit engagement with patients and help establish a fuller formulation of their problems.

Refugees and loss

Refugees face a multitude of potential losses. These include childhood family and friends, their home with all its embedded memories, material possessions and memorabilia, their social status and role in a community, a common language, and shared culture. Some losses are felt immediately and others, such as the loss of shared values or old friends, may have their impact only later. Whilst material possessions can be replaced with time, the embedded memories they contained cannot.

Models of grief

Western constructs of bereavement may prove to be of only partial or limited value in explaining symptoms of grief when applied to people from other cultures; however, this is an area worth further study. Bereavement is universally experienced but the ways in which it is expressed and the socially sanctioned rituals associated with it are determined by culture. Of the established models of grief, perhaps the most well known is that of Elizabeth Kübler-Ross (Kübler-Ross, 1969). Her five-stage model is however based on work with people coming to terms with their own terminal diagnosis. John Bowlby, a child psychiatrist and psychoanalyst, developed a four-stage model from work with children experiencing loss. These four stages were numbness or protest; yearning and searching; disorganization and despair; reorganization (Bowlby, 1980). Sigmund Freud described the role of the unconscious and ambivalence in grief; abnormal grief reactions are unconsciously driven and involve ambivalent feelings to the lost object with resultant depressive symptoms including significant decline in self-esteem (Freud, 1953). In normal grieving it is common to exhibit depressive symptoms and these may cross a threshold where treatment is merited, but with the background of grief borne clearly in mind. Pseudo-hallucinations, experiences of hearing the lost person or seeing them in the street, are now acknowledged to be a part of the normal spectrum of the grief experience, and in some cultures these can be very vivid and visitations from ghosts can continue for many years (among Hopi Indians, for example (Matchett, 1972)). All societies have conventions around how grief should be displayed and how long it should last. Grief that goes beyond these conventions by lasting too long, or that is unusually displayed, may be regarded as abnormal or as complicated bereavement (DSM-IV, 1994). Abnormal grief can be accompanied by guilt, feelings of hopelessness, and persistent hallucinations. It may manifest with apparently incongruous behaviours or dramatic somatization, such as weakness of a limb mimicking where the deceased had had a stroke. Other phenomena include mummification, where possessions and the room or house the person inhabited are preserved in stasis by the bereaved.

The relationship between bereavement and depression is well recognized but perhaps not clearly understood. By DSM convention, a major depressive episode is diagnosed, instead of bereavement, if symptoms of depression are present two or more months after the loss, or the following symptoms are present: a) guilt about things other than actions taken or not taken by the survivor at the time of the death; b) thoughts of death other than the survivor feeling that he or she would be better off dead or should have died with the deceased person; c) morbid preoccupation with worthlessness; d) marked psychomotor retardation; e) prolonged and marked functional impairment; and f) hallucinatory experiences other than thinking that he or she hears the voice of, or transiently sees the image of, the deceased person. But as Bhugra and Becker (2005) note, the point at which grief is considered to have crossed the threshold to acquire the attributes of a depressive illness is largely based on a Western construct for the diagnosis of abnormal grief and as such does not take into account different cultural expressions of bereavement. The importance of placing these expressions of grief in the appropriate cultural context is essential in differentiating between abnormal and normal reactions to loss.

For example, in a study of the palliative care experience of Bangladeshi patients and their carers in east London, recent migration, linguistic barriers, religious beliefs, and financial issues impacted the ability to optimize pain control in patients and the grieving process of family members; burial of the deceased in Bangladesh and social support from family and friends were potentially helpful in the grieving process (Spruyt, 1999). Another illustration of the importance of culture in the expression of grief comes from a case report of bereavement in an Ethiopian female refugee. Her symptoms of grief were complicated by her inability to perform her culturally sanctioned purification rituals because of her relocation. Compounding her problem, she was erroneously diagnosed at various times due to the use of Western derived diagnostic criteria and a lack of appreciation of the cultural differences in the presentation of grief by clinicians (Schreiber, 1995).

Abnormal grief and mental illness

Risk factors for abnormal grief reactions include prior mental health problems; sudden or unexpected death and circumstances where grieving is suppressed (for example, because of needing to appear strong for the sake of one's children). Many migrants will have been exposed to these and similar circumstances including frankly traumatic circumstances such as war (e.g. Somalia 1991–1993), genocide (Rwanda 1994), discrimination against an ethnic or religious group (Kurds in Iraq), famine, or the fear of political persecution. The process of migration itself can be a significant source of distress, the migrant having to endure long journeys marred by the uncertainty of when one might be turned back and physical hardship.

All of these add up to a considerably increased risk for abnormalities in the grieving process as well as for the risk of all forms of mental illness. A systematic review found refugees to be ten times more likely to suffer PTSD (Fazel *et al.*, 2005). A US study of mental health in Cambodian refugees 20 years after resettlement found that rates of PTSD and depression were still much above the population average (Marshall *et al.*, 2005). This diagnosis may be necessary but not sufficient for a full formulation and appropriate intervention. Diagnoses such as PTSD are to some degree culture-bound themselves, and caution needs to be exercised when applying them across cultural borders. The diagnosis does not account for either the culture-specific modes of communicating distress and seeking help, or for patterns of grief. Indeed, it necessarily carries assumptions about what behaviour is normal. This has been termed the 'category fallacy' by Arthur Kleinman, a psychiatrist and anthropologist (Kleinman, 1977), whilst others contest the validity if not reliability of PTSD (Rosen *et al.*, 2008).

Besides depression, bereavement has been associated with anxiety and other mood disorders, and even with psychotic illness; again, misinterpretation of the cultural expressions of grief by Western trained clinicians and their diagnostic criteria of psychiatric disorders can lead to misdiagnosis. Undoubtedly, people who have migrated due to political upheaval or war may have witnessed or participated in combat and torture; thus, affected individuals may have PTSD and bereavement, as these diagnoses are not mutually exclusive. Patterns of grief from other cultures may resemble the presentation of major mental illness, but equally grief may trigger it.

Cultural bereavement

Maurice Eisenbruch, an Australian psychiatrist and anthropologist, coined the term 'cultural bereavement' following his experiences of working with Southeast Asian refugees in the USA and Australia. In his words, 'many victims manifest a pervasive suffering that can have a widespread effect on personality and behaviour. It is not simply a result of 'stress' or psychiatric disorder but seems to arise from their feelings of massive loss'. He defined cultural bereavement as:

> 'the experience of the uprooted person – or group – resulting from loss of social structures, cultural values and self-identity: the person – or group – continues to live in the past, is visited by supernatural forces from the past while asleep or awake, suffers feelings of guilt over abandoning culture and homeland, feels pain if memories of the past begin to fade, but finds constant images of the past (including traumatic images) intruding into daily life, yearns to complete obligations to the dead, and feels stricken by anxieties, morbid thoughts, and anger that mar the ability to get on with daily life'.
>
> (Eisenbruch, 1990)

Describing how this was an important concept in his understanding of the experience of Cambodian refugees, Eisenbruch argues that cultural bereavement complements diagnoses such as PTSD, by adding depth to the formulation and clarifying where psychopathology may in fact be an understandable response to massive loss (Eisenbruch, 1991).

Our hypothesis is that the migrant experience is mediated through and influenced by cultural and ethnic identity (also see Ruiz *et al.* in this volume). Cultural bereavement is not only helpful in drawing attention to the grief felt over what has been left behind, but it is also helpful in thinking about local resources in the host country that can help assuage it. Just as the bereaved individual must 'move on' to a new role so too must the culturally bereft find a balance between letting go of the past and embracing the present.

Cultural identity and assimilation

One key term to describe the adjustment from one culture to another is that of cultural assimilation (Berry, 2007). It encompasses the notion of a shift in cultural identity to incorporate more or less of the cultural characteristics of the host nation and 'to do, when in Rome as the Romans do'. But to consider this, we must first clarify what is meant by cultural identity.

Cultural identity itself is a complex construct. It describes the many facets of someone's identity which are informed by the values of a particular culture or cultures. This may include aspects of religious beliefs, customs around food, and leisure preferences, and less clearly aspects of behaviour and character (see later). Such values, when shared, can preserve the identity of a minority community and foster a sense of belonging, often reinforced particularly by religion and rites of passage.

Bhugra (2004a) writes of the importance of linguistic competence and economic stability as determinant factors prompting individuals to eventually leave their non-dominant cultural group, which typically is geographically bound, and venture into the dominant culture. Returning to models of individual development, this draws parallels with Bowlby's theory of a 'secure base': a stable, safe attachment, which gives an infant security from which to venture out and explore (Bowlby, 2005).

Whilst a strong cultural identity within a community can be helpful in this way, cultural differences can be stressful and result in problems with self-esteem and resulting depression. Cultural bereavement may be one factor in post-migration stresses with accompanying cultural confusion, increased feelings of alienation, and depression. New societies' attitudes to refugees and degrees of relative and absolute disadvantage may further compound the risk of mental disorder (Bhugra and Becker, 2005).

Ethnic density and social capital

Successful adaptation is likely to be influenced by the similarity between the culture of origin and new culture, acceptance by the new culture, and access to an expatriate community that the person can relate to. The ethnic density hypothesis predicts that in geographical areas where an immigrant lives in close proximity to a large number of people from the same minority, shared values and health communication styles increase this informal support and reduce morbidity. Research findings are mixed, but interestingly a recent study based on UK Census data found that perceived rather than actual measured ethnic density was associated with lower levels of ill health (Stafford *et al.*, 2009). Developing the concept of ethnic density further, *social capital* is defined as the norms and networks that enable collective action (Putnam, 1993). The network relationships are sometimes referred to in terms of 'bonding' and 'bridging' ties between people. Bonding ties are those that strengthen the cohesion of a social group, typified by high levels of mutual trust, loyalty, and shared responsibility.

The benefits include caring for vulnerable members of the group, but the other side of the coin are more negative characteristics of intolerance of those who do not 'fit in' to the structures and rules of the group. Bridging ties, on the other hand, describe the wider links between diverse groups, including broad networks of friends and acquaintances and business partners' wider community. It is thought to promote social inclusion and is generally viewed as positive. Again, whilst this has good construct validity, research findings are complex. A large study of South London communities, for example, found a non-linear relationship between rates of psychosis and measures of social cohesion, trust, and social disorganization, suggesting that although some cohesion provides support and regulates stress, it can also be toxic for the few people who for whatever reason are cast out and excluded (Kirkbride *et al.*, 2008).

Collective and individualistic cultures

Cultures have been described as collective or individualistic (Hofstede, 1980). A society which is collective or socio-centric, values shared responsibility, group solidarity, and emotional inter-dependence (e.g. China, Vietnam). One which is individualistic or ego-centric values more highly self-determination, emotional independence, and autonomy (e.g. USA, Australia). Bhugra (2004b) has previously observed that the move from a collective to an individualistic culture is more likely to be experienced as difficult by socio-centric individuals and that cultural congruity rather than ethnic density factors alone may be particularly important in buffering against the dissonance that can result from the clash between the individual's and broader cultural values. On the other hand, someone who is egocentric and driven by self-determined goals may thrive on moving to an individualistic culture from a collectivist one.

Finally, the distinction between cultural values and lay beliefs about national character should be made. Whilst different cultures value different behaviours and attitudes, shared beliefs about national identity may hold up the notion of a national character, which exemplifies these. In a study of 4000 people from 49 countries, beliefs about national character were found to be reliable but unrelated to actual measured personality profiles of individuals from different countries. In other words, this suggests that whilst people may hold different values and communicate differently, actual personality traits do not differ with nationality (Terracciano et al., 2005). Perhaps cultural factors can be misconstrued as personality.

Help-seeking, assessment, and the provision of care

How people present emotional distress and who they choose to consult is strongly influenced by culture (Rogler and Cortes, 1993). People from the Indian subcontinent or China may, for example, consult doctors with physical symptoms at times of stress when a presentation of anxiety or depression may be expected in Western cultures. Not being familiar with such differences can lead to misdiagnosis and sub-optimal treatment, and indeed it can be argued that this can happen on a public health level, such as the WHO's policy on treating Indian women presenting with abnormal vaginal discharge with empirical antibiotics when in fact psychosocial interventions are called for in the majority of cases (Patel et al., 2005).

The term *cultural competence* describes the ability of practitioners to recognize and work with cultural variants of ill health. It in turn overlaps with the *ecological approach* to thinking about a patient in their environment, the resources they can access in their community, and working with community leaders or culture-specific healers.

Cultural competence in assessment includes determining how experiences of loss may be contributing to a refugee's mental distress. Eisenbruch (1990) proposed a semi-structured interview to serve as a framework which clinicians can use to approach some understanding of cultural bereavement. The interview takes into account the language and cultural constructs of the bereaved individual and explores the following, which are further described later: a) memories of family and the past; b) communication with the past, including experiencing ghosts and spirits; c) survivor guilt, including its expression through dreams, and impact upon recollection of the past; d) experiences of death; and e) anger and ambivalence (Eisenbruch, 1990). It also incorporates exploration of religious belief and practice, stressing the potential benefit of help seeking through 'traditional' treatments.

Memories of the past

In carrying out such an assessment, one can explore first preoccupation with the past and feelings around it. How much does the person find themselves preoccupied by the past? What triggers those thoughts? What feelings or emotions are elicited? This begins to explore the person's memories of their former home. One can then proceed to enquire after intrusions of the past into the present, be it misperceptions, feelings of a presence in the room, or hallucinations and ghosts. The behaviour and apparent motives of any ghosts or visitations should be enquired after. What do they say? Are they helpful or do they goad and beckon the person towards death? If flashbacks of a traumatic experience are volunteered, PTSD symptoms can be gently explored further.

Dreams are often not explicitly discussed or volunteered but can also be useful inroads into the patient's experience and should be explored fully—the sequence, the people who feature in it, death, salvation, or religious themes. Dissociative symptoms such as derealization, dream-like states, may be culturally sanctioned and judged normal and appropriate.

Preservation of the past

In her work with Chilean exiles in the UK, Liliana Muñoz, an anthropologist, described the theme of the fear of losing one's culture and memories by displacement as the new cultural norms are learned (Muñoz, 1980). She draws a parallel between the effects of exile she observed and atypical grief. Fear of losing the past, and indeed fear of the new, can lead to idealization and mummification of the lost home, where fading memories are rehearsed, preserved, and distorted and the homeland progressively idealized by comparison with the new culture. Questions about the person's feelings about their future, fears of forgetting their previous home, current memories, and whether they are fading can steer the interview in this direction. It should be noted that, in common with atypical grief, some refugees appear to relish their new environment and engage it with zeal, difficulties relating to identity and belongingness becoming manifest only much later.

Guilt, anger, and reproach

Refugees from conflict and famine can be haunted by survivor guilt, whether for friends and relatives who did not survive, or who were left behind. They can also feel angry in the same way—that somebody didn't survive or make the journey. Their own survival may be experienced as arbitrary and a fluke. The most difficult emotions are dissonant ones, where feelings of grief and sadness have to be carried with conflicting feeling of anger or reproach, relief, and guilt about feeling relieved. Exploring feelings about home, conflicts between seeing it as good and bad, relatives left behind, should be done with tact and if there is sufficient engagement some attempt can be made to normalize dysphoric experiences of conflicting emotions by describing how they can commonly occur in grief.

Guilt deserves special mention because it has distinctly different currency in other cultures. Within Christian, individualistic traditions it is very common in depression as part of self-reproach and reduced attribution bias (the normal psychological mechanism by which people attribute successes to their own actions and failure to those of others). However, for example, in Buddhist cultures there is a core belief in events being interconnected, and so if one does something bad, compensatory events can be expected to naturally counterbalance it. Guilt is not tied to self-blame and self-criticism in the same way, it is not as common in depression. Importantly, when it is mentioned, one cannot assume to know its object, but the explicit cause should be explored, lest it be on behalf of someone else, on behalf of a rejecting host community, or other collective notions.

Having elicited symptoms and difficulties, the interviewer can gather information on cultural norms and protective or healing rituals. These may become relevant if support can be accessed locally and help the person consolidate their memories and experience.

Religious beliefs, leave-taking ceremonies, and rituals of grief in the homeland

Religious or spiritual practices and rituals can serve as protective factors, but may rely in part on a cohesive group or community which may be absent. However, in some instances refugees are able to access healers or religious leaders from their background in their host community. In such cases collaboration can be very fruitful. Cultural expectations for coping with loss and grief can be enquired after from the person or an informant. This can help ascertain which symptoms are culturally normal.

Current (potential) supports and resources

Finally, explicit consideration should be given to the potential for accessing local supports if there is a local community with a background shared with that person. Creating links with informal community leaders and religious centres is perhaps an uncomfortable proposition but adds a great deal to creating a management plan which is meaningful to the patient (Miller and Rasco, 2004).

Other examples

Given the origins of this model in work with East Asian refugees in Western countries, one could speculate whether it is not in some way culture-bound itself. A broader reading, however, finds recognizable themes in case reports and writing from a broad range of geographies and backgrounds. Below are examples taken from internal displacement in the USA, and writing on exile.

Internal displacement

'It feels as though my skin has been ripped off and I am exposed, just dangling there, lost amidst a group of people. I do not know as I search for my place, my new skin. I fervently try to sew together ripped shards of the old me, hoping they will hold. To my dismay they never do and so I continue my search for my new skin' (Dugan, 2007).

Reading this, one can recognize the suggestion of a dissociative experience or post-traumatic shock. However, it is the subjective report of displacement, which, on a full reading, stresses the process of mourning for a lost home. The author was (at that time) a nursing student displaced by hurricane Katrina from New Orleans, USA, in 2005. She transferred to a nearby city and did not suffer the more total loss experienced by international refugees, but nonetheless struggled to come to terms with her feelings, specifically those of loss.

The long-term impact of displacement and exile

'Exile is strangely compelling to think about but terrible to experience. It is the unhealable rift between a human being and a native place, between the self and its true home: its essential sadness can never be surmounted' (Said, 2000).

Edward Said, a Palestinian brought up in Egypt for much of his childhood before moving to the USA, was a historian well known for his writing on Western ideas of the East and the concept of otherness. In an essay on exile, he cites the work of Joseph Conrad, a Polish writer exiled in Britain, whose novels are populated by characters who cannot quite fully integrate with those around them. Reflecting, he writes that he did not recognize how much he identified with them until an (ultimately terminal) diagnosis late in his middle age caused deep anxieties about his scattered, restless life to resurface. He found himself writing an autobiographical letter to his mother, deceased some two years previously, to consolidate his own feelings of rootlessness (Said, 1997).

Joseph Conrad, whilst patriotic about the idea of Poland, did not return there when it was reinstated following WWI. Similarly, other displaced people find that following a prolonged absence, the sense of loss is not remedied by returning home even if that is a possibility. This is in part because memories of home are static, whereas life carries on, communities and countries change. For example, Dominican economic migrants returning home from the UK after decades away report an ambivalent experience. Whilst not discounting the positive aspects of return, often there is a sense that they do not belong in the Dominican Republic just as they did not belong in the UK (Sorhaindo and Pattullo, 2009). Similarly, a recent study of refugees in Germany who were forced to return once it was safe to do so, demonstrated increased psychiatric morbidity (von Lersner *et al.*, 2008).

Conclusions

In seeing patients, the importance of empathy, engagement, and reaching a shared understanding of their difficulties has long been appreciated. Cultural and language differences make this a more challenging task for the clinician, but in addition to these, the sense of loss that refugees experience can be an unrecognized domain. Being mindful of this by applying the familiar concept of grief and bereavement aids a fuller formulation.

Familiar presentations of atypical grief can be observed, whether the mummification of the past, delayed presentation of grief and depressive symptoms, or prolonged feelings of a lost attachment. The symptoms themselves are modulated by cultural factors with the result that phenomena such as visitations by ghosts, or somatization, are not uncommonly encountered. The sources for much of this material come from not psychiatry but anthropology, sociology, and literature. Remembering that all knowledge comes from experience, the clinician may apply simple questions directed around loss and the idioms of distress in that person's culture. These may reveal themes that will otherwise be missed.

References

Alighieri, D. (2007). *Paradiso*. New York: Doubleday.

Berry, J.W. (2007). Acculturation and identity. In D. Bhugra and K. S. Bhui (Eds.), *Textbook of Cultural Psychiatry*. Cambridge: Cambridge University Press.

Bhugra, D. (2004a). Migration, distress and cultural identity. *British Medical Bulletin* **69**: 129–141.

Bhugra, D. (2004b). Migration and mental health. *Acta Psychiatrica Scandinavia* **109**: 243–258.

Bhugra, D. and Becker, M.A. (2005). Migration, cultural bereavement and cultural identity. *World Psychiatry* **4**: 18–24.

Bowlby, J. (1980). *Attachment and Loss*. New York: Basic Books.

Bowlby, J. (2005). *A Secure Base*. London: Routledge.

Dugan, B. (2007). Loss of identity in disaster: How do you say goodbye to home? *Perspectives in Psychiatric Care* **43**: 41–46.

DSM-IV. (1994). *Diagnostic and Statistical Manual of Mental Disorders, 4th ed*. Washington DC: American Psychiatric Press.

Eisenbruch, M. (1990). The cultural bereavement interview: A new clinical research approach for refugees. *Psychiatrical Clinics of North America* **13**: 715–735.

Eisenbruch, M. (1991). From post-traumatic stress disorder to cultural bereavement: diagnosis of Southeast Asian refugees. *Social Science and Medicine* **33**: 673–680.

Fazel, M., Wheeler, J., and Danesh, J. (2005). Prevalence of serious mental disorder in 7000 refugees resettled in western countries: A systematic review. *Lancet* **365**: 1309–1314.

Freud, S. (1953). Mourning and melancholia. In *The Standard Edition of the Complete Psychological Works of Sigmund Freud, Vol* 14. London: Hogarth Press and Institute of Psycho-Analysis.

Hofstede, G. (1980). *Culture's Consequences: International Differences in Work-Related Values*. Newbury Park, CA: Sage.

Kirkbride, J.B., Boydell, J., Ploubidis, G.B., *et al.* (2008). Testing the association between the incidence of schizophrenia and social capital in an urban area. *Psychological Medicine* **38**: 1083–1094.

Kleinman, A.M. (1977). Depression, somatization and the 'new cross-cultural psychiatry'. *Social Science and Medicine* **11**: 3–10.

Kübler-Ross, E. (1969). *On Death and Dying*. New York: Macmillan.

Marshall, G.N., Schell, T.L., Elliott, M.N., Berthold, S.M., and Chun, C.A. (2005). Mental health of Cambodian refugees 2 decades after resettlement in the United States. *Journal of American Medical Association* **294**: 571–579.

Matchett, W.F. (1972). Repeated hallucinatory experiences as a part of the mourning process among Hopi Indian women. *Journal for the Study of Interpersonal Processes* **35**: 185–194.

Miller, K.E. and Rasco, L.M. (Eds.). (2004). *The Mental Health of Refugees: Ecological Approaches to Healing and Adaptation*. Mahwah, NJ: Lawrence Erlbaum Associates.

Muñoz, L. (1980). Exile as bereavement: socio-psychological manifestations of Chilean exiles in Great Britain. *British Journal of Medical Psychology* **53**: 227–232.

Patel, V., Pednekar, S., Weiss, H., *et al.* (2005). Why do women complain of vaginal discharge? A population survey of infectious and pyschosocial risk factors in a South Asian community. *International Journal of Epidemiology* **34**: 853–862.

Putnam, R.D. (1993). *Making Democracy Work: Civic Traditions in Modern Italy*. Princeton, NJ: Princeton University Press.

Rogler, L.H. and Cortes, D.E. (1993). Help-seeking pathways: A unifying concept in mental health care. *American Journal of Psychiatry* **150**: 554–561.

Rosen, G.M., Spitzer, R.L., and McHugh, P.R. (2008). Problems with the post-traumatic stress disorder diagnosis and its future in DSM V. *British Journal of Psychiatry* **192**: 3–4.

Said, E. (1997). No reconciliation allowed. In A. Aciman, C. Simic, B. Mukherjee, E. Said, and E. Hoffman (Eds.), *Letters of Transit: Reflections on Exile, Identity, Language, and Loss*, pp. 87–115, NY: New Press.

Said, E. (2000). Reflections on Exile. In *Reflections on Exile and Other* Essays. Cambridge, MA: Harvard University Press, pp. 173–187.

Schreiber, S. (1995). Migration, traumatic bereavement and transcultural aspects of psychological healing: Loss and grief of a refugee woman from Begameder county in Ethiopia. *British Journal of Medical Psychology* **68**: 135–142.

Sorhaindo, C. and Pattullo, P. (2009). *Home Again: Stories of Migration and Return*. Dominica and London: Papillote Press.

Spruyt, O. (1999). Community-based palliative care for Bangladeshi patients in east London. Accounts of bereaved carers. *Palliative Medicine* **13**: 119–129.

Stafford, M., Becares, L., and Nazroo, J. (2009). Objective and perceived ethnic density and health: findings from a United Kingdom general population survey. *American Journal of Epidemiology* **170**: 484–493.

Terracciano, A., Abdel-Khalek, A.M., Adam, N., *et al.* (2005). National character does not reflect mean personality trait levels in 49 cultures. *Science* **310**: 96–100.

Von Lersner, U., Elbert, T., and Neuner, F. (2008). Mental health of refugees following state-sponsored repatriation from Germany. *BioMed Central Psychiatry* **8**: 88.

Chapter 16

Child refugees and refugee families

Julia Huemer and Panos Vostanis

Introduction

The impact of large-scale population displacement, migration, conflicts, and disasters leading to humanitarian crises across the globe is attracting increasing attention by the public, media, legislation, and welfare policy (Seaman and Maguire, 2005). The rapid increase of unaccompanied minors and children of asylum seeking and refugee families has often taken Western governments and services by surprise, because of the unprecedented extent, multiplicity, and nature of needs of these young people. The emerging evidence from epidemiological and service-based studies is just beginning to inform interventions and service models. This chapter discusses the mental health and related needs of refugee children and their parents, in the context of research, practice, and service development.

Definitions and extent of the problem

There are currently 31.7 million people under the protection of the United Nations High Commissioner for Refugees (UNHCR), nearly 44% of them are under 18 years of age, and 10% are under the age of 5 (UNHCR, 2008). A counted 192 countries are situated in the region of armed conflicts ongoing in the world (The Ploughshares Monitor, 2008), making the challenge of addressing the needs of refugees a global phenomenon. The UNHCR's founding mandate defines refugees as people who are outside their country, and cannot return owing to a well-founded fear of persecution because of their race, religion, nationality, political opinion, or membership of a particular social group. When people flee their own country and seek sanctuary in another state, they often have to apply for 'asylum'—the right to be recognized as bona fide refugees, and to receive legal protection and material assistance (UNHCR, 2008).

The word 'child' is used in the Guidelines on the Formal Determination of the Best Interests of the Child (Formal Determination of the Best Interests of the Child, 2008) in accordance with the definition contained in Article 1 of the Convention on the Rights of a Child (CRC – United Nations Convention on the Rights of a Child, 2008). In line with the CRC, 'a child means every human being below the age of 18 years unless, under the law applicable to the child, majority is attained earlier'.

Policies in terms of asylum seeking as well as legislative frameworks differ considerably throughout Europe. The idea of a common European policy on immigration was first discussed at the Seville European Council in 2002, based on The Amsterdam Treaty, which has been in force since 1999, by recognizing that immigration and asylum questions could not be solved purely at national level. As of now, when refugees in Europe have their asylum applications rejected, they remain in custody pending deportation. Taking into account that this can last up to several years, this long time span of insecurity prevents naturalization and is especially traumatic for children. The EU is now trying to improve this problem by implementing a new legislative framework, the 'return' directive, which lays down a maximum period of custody and a ban on re-entry into the EU by deportees. This would be one part of the common immigration policy that the European Union is planning to achieve. Other basic principles should involve measures to promote legal immigration by skilled workers (the Blue Card directive), and a third directive that would penalize employers of illegal immigrants and therefore discourage clandestine working (European Parliament, 2008).

Mental health problems among children and young people

The experiences of war and political violence have considerable impact on the psychosocial well-being and mental health of children and adolescents, as has been documented by previous research. Among mental health problems of refugee children and adolescents, PTSD and its comorbidity spectrum have been most extensively examined. Refugee children and adolescents are described to suffer from anxiety and depression, anger and violence, psychic numbing, paranoia, insomnia, and an increased awareness of death (Garbarino and Kostelny, 1996). They are at high risk of developing PTSD and depressive disorders, which are often comorbid (Thabet et al., 2004). Trauma severity is a significant predictor of trauma response (Thabet and Vostanis, 1999; Shaw, 2003). Other factors such as the poor mental health of parents (Ajdukovic and Ajdukovic, 1993), and female gender (Smith et al., 2002) have been negatively associated with the mental health of refugee adolescents. Pre-trauma psychopathology has been found to predict the development of PTSD (Engelhard et al., 2003). Felsman et al. (1990), though, pointed out that there is no way of truly determining if the psychological distress that is experienced by refugee adolescents is caused by pre-departure difficulties and experiences, departure stress, transitional stress, post-arrival stress (adaptation to new life), or the cumulative effect of all these factors.

As a point of critical consideration, research on development and psychopathology must take into account culturally embedded aspects (Vostanis, 2007). Additionally, assessments of war-affected youths measure, in most cases, loss and adversity (Lustig *et al.*, 2004). This perspective may sometimes ignore child refugees' resilience and coping strategies (Betancourt and Khan, 2008). In addition, other aspects beyond the assessment of trauma and loss must be integrated into future research and service agendas. These include neurobiological influences, assessment of the whole range of psychopathology, the interface between personality and psychopathology, the influence of legislative factors on mental health problems, prevalence of psychopathology examining the pathway from trauma to aggression, post-migratory stressors, and resilience-related aspects. In terms of study designs, the implementation of interventional and longitudinal studies is of great importance.

Vulnerability factors

Mental health problems and disorders in childhood and young life are associated with a range of environmental factors, both chronic and acute, within the child's family, school, and wider community. Such factors may interact with a child's intrinsic characteristics, in predicting severity and continuation of mental health problems in later life (Rutter, 2005). These can be counteracted by protective factors, which also offer escape routes for every child and young person. Although it is difficult to determine the extent of children's vulnerability, some young population groups often stand out in their exposure to trauma, which consists of severe and ongoing adversities such as physical, sexual, and/ or emotional abuse and neglect; experience of domestic violence within the family; and family conflict or breakdown (Vostanis, 2004). These traumatic experiences have not only a direct impact on their mental health and well-being, but also indirect effects through secondary difficulties (for example, offending, school exclusion, or substance abuse), and multiple changes in their life circumstances such as being placed in public care or becoming homeless. Certain factors are of prominent risk for refugee children, and these are related to both their previous experiences and their adjustment to a new society (Hodes, 2000).

The impact of war and related trauma on children has been widely studied in recent years (Shaw, 2003; Barenbaum *et al.*, 2004). Earlier research on the links between traumatic events and child psychopathology, predominantly

PTSD and other emotional presentations (Thabet and Vostanis, 1999; Thabet *et al.*, 2002), has been followed by attempts at understanding the mechanisms that underpin this association, hence better inform future interventions (Thabet *et al.*, 2008a). Such factors are predominantly related to the impact of war on the family and wider community systems, and may vary in different circumstances, including the meaning given to different types of conflict (Jones and Kafetsios, 2005). Lack of basic needs, displacement of communities, collapse of social support networks, and internal migration, affect adults and children (Paardekooper *et al.*, 1999; Yurtbay *et al.*, 2003). The same applies to exposure to violence by witnessing or hearing about deaths, injuries, and torture in their immediate and extended group. Longstanding deprivation and poverty in refugee camps accentuate the acute impact of war trauma. In some conflicts, exposure to ongoing trauma mitigates against the introduction of protective factors (Altawil *et al.*, 2008). Mental health problems such as PTSD have been found to persist or recur well after children's move to a different country (Almqvist and Brandell-Forsberg, 1997; Ahmad *et al.*, 2008).

Children's cognitive capacity is important in processing the threat of conflict and violence, which in turn impact on their mental health (Carlton-Ford *et al.*, 2008). Parents' experiences and perceptions of trauma have consistently been found to both precipitate and sustain child mental health problems. Parental morbidity may have a number of effects, particularly through impairing their parenting skills (Qouta and Odeb, 2005; Thabet *et al.*, 2008b), conversely parental support has been found to exert a moderating effect (Thabet *et al.*, 2009).

Refugee children are also largely affected by socioeconomic adversities and social exclusion following immigration. A number of studies have established risk factors such as long-term parental unemployment (Tousignant *et al.*, 1999), low support living arrangements (Hodes *et al.*, 2008), discrimination (Oppedal *et al.*, 2005), and associated physical ill health (Ackerman, 1997). The latter can particularly affect unaccompanied minors, who may have to live in children's homes, hostels, semi- or independent lodgings, or with foster carers of usually different backgrounds and experiences (Papageorgiou *et al.*, 2000). Acquiring a new language and the social aspects of communication are of importance (Leavey *et al.*, 2004), and can compound both academic achievement and social integration (Kolaitis *et al.*, 2003). Cultural and religious beliefs often underpin coping and disenfranchising mechanisms, in relation to the children's country of origin and the receiving society, although practitioners should remain open and not stereotype largely heterogeneous refugee groups (Whittaker *et al.*, 2005).

Resilience and protective factors

Resilience is a 'dynamic state that enables an individual to function adaptively despite significant stressors, by utilizing certain protective factors to moderate the impact of certain risk factors' (Rutter, 1985). Three components of resilience are described, accounting for the fact that children and adolescents display reactions, ranging from severe PTSD to the absence of any mental health problem when facing adversity (Werner and Smith, 1982; Yehuda *et al.*, 2006); individual characteristics (such as shown by Garmezy, 1991; and Tugade and Fredrickson, 2004); family protective factors (Cowen, 1988); and community protective factors (Hechtman, 1991). Although to date there has been limited evidence on resilience mechanisms among war-affected children, several studies report findings which support the concept mentioned earlier.

Adequate emotional expression, supportive family relations, good peer relations, and pro-sociality were described as the main indicators of resilience in a sample of refugee children whose parents had been traumatized and were suffering from PTSD (Daud *et al.*, 2008). Among a sample of 57 young Khmer who had resettled in Montreal as a consequence of the Khmer Rouge regime and were followed from early to late adolescence, Rousseau *et al.* (2003) found that the preservation of traditional values might have contributed to explain the association between the families' exposure to political violence and the adolescents' psychosocial adjustment in the host country. Kanji *et al.* (2007) described absolute faith in Allah (God), family support, and community support as protective factors among war-affected Afghan families. Among unaccompanied refugee minors, Goodman (2004) identified four coping strategies in a qualitative study design, i.e. collectivity, suppression and distraction, making meaning, and the notion of hope after the stressful past.

A further example in terms of community factors was provided by Hodes *et al.* (2008), who stated that unaccompanied separated children might have less psychological distress if supported by high-support living arrangements and general support as they approach the age of 18 years. Qouta and Odeb (2005) emphasized the importance of the home and family surrounding for adaptive child development. This protection is destroyed by war, as exemplified in a sample of Palestinian children.

When analysing resilience in war-affected children and adolescents, particular factors need to be outlined and should be incorporated in future studies. Betancourt and Khan (2008) argued in a recent publication that the emphasis on trauma alone resulted in inadequate attention to factors associated with resilient mental health outcomes in war-affected youth. It was suggested that further research on war-affected children should pay particular attention to coping and meaning at individual level, role of attachment relationships, caregiver health, resources and connection in the family, and social support available in peer and extended social networks. Additionally, cultural and community influences such as attitudes towards mental health and healing, as well as the meaning given to the experience of war itself should be included in the consideration on resilience. This last mentioned directive is in line with Rousseau *et al.*'s (2003) findings, which suggest that the individual meaning of experiencing adversity needs to be mapped on to the collective meaning of experiencing stressful life events, thus emphasizing the importance of the cultural embeddedness of protective factors. Additionally, reflection on resilience should analyze, according to Rousseau *et al.* (1998), the origins where strategies were learned and developed. Furthermore, since war affection, and becoming refugee in childhood form a sequential traumatization process, research on resilience needs to take into account that this construct is partly heritable, and that protective processes operate through both genetic and environmental effects (Kim-Cohen *et al.*, 2004). Eventually, a considerable lack in research on resilience among refugee children and adolescents concerns the analysis of personality factors and its links to psychopathology.

Specific issues of unaccompanied refugee minors

Among the total population of child and adolescent refugees, one group is of particular interest, since it is exposed to cumulative traumatization and a high degree of vulnerability—*unaccompanied refugee minors*. Unaccompanied children and adolescents (or URMs—according to the Convention on the Rights of the Child) (United Nations Convention on the Rights of a Child, 2008) are children and adolescents who have been separated from both parents and relatives, and are not being cared for by an adult who, by law or custom, is responsible for doing so. Previous literature on mental health issues among this group is to a certain extent limited, since it had a considerable emphasis on the assessment of PTSD symptoms (Huemer *et al.*, in submission). Most of these studies revealed higher levels of PTSD symptoms in comparison to the general population and to accompanied refugee children (Huemer *et al.*, in submission).

Unaccompanied refugee children come from a variety of ethnic backgrounds and leave their home countries for diverse reasons. All of them, though, lack close contact to their primary caregiver and have faced sequential stressful life events in the past (war, obstacles of flight), before arriving in a country, where, again, they are confronted with cultural differences and new hurdles of legislative and social systems. Throughout Europe, unaccompanied refugee minors are exposed to an additional institutional conflict. They are treated according to their refugee or asylum seeking status, not primarily as children and adolescents, thus neglecting their needs during a crucial developmental period (Derluyn *et al.*, 2008).

Besides multimodal (Steiner, 2004) and culturally sensitive (Vostanis, 2007) approaches, interventions should take into account that the vulnerability of their age, combined with the adverse events these most unfortunate youths have faced, need to outweigh their legal status. Internationally established guidelines in terms of legislation and interventions are needed, especially when considering children's vulnerability for antisocial trajectories such as prostitution in girls, and drugs and violence in boys (Steiner *et al.*, 1997). Overall, challenges refer to the integration of URMs in a social system, foster or residential care, access to language classes and education, involvement in an employment structure, and prospects after the age of 18. Lack of activity, which is, in many settings, due to the lengthy asylum process, combined with social isolation (being torn away from their cultural and familial systems), does not foster resilience or coping; on the contrary, it places these youths even at more considerable risk for psychiatric morbidity.

Specific issues of children of refugee parents

Similar vulnerability and protective factors operate for asylum seeking and refugee families. In addition, parent- and family-related factors and mechanisms need to be taken into consideration. These include parents' response to trauma and immigration; their mental health status; parenting and rearing attitudes; cultural perceptions of child mental health problems; and the interaction of all these with their new environment.

The association between parental and child psychiatric disorders is well established in different societies (Ramchandani and Stein, 2003). Children of mentally ill parents are at high risk of a range of emotional, behavioural, cognitive, and social difficulties (Leverton, 2003). This relationship between parental and child psychopathology has been found to be confounded by family discord (Rutter and Quinton, 1984) and socioeconomic adversity (Canino *et al.*, 1990). Exposure to external trauma such as war and political conflict may impact interactively on both parents and children, and this interaction can sustain child psychopathology (Thabet *et al.*, 2008b).

Child mental health problems are predicted by negative parenting attitudes, which themselves are associated with previous life events and adversities (Johnson *et al.*, 2001; Vostanis *et al.*, 2006). Attitudes to child rearing and expectations of children's behaviour have been found to differ between cultural groups (Dogra *et al.*, 2005). Moreover, cross-cultural differences appear to be linked to reporting of either more internalizing problems such as withdrawal, somatic complaints, and anxiety/depression symptoms in non-Western child populations, or externalizing problems such as attention problems and delinquent and aggressive behaviour in Western groups (Crinjen *et al.*, 1997). Culture is not the only factor accounting for these differences. For example, child psychopathology may be mediated by socioeconomic adversity across all cultural groups (Stansfield *et al.*, 2004). Cross-cultural differences appear to endure when people immigrate to other societies. For example, there seem to be differences in parents' reporting of children's problems between the indigenous population and the ethnic minorities living in Western countries (Bengi-Arslan *et al.*, 1997). Consequently, refugee families' perceptions and expectations of Western child mental health services usually vary (Thabet *et al.*, 2006). All the previous factors need to be considered in a service, cultural, and ethics context by clinicians involved in the care of refugee children and their parents; for example, which rearing attitudes are deemed acceptable, and when do others cross the child protection boundaries?

Nurturing parenting and strong family supports also play a protective role across all cultures, as discussed earlier in the chapter. Among Palestinian children exposed to political conflict, the risk was moderated if it was faced in the context of a fully functioning family system (Garbarino and Kostelny, 1996). Although war and political conflict by their nature can disturb and break up family life, it has also been found that parents can exert beneficial effects (Virginia *et al.*, 2004); in particular, parental support to children exposed to war trauma (Khamis, 2008; Thabet *et al.*, 2009).

Clinical implications

Assessment

The clinical process can not be separated from its service context, as the latter will determine the route and nature of referrals, clarity, and expectations from a mental health service, and its links and integration to other agencies and their input. As refugee children usually present with multiple needs and require a range of support systems in place, it is essential that care pathways are clear and that agency roles are defined from the outset. Otherwise, it is likely that these will become enmeshed with those of mental health practitioners and services. Consistent information to and training of referrers will help in this direction, although this would be more cost-effective if targeted, i.e. when refugee children are referred by a relatively small group of referrers, and/or have a focal access point to services such as through a refugee organization (statutory or voluntary). In addition to constraints facing referrals of other groups of vulnerable children, requests for a mental health assessment of refugee children are often influenced by their previous history, which can be unknown, hence emotional problems missed if only relying on observations; or, over-attribution of mental difficulties to past trauma without taking into consideration their current circumstances and psychosocial adjustment.

Pending attendance at a child mental health service should be clearly discussed with any child or young person, in order to alleviate their anxieties and address any misperceptions. A number of factors are particularly likely to operate in this group of children, and these should be discussed with their principal carer. Such factors include their completely different understanding and experience of services; mental health concepts; communication barriers; and fears of deportation, which is a common reason for both disengagement (in case it threatens their asylum status) and misunderstanding of the referral (to assist their application) (Herlihy and Turner, 2007). Either way, these thoughts will be prominent in their mind, and should be checked again at the beginning of the assessment (Tufnell, 2003). The importance of ethical issues such as consent and confidentiality can not be stated enough in any contact with refugee children, especially unaccompanied minors (Engebrightsen, 2003).

The mental health practitioner should judge whom to involve in the first session. Corroborative information is valuable, so is the reassuring presence of adults already known to an unaccompanied child (usually a social worker or foster carer, but also a teacher or youth worker). Cultural factors may affect who attends in the case of refugee families. If one considers the interpreter, the number of significant adults, and sensitive issues to be explored, such a setting can be over-bearing and counterproductive by making the child (and potentially their parents) even more anxious and defensive. In such situations, separate meetings or means of collecting information should be sufficient in maximizing clinical engagement and effectiveness.

Interpreters vary in their awareness of mental health issues and degree of involvement, for example when the child becomes distressed. Again, the practitioner should formulate an opinion before and throughout the assessment (or subsequent intervention), so that the child is not exposed to additional stressors that will inhibit their engagement (Raval, 2005). Children's readiness to do so should lead the clinician (rather than the other way round) when to ask difficult questions about their experiences or their uncertain future. Asking many, unstructured, and potentially insensitive questions can result in a poor assessment and put the child off attending in the future. Similarly, avoiding difficult areas will ultimately deprive the child of a rare opportunity to share their thoughts and emotions. What is of ultimate importance is, to place the child's emotional safety first, constantly follow their clues, including their non-verbal behaviours, and consider their history, before deciding how to handle a particular clinical interview. Refugee parents' own worries, perceptions, and values, as well as the child's developmental stage and cognitive capacity, should also be taken into consideration. The latter can be extremely difficult to establish at the beginning, because of communication difficulties, while the history can be fragmented or even missing, with the assessing clinician needing to adjust throughout this process.

When engaged, children have an accurate recollection of trauma, including direct exposure (seeing somebody being killed or dead bodies; witnessing shelling); impact on family and community (forced to leave village or town, separated from family); and cognitive or emotional impact (thought s/he would be killed or die from cold) (Papageorgiou *et al.*, 2000; Yurtbay *et al.*, 2003). The interpretation of children's reported symptoms and mental state, hence the differential psychiatric diagnosis, can be affected by a number of the previously stated factors, as well as by cultural presentations and expression of distress (Weine *et al.*, 1995; Papadopoulos and Hildebrand, 1997). It may, therefore, require more than one assessment and other kinds of observation or information (Rousseau and Drapeau 1998) before establishing the post-traumatic, grief, depressive, somatizing or psychotic nature of the underlying symptoms, or a combination of them (Eisenbruch, 1991). This should lead to an evidence-based treatment plan, usually defining the remit of other supporting agencies.

Service models and interventions

The trend of continuing increase in numbers of asylum seeking and refugee children is likely to continue. Commissioners and planners of welfare, public and mental health services should, therefore, remain regularly informed of service patterns, impact on existing service provision, and the extent to which children's needs are met. In most cases, adjustment of existing mental health services, both in terms of resources and ways of working, should be sufficient, even in inner-city areas. If, however, there is indication of clusters of children and families, for example through the establishment of entry, assessment, or other centres in a particular area, designated service models may be more appropriate. These should be sustainable and mainstreamed into public health funding rather than relying on short-term charity-funded initiatives. The latter can instead be useful in complementing local and central government funds during transitional periods such as the early phase of a refugee centre, and in providing additional educational, social, and leisure activities.

In both scenarios, principles of service provision for other groups of vulnerable children should be followed (Elliott, 2007). These include joint commissioning and care pathways with welfare agencies; establishment of inter-agency networks; joint working between frontline (social care, education, non-statutory) and specialist services to rationalize skills and resources, through consultation and training; preferably direct referral routes; training and continuity of interpreters; and development of applied therapeutic interventions which integrate existing knowledge and evidence with the characteristics of refugee children and young people (Howard and Hodes, 2000; Christie, 2003).

As most studies in recent years have addressed refugee children's needs, there is so far limited evidence on the effectiveness and specificity of therapeutic interventions, other than description of innovative programmes (Brymer *et al.*, 2008). Practice can, however, be informed by the application of interventions for other groups of children who suffered trauma (Vostanis, 2007); from emerging findings with refugee children and young people (Enholt and Yule, 2006); and from studies with adult refugees discussed in previous chapters. Issues that need to be taken into consideration include the integration of mental health treatment with other aspects of the care plan such as housing, education, and the legal process; flexibility, cultural appropriateness, and sensitivity of interventions; children's engagement; and ethics (Cemlyn and Briskman, 2003; Saltzman *et al.*, 2003).

Barnebaum *et al.* (2004) make an interesting distinction between non-specific interventions that promote resilience (such as the important role of education, social and family networks, and working with local communities) and specific individual or group therapeutic techniques. An example of a non-specific resilience-building programme was reported by Harris (2007) on the effects of a psychosocial intervention on group cohesion among African adolescent survivors of war and organized violence. This study established a decrease in symptoms of anxiety, depression, intrusive recollection, and aggression. School belonging was found to be associated with self-efficacy among Somali adolescent refugees resettled in the United States (Kia-Keeting and Ellis, 2007).

Psychotherapeutic modalities should have clear objectives in enhancing the normalization of emotions, exploration and understanding of experiences, or problem-solving and coping strategies (Elliott, 2007; Murray *et al.*, 2008). Enholt and Yule (2006) propose a phased model of intervention in the context of a holistic approach. In their review of existing evidence, the authors detect promising findings from studies of cognitive–behavioural therapy, testimonial psychotherapy, narrative exposure therapy, and eye movement desensitization and reprocessing (EMDR). Therapists should keep an open mind whether children from non-Western cultures can utilize 'talking' techniques, or whether other means may be preferable, at least at the beginning. It is always useful to follow children's clues and definition of difficulties (Montgomery, 2005).

Indeed, there is emerging evidence that refugee children have a range of mental health treatment needs, and that trauma-focused therapy is not always the indicated intervention (Kinzie *et al.*, 2006). The presence of interpreters and parents' perceptions may affect children's ability or willingness to share difficult feelings, and sometimes this may need to be deferred until a later period, when they feel safer, the families are engaged, and their communication/language has improved.

Methodological implications

When conceptualizing research with refugee children and adolescents, several methodological considerations need to be taken into account. These considerations are iteratively and interdependently related to research ethics with particularly vulnerable young populations (Dyregrov *et al.*, 2000). Directives for conducting ethical research have been described through documents such as the American Psychological Association (APA) ethics code (APA 2002), the Belmont Report (National Commission for the Protection of Human Subjects of Biomedical and Behavioral Research 1979) and the Nuremberg Code (1949). These standards should be critically analyzed, particularly when examining groups who are culturally divergent from a European-American-inspired viewpoint, represent a potentially traumatized population, and who are under the age of 18 years. These children and adolescents come from very diverse ethnic backgrounds and cultural systems. This makes it hard to apply culturally sensitive methods; even tools in the mother tongue of the children and adolescents are often not available. Additionally, factors such as obtaining informed consent may turn out as a major challenge.

In terms of cultural sensitivity, it is of great importance to study more profoundly the educational and familial systems in which these youths have been brought up. These factors may considerably influence concepts of personality, psychosocial functioning, and resilience. When looking at it exclusively from an ethical viewpoint, the research design necessitates an analysis of cultural values and norms of that cultural group. Apart from this methodological and ethical approach, feasibility in terms of tracing these youth is frequently a major obstacle. Refugee populations are heterogeneous and often difficult to access, and limited statistical data may make it difficult if a sample is representative, and thus lead to generalizable findings (Spring *et al.*, 2003).

The fact that these children and adolescents can be severely traumatized must be taken into account when organizing a research design. Generally, one risk involves that the participants of the study experience further emotional suffering as a consequence of revisiting traumatic events (Newman and Kaloupek, 2004). In this context, factors such as timing and consequence for each individual are important mediators to analyze vulnerability to distress and outcomes (Beiser and Wickrama, 2004). It is, therefore, of utmost importance to offer immediate as well as long-term mental health support in cases of upcoming behavioural problems or the re-experiencing of traumatic events during the encounter. On an even larger scale, more interdisciplinary and internationally operating research teams should be formed to adequately address the needs of refugee children and adolescents.

Conclusions

In recent years, there has been a dramatic increase in the numbers of refugee and asylum seeking children and young people in Western societies, with a substantial proportion of them being unaccompanied. A growing body of evidence has established that these children have complex and multiple needs, which are related to high prevalence rates of mental health problems. Psychopathology has been found to be associated to vulnerability factors arising both from the children's traumatic experiences in their countries of origin and their immigration circumstances. Parents' responses and mental state play a major role in children's adjustment. These mechanisms also highlight opportunities for future interventions by strengthening resilience, family and social networks, education, and social integration. Despite some favourable policies and interest in meeting refugee children's mental health, their access to appropriate services remains limited and there is scarce knowledge of effective interventions and services. Descriptive studies and evidence from services for other groups of vulnerable children indicate that the development of such services should be needs-led, jointly commissioned and planned between health and social welfare agencies, culturally sensitive, and offering flexible and applied therapeutic interventions.

References

Ackerman, L. (1997). Health problems of refugees. *Journal of the American Board of Family Practice* **10**: 337–348.

Ahmad, A., Von Knorring, A.L., and Sundelin-Wahlsten, V. (2008). Traumatic experiences and post-traumatic stress symptoms in Kurdish children in their native country and exile. *Child and Adolescent Mental Health* **13**: 193–197.

Ajdukovic, M. and Ajdukovic, D. (1993). Psychological well-being of refugee children. *Child Abuse and Neglect* **17**(6): 843–854.

Almqvist, K. and Brandell-Forsberg, M. (1997). Refugee children in Sweden: Post-traumatic stress disorder in Iranian preschool children exposed to organised violence. *Child Abuse and Neglect* **21**: 351–366.

Altawil, M., Harrold, D., and Samara, M. (2008). Children of war in Palestine. *Children in War* **1**: 5–11.

Barenbaum, J., Ruchkin, V., and Schwab-Stone, M. (2004). The psychosocial aspects of children exposed to war: Practice and policy initiatives. *Journal of Child Psychology and Psychiatry* **45**: 41–62.

Beiser, M. and Wickrama, K. (2004). Trauma, time and mental health: A study of temporal reintegration and Depressive Disorder among Southeast Asian refugees. *Psychological Medicine* **34**: 899–910.

Bengi-Arslan, L., Verhulst, F., Van der Ende, J. and Erol, N. (1997). Understanding childhood (problem) behaviours from a cultural perspective: Comparison of problem behaviours and competencies in Turkish immigrant, Turkish and Dutch children. *Social Psychiatry and Epidemiology* **32**: 477–484.

Betancourt, T. and Khan, K. (2008). The mental health of children affected by armed conflict: Protective processes and pathways to resilience. *International Review of Psychiatry* **20**: 317–328.

Brymer, M., Steinberg., Sornborger, J., Layne, C., and Pynoos, R. (2008). Acute interventions for refugee children and families. *Child and Adolescent Psychiatric Clinics of North America* **17**: 625–640.

Canino, G., Bird, H., Rubio-Stipec, M., Bravo, M., and Alegria, M. (1990). Children of parents with psychiatric disorders in the community. *Journal of the American Academy of Child and Adolescent Psychiatry* **29**: 398–406.

Carlton-Ford, S., Ender, M., and Tabatabai, A. (2008). Iraqi adolescents: Self-regard, self-derogation, and perceived threat in war. *Journal of Adolescence* **31**: 53–75.

Cemlyn, S. and Briskman, L. (2003) Asylum, children's rights and social work. *Child and Family Social Work* **8**: 163–178.

Christie, A. (2003). Unsettling the 'social' in social work: Responses to asylum seeking children in Ireland. *Child and Family Social Work* **8**: 223–231.

Crinjen, A., Achenbach, T., and Velhurst, F. (1997). Comparison of problems reported by parents of twelve cultures: Total problems externalizing and internalizing. *Journal of the American Academy of Child and Adolescent Psychiatry* **36**: 1269–1277.

Cowen, E.L. and Work, W.C. (1988). Resilient children, psychological wellness, and primary prevention. *American Journal of Community Psychology* **16**: 591–607.

Daud, A., Af Klinteberg, B., and Rydelius, P. (2008). Resilience and vulnerability among refugee children of traumatized and non-traumatized parents. *Child and Adolescent Psychiatry and Mental Health* **2**: 7.

Derluyn, I. and Broekaert, E. (2008). Unaccompanied refugee children and adolescents: the glaring contrast between a legal and a psychological perspective. *International Journal of Law and Psychiatry* **31**: 319–330.

Dogra, N., Vostanis, P., Abuateya, H., and Jewson, N. (2005). Understanding of mental health and mental illness by Gujarati young people and their parents. *Diversity in Health and Social Care* **2**: 91–98.

Dyregrov, K., Dyregrov, A., and Raundalen, M. (2000). Refugee families' experience of research participation. *Journal of Traumatic Stress* **13**: 413–426.

Eisenbruch, M. (1991). From post traumatic stress disorder to cultural bereavement: Diagnosis of Southeast Asian refugees. *Social Science and Medicine* **33**: 673–680.

Elliott, V. (2007). Interventions and services for refugee and asylum seeking children and families. In P. Vostanis (Ed.), *Mental Health Interventions and Services for Vulnerable Children and Young People,* London: Jessica Kingsley Publishers.

Engebrightsen, A. (2003). The child's – or the state's – best interests? An examination of the ways immigration officials work with unaccompanied asylum seeking minors in Norway. *Child and Family Social Work* **8**: 191–200.

Engelhard, I., Van Den Hout, M., and Kindt, M. (2003). The relationship between neuroticism, pre-traumatic stress, and post-traumatic stress: A prospective study. *Personality and Individual Differences*, **35**: 381–388.

Entholt, K. and Yule, W. (2006). Assessment and treatment of refugee children and adolescents who have experienced war related trauma. *Journal of Child Psychology and Psychiatry* **47**: 1197–1210.

European Parliament. Available at: http://www.europarl.europa.eu/sides/getDoc. do?language=EN&type=IM-PRESS&reference=20080609BKG31068 (accessed December 14, 2008).

Felsman, J.K., Leong, F.T., Johnson, M.C., and Felsman, I.C. (1990). Estimates of psychological distress among Vietnamese refugees: adolescents, unaccompanied minors and young adults. *Social Science and Medicine* **31**(11): 1251–1256.

Formal Determination of the Best Interests of the Child. Available at: www.unhcr.org (accessed November 15, 2008).

Garbarino, J. and Kostelny, K. (1996). The effects of political violence on Palestinian children's behaviour problems: A risk accumulation model. *Child Development* **67**: 33–45.

Garmezy, N. (1991). Resilience in children's adaptation to negative life events and stressed environments. *Pediatrics Annals* **20**: 459–460.

Goodman, J. (2004). Coping with trauma and hardship among unaccompanied refugee youths from Sudan. *Qualitative Health Research* **14**: 1177–1196.

Harris, D. (2007). Dance/movement therapy approaches to fostering resilience and recovery among African adolescent torture survivors. *Torture* **17**: 134–155.

Hechtman, L. (1991). Resilience and vulnerability in long term outcome of attention deficit hyperactive disorder. *Canadian Journal of Psychiatry* **36**: 415–421.

Herlihy, J. and Turner, S. (2007). Asylum claims and memory of trauma: sharing our knowledge. *British Journal of Psychiatry* **191**: 3–4.

Hodes, M. (2000). Psychologically distressed refugee children in the United Kingdom. *Child Psychology and Psychiatry Review* **5**: 57–68.

Hodes, M., Jagdev, D., Chandra, N., and Cunniff, A. (2008). Risk and resilience for psychological distress amongst unaccompanied asylum seeking adolescents. *Journal of Child Psychology and Psychiatry* **49**: 723–732.

Howard, M. and Hodes, M. (2000). Adversity and service utilization of young refugees. *Journal of the American Academy of Child and Adolescent Psychiatry* **39**: 368–377.

Huemer, J., Karnik, N., Voelkl-Kernstock, S., *et al.* (2009). Mental health issues in unaccompanied refugee minors. *Child and Adolescent Psychiatry and Mental Health* **3**(1): 13.

Johnson, J., Cohen, P., Kasen, S., Smailes, E., and Brook, J. (2001). Association of maladaptive parental behaviour with psychiatric disorder among parents and their offspring. *Archives of General Psychiatry* **58**: 453–460.

Jones, L. and Kafetsios, K. (2005). Exposure to political violence and psychological well-being in Bosnian adolescents. *Clinical Child Psychology and Psychiatry* **10**: 157–176.

Kanji, Z., Drummond, J., and Cameron, B. (2007). Resilience in Afghan children and their families: a review. *Paediatric Nursing* **19**: 30–33.

Khamis, V. (2008). Post-traumatic stress and psychiatric disorders in Palestinian adolescents following intifada-related injuries. *Social Science and Medicine* **67**: 1199–1207.

Kia-Keating, M. and Ellis, H. (2007). Belonging and connection to school in resettlement: young refugees, school belonging, and psychosocial adjustment. *Clinical Child Psychology and Psychiatry* **12**: 29–43.

Kim-Cohen, J., Moffitt, T., Caspi, A., and Taylor, A. (2004). Genetic and environmental processes in young children's resilience and vulnerability to socioeconomic deprivation. *Child Development* **75**: 651–668.

Kinzie, J., Cheng, K., Tsai, J., and Riley, C. (2006). Traumatized refugee children: The case for individualized diagnosis and treatment. *Journal of Nervous and Mental Disease* **194**: 534–537.

Kolaitis, G., Tsiantis, J., Madianos, M., and Kotsopoulos, S. (2003). Psychosocial adaptation of immigrant Greek children from the former Soviet Union. *European Child and Adolescent Psychiatry* **12**: 67–74.

Leavey, G., Hollins, K., King, M., Barnes, J., Papadopoulos, C., and Grayson, K. (2004). Psychological disorder amongst refugee and migrant schoolchildren in London. *Social Psychiatry and Psychiatric Epidemiology* **39**: 191–195.

Leverton, T. (2003). Parental psychiatric illness: the implications for children. *Current Opinion in Psychiatry* **16**: 395–402.

Lustig, S., Kia-Keating, M., Knight, W., *et al.* (2004). Review of child and adolescent refugee mental health. *Journal of the American Academy of Child and Adolescent Psychiatry* **43**: 24–36.

Montgomery, E. (2005). Traumatized refugee families: the child's perspective. In P. Berliner, A.G. Julio and J.O. Haagensen (Eds.), *Torture and Organized Violence: Contributions to a Professional Human Rights Response*. Virum: Dansk Psykologisk Forlag.

Murray, L., Cohen, J., Ellis, B., and Mannarino, A. (2008). Cognitive behavioural therapy for symptoms of trauma and traumatic grief in refugee youth. *Child and Adolescent Psychiatric Clinics of North America* **17**: 585–604.

Newman, E. and Kaloupek, D. (2004). The risks and benefits of participating in trauma-focused research studies. *Journal of Traumatic Stress* **17**: 383–394.

Oppedal, B., Roysamb, E., and Heyerdahl, S. (2005). Ethnic group, acculturation, and psychiatric problems in young immigrants. *Journal of Child Psychology and Psychiatry* **46**: 646–660.

Paardekooper, B., De Jong, J., and Hermanns, J. (1999). The psychological impact of war and the refugee situation on south Sudanese children in refugee camps in northern Uganda. *Journal of Child Psychology and Psychiatry* **40**: 529–536.

Papadopoulos, R. and Hildenbrand, J. (1997). Is home where the heart is? Narratives of oppositional discourses in refugee families. In R. Papadopoulos and J. Byng-Hall (Eds.), *Narratives in Systemic Family Therapy*, pp. 206–236, London: Tavistock Clinic Series.

Papageorgiou, V., Frangou-Garunovic, A., Ioardanidou, R., Yule, W., Smith, P., and Vostanis, P. (2000). War trauma and psychopathology in Bosnian refugee children. *European Child and Adolescent Psychiatry* **9**: 84–90.

Qouta, S. and Odeb, J. (2005). The impact of conflict on children: The Palestinian experience. *ournal of Ambulatory Care and Management* **28**; 75–79.

Ramchandani, P. and Stein, A. (2003). The impact of parental psychiatric disorder on children: Avoiding stigma, improving care. *British Medical Journal* **327**: 242–243.

Raval, H. (2005). Being heard and understood in the context of seeking asylum and refuge: Communicating with the help of bilingual co-workers. *Clinical Child Psychology and Psychiatry* **10**: 197–216.

Rousseau, C. and Drapeau, A. (1998). Parent–child agreement on refugee children's psychiatric symptoms: A transcultural perspective. *Journal of the American Academy of Child and Adolescent Psychiatry* **37**: 629–636.

Rousseau, C., Said, T., Gagne, M., and Bibeau, G. (1998). Resilience in unaccompanied minors from the north of Somalia. *Psychoanalysis Review* **85**: 615–637.

Rousseau, C., Drapeau, A., and Rahimi, S. (2003). The complexity of trauma response: A 4-year follow-up of adolescent Cambodian refugees. *Child Abuse and Neglect* **27**: 1277–1290.

Rutter, M. (1985) Resilience in the face of adversity: Protective factors and resistance to psychiatric disorder. *British Journal of Psychiatry* **147**: 598–611.

Rutter, M. (2005). Environmentally mediated risks for psychopathology: Research strategies and findings. *Journal of the American Academy of Child and Adolescent Psychiatry* **44**: 3–18.

Rutter, M. and Quinton, D. (1984). Parental psychiatric disorder: Effects on children. *Psychological Medicine* **14**: 853–880.

Saltzman, W., Layne, C., Steinberg, A., Arslanagic, B., and Pynoos, R. (2003). Developing a culturally and ecologically sound intervention programme for youth exposed to war and terrorism. *Child and Adolescent Psychiatric Clinics of North America* **12**: 319–342.

Seaman, J. and Maguire, S. (2005). ABC of conflict and disaster: The special needs of children and women. *British Medical Journal* **331**: 34–36.

Shaw, J. (2003). Children exposed to war/terrorism. *Clinical Child and Family Psychology Review* **6**: 237–246.

Spring, M., Westermeyer, J., Halcon, L., *et al.* (2003). Sampling in difficult to access refugee and immigrant communities. *Journal of Nervous and Mental Disease* **191**: 813–819.

Stansfield, S., Haines M., Head, J., *et al.* (2004). Ethnicity, social deprivation and psychological distress in adolescents. *British Journal of Psychiatry* **185**: 233–238.

Steiner, H. (2004). *Handbook of Mental Health Interventions in Children and Adolescents: An Integrated Developmental Approach*. San Francisco: Jossey-Bass.

Steiner, H., Garcia, I., and Matthews, Z. (1997). Posttraumatic stress disorder in incarcerated juvenile delinquents. *Journal of the American Academy of Child and Adolescent Psychiatry* **36**: 357–365.

Thabet, A. and Vostanis, P. (1999). Child post-traumatic stress reactions in children of war. *Journal of Child Psychology and Psychiatry* **40**: 385–392.

Thabet, A.A., Abed, Y., and Vostanis, P. (2002). Emotional problems in Palestinian children living in a war zone. *The Lancet* **359**: 1801–1804.

Thabet, A.A., Abed, Y., and Vostanis, P. (2004). Comorbidity of PTSD and depression among refugee children during war conflict. *Journal of Child Psychology and Psychiatry* **45**: 533–542.

Thabet, A.A., El Gammal, H., and Vostanis, P. (2006). Palestinian mothers' perceptions of child mental health problems and services. *World Psychiatry* **5**: 108–112.

Thabet, A.A., Tawahina, A., El Sarraj, E., and Vostanis, P. (2008a). Children exposed to political conflict: Implications for health policy. *Harvard Health Policy Review* **8**: 158–165.

Thabet, A.A., Tawahina, A., El Sarraj, E., and Vostanis, P. (2008b). Exposure to war trauma and PTSD among parents and children in the Gaza Strip. *European Child & Adolescent Psychiatry* 17: 191–199.

Thabet, A.A, Ibraheem, A., Shivram, R., Van Milligen, E., and Vostanis, P. (2009). Parenting support and PTSD in children of a war zone. *International Journal of Social Psychiatry* 55: 226–237.

The Ploughshares Monitor. Available at: http://www.ploughshares.ca/libraries/monitor/monj08j.pdf (accessed November 15, 2008).

Tousignant, M., Habimana E., Biron, C., Malo, C., Sidoli-LeBlanc, E., and Bendris, N. (1999). The Quebec Adolescent Refugee Project: Psychopathology and family variables in a sample from 35 nations. *Journal of the American Academy of Child and Adolescent Psychiatry* 38: 1426–1432.

Tufnell, G. (2003). Refugee children, trauma and the law. *Clinical Child Psychology and Psychiatry* 8: 1359–1045.

Tugade, M. and Fredrickson, B. (2004). Resilient individuals use positive emotions to bounce back from negative emotional experiences. *Journal of Personality and Social Psychology* 86: 320–333.

UNHCR. 2007, Global Trends: Refugees, Asylum-Seekers, Returnees, Internally Displaced and Stateless Persons. Available at: www.unhcr.org (accessed November 15, 2008).

United Nations Convention on the Rights of the Child. Available at: www.unhcr.org (accessed November 15, 2008).

Virginia, G., Holman, E., and Silver, R. (2004). Adolescent vulnerability following the September 11th terrorist attacks: a study of parents and their children. *Applied Developmental Science* 8: 130–142.

Vostanis, P. (2004). Impact, psychological sequelae and management of trauma affecting children. *Current Opinion in Psychiatry* 17: 269–273.

Vostanis, P. (2007). *Mental Health Interventions and Services for Vulnerable Children and Young People.* London: Jessica Kingsley Publishers.

Vostanis, P., Graves, A., Meltzer, H., Goodman, R., Jenkins, R., and Brugha, T. (2006). Relationship between parental psychopathology, parenting strategies and child mental health. *Social Psychiatry and Psychiatric Epidemiology* 41: 509–514.

Weine, S., Becker, D., Mc Glashan, T., *et al.* (1995). Psychiatric consequences of 'ethnic cleansing': clinical assessments and trauma testimonies of newly resettled Bosnian refugees. *Journal of the American Academy of Child and Adolescent Psychiatry* 152: 536–542.

Werner, E. and Smith, R. (1982). *Vulnerable but Invincible: A Longitudinal Study of Resilient Children and Youth.* New York: McGraw-Hill.

Whittaker, S., Hardy, G., Lewis, K., and Buchan, L. (2005). An exploration of psychological well-being with young Somali refugee and asylum-seeker women. *Clinical Child Psychology and Psychiatry* 10: 177–196.

Yehuda, R., Flory, J., Southwick, S., and Charney, D. (2006). Developing an agenda for translational studies of resilience and vulnerability following trauma exposure. *Annals of the New York Academy of Science* 1071: 379–396.

Yurtbay, T., Alyanak, B., Abali, O., Kaynak, N., and Durukan, M. (2003). The psychological effects of forced emigration on Muslim Albanian children and adolescents. *Community Mental Health Journal* 39: 203–212.

Chapter 17

Sexual violence and refugees

Gill Mezey and Ajoy Thachil

Introduction

This chapter will focus on experiences of sexual violence in refugees and asylum seekers. Many refugees and asylum seekers experience rape and sexual violence, because they are fleeing armed conflict and civil unrest, or because they come from societies and communities in which gender based violence (including homophobic violence) and oppression are common. Sexual violence is only one form of persecution, trauma, and losses (including dislocation) reported by asylum seekers, which cumulatively impact on the individual's health and social functioning. The adverse impact on health ranges from the immediate to the long term, with victims experiencing problems with both physical and mental health.

Definitions

In its World Report on Violence and Health (Krug *et al.*, 2002) the World Health Organization defines *violence* as the 'intentional use of physical force or power, threatened or actual, against oneself, another person, or against a group or community, that either results in or has a high likelihood of resulting in injury, death, psychological harm, maldevelopment or deprivation'.

This definition of violence encompasses three domains:

(a) Self-directed violence or suicidal behaviour;

(b) interpersonal violence; and

(c) collective violence consisting of violence committed by larger groups of individuals or states (e.g. hate crimes committed by organized groups, terrorist acts, mob violence, and war).

Of these, the interpersonal domain is further divided into four categories: 1) physical violence; 2) sexual violence; 3) psychological violence; and 4) deprivation or neglect.

The World Health Organisation defines *sexual violence* as 'any sexual act, attempt to obtain a sexual act, unwanted sexual comments or advances, or acts to traffic, or otherwise directed, against a person's sexuality using coercion, by any person regardless of their relationship to the victim, in any setting, including but not limited to home and work' (Krug *et al.*, 2002). Within this definition, *coercion* is defined as including physical force, psychological intimidation, blackmail, or other threats, or taking advantage of an individual who is incapable of giving consent because they are drunk, drugged, asleep, or mentally incapable of understanding the situation (Jewkes *et al.*, 2002). *Rape* is defined as oral, vaginal, or anal penetration with a penis, when the individual did not consent. Penetration with an object other than a penis is assault by penetration (Home Office, 2003).

This public health definition of *sexual violence* includes sexual abuse of mentally or physically disabled people and sexual abuse of children, which are defined as violations of the criminal code in virtually all jurisdictions. However, it also includes a number of other acts that are either not violent or are not classified as sexual violence in the criminal codes of many jurisdictions, for example, forced marriage or cohabitation, sexual harassment, and denial of the right to use contraception or to adopt other measures protecting against sexually transmitted diseases (Jewkes *et al.*, 2002).

The UN Declaration on the Elimination of Violence against Women (Article 1) defines gender based violence as violence that results in, or is likely to result in, physical, sexual, or psychological harm or suffering to women. Gender based violence represents an attack on the victim's sexuality and sexual integrity (male or female) even if they do not involve actual sexual assault. This includes, for instance, being held naked, being taunted, being subjected to sexualized comments, assaults on genitals (including electric shocks), and withholding of sanitary protection (e.g. Asgary *et al.*, 2006). Trafficking for the purpose of sexual exploitation and forced prostitution, including coercing a woman into a sexual act as a condition for allowing or arranging her migration, are also examples of gender based violence.

Although men and boys may be sexually abused and assaulted, the majority of victims are female. Throughout this chapter the pronoun 'she' will be used, although we recognize that the effects of sexual violence are likely to be serious and long lasting for all victims, regardless of gender.

Epidemiology of sexual violence

Women are at greater risk of sexual abuse than men throughout their lives (Gilbert *et al.*, 2008). Between 5 and 10% of girls and 1 and 5% of boys worldwide are exposed to penetrative sexual abuse during childhood. The prevalence is much higher if non-penetrative forms of sexual abuse are included

(Andrews *et al.*, 2004; Gilbert *et al.*, 2008). International comparisons are difficult, partly because of differing definitions of rape and sexual violence. However, in the UK, around 1 in 20 women (4.9%) women claim to have been sexually assaulted at least once since the age of 16, compared with 1 in 200 men (Myhill and Allen, 2002; Walby and Allen, 2004).

Sexual violence against refugees

Sexual violence against refugees is recognized as a serious global problem. Refugees who are most at risk of being subjected to sexual violence are: unaccompanied women and children, children in foster care arrangements, and individuals who are in detention or detention-like situations (UNHCR, 1995).

For many refugees and asylum seekers, the experience of rape and sexual assault occurs on a background of oppression, restricted freedoms, and gender based discrimination, often starting from early childhood (Agger, 1994). Women and girls who are most vulnerable to sexual violence in war are also at greatest risk of various forms of sexual violence in peacetime, such as early or forced marriage, forced cohabitation, abuse by partners, child sexual abuse, forced or coerced prostitution, other forms of sexual exploitation, and sex trafficking, as a consequence of their subordinate role within their cultures (Ward and Vann, 2002).

Refugees and asylum seekers remain vulnerable to sexual victimization and exploitation, even as arrivals in supposedly safe host countries, because of communication difficulties and social exclusion (e.g. poverty, inadequate housing, etc.), which make it more difficult for them to access, or even know about different sources of help and support, including legal advice. Another factor that contributes to this vulnerability is the association between childhood sexual abuse, sex trading in adolescence or adulthood, and sexual risk taking (Senn *et al.*, 2007; Gilbert *et al.*, 2008).

Sexual violence in war and conflict

Sexual violence in war and armed conflict can be classified into two types (Ward and Vann, 2002). The first and most common type is often arbitrary, spontaneous, and random, and is a by-product of a general breakdown in community support systems, social norms, and laws. The second type is planned and systematic, when it is used to destabilize populations, advance ethnic cleansing, express hatred for the enemy, or supply combatants with sexual services.

The widespread use of sexual violence and abuse as a 'weapon of war' has been described in armed conflicts worldwide including: Darfur in Sudan,

Colombia, Algeria, Rwanda, Uganda, Sri Lanka, Somalia, India, Liberia, and Congo, figures of between 40,000 and 50,000 rapes of women have been estimated, during the current conflict (Krug *et al.*, 2002; Wakabi, 2008; Henttonen *et al.*, 2008). Sexual violence may be directly experienced or witnessed by victims. Within some communities, the mere threat of sexual violence and abuse may lead to families and whole communities dispersing, or individuals committing suicide, to avoid what is commonly regarded as a 'fate worse than death' (Beevor, 2003). Mass rapes of women in Berlin by Russian soldiers were documented during the 1945 campaign, which Red Army officers 'had neither the will nor inclination to stop'. Of the 130,000 women who were raped, it is estimated that around 10% subsequently committed suicide. The remainder were so traumatized by their ordeal that most never spoke about or referred to the experience ever again, retreating behind a wall of silence (Beevor, 2003). In the former Yugoslavia, sexual abuse was regarded as a form of ethnic cleansing (Mezey, 1994).

Women and girls are particularly vulnerable to all types of sexual violence in war and conflict situations. This may occur in the midst of fighting, while escaping from their homes, or inside refugee camps. Families may become separated during the chaos of flight. Men may have to leave their families to fight, leaving women to look after their families on their own and vulnerable to predatory men. At border crossings, women may be forced to endure rape as a 'price of passage'. Even refugee camps may offer little protection, as women's lack of economic power can leave them open to sexual exploitation and coercion. Women in such situations find themselves living without protection in a culture of violence and social chaos (Shanks and Schull, 2000). They may be subject to sexual extortion, in connection with the granting of basic necessities, personal documentation, or refugee status (UNHCR, 1995).

Home Office/legal aspects

Refugees and asylum seekers are likely to experience considerable difficulties in disclosing sexual assault during Home Office interviews, because of the traumatic and shameful nature of these experiences. Crime surveys repeatedly refer to the under-reporting of rape and sexual assault and the attrition of cases throughout the Criminal Justice System, leading to only about 5% of all reported cases ending with a successful conviction (Kelly *et al.*, 2005). The British Crime Survey found that the police came to know what had happened in less than one in seven cases of sexual assault (Walby and Allen, 2004). Male victims of rape and sexual assault may find it even more difficult to disclose sexual violence and abuse (Mezey and King, 1989).

It is therefore not surprising that refugees and asylum seekers tend not to disclose sexual violence to the police or to authorities, or often end up reporting such violence only at a later stage of their claim, or end up disclosing partial accounts of what happened (Cenada and Palmer, 2006). However, late or piecemeal disclosure of sexual violence by an asylum seeker is often used to discredit and undermine the asylum seeker's credibility. A further problem is that victims of sexual violence and abuse rarely have any physical evidence to support their account (unlike claims involving physical torture). The experience of being subjected to a Home Office interrogation, no matter how sensitively conducted, is likely to provoke anxiety and a sense of intimidation in the victim, particularly if female rape victims find themselves being interviewed by a male interviewer. Individuals with post-traumatic stress disorder may psychologically re-live their experience, be overwhelmed by anxiety, or dissociate during the interview, giving the impression of being vague, inconsistent, or evasive, thus further undermining their credibility (Bogner *et al.*, 2007).

Women are often granted asylum or refugee status based on their husband's claim and may not realize they can claim asylum in their own right. Their lack of independence and power makes them particularly vulnerable to abuse and exploitation after arriving in the UK and less able to disclose domestic and sexual abuse, or access services, as they then risk losing their home and jeopardizing their immigration status (Wilson *et al.*, 2007).

The Home Office has now adopted guidelines to ensure that gender issues are considered when assessing accounts of persecution by female asylum seekers (Home Office, 2004; Cenada and Palmer, 2006). The guidance has recommended that, when assessing claims, case workers should consider gender related harm, e.g. marriage related harm, violence within the family or community, domestic slavery, and female genital mutilation as legitimate grounds for claiming asylum. There has also been recognition by the Home Office that trafficking is a form of harm, which may constitute persecution. Thus, if a woman can be shown to have a well-founded fear of being re-trafficked for sexual exploitation, she may be granted humanitarian protection (Home Office and Scottish Executive, 2007).

Effects of sexual violence

In some communities, sexual violation results in rejection and ostracization by partners and communities. This represents a form of social death. Women who have been raped may be regarded as so damaged and defiled, as to render them permanently unmarriageable, which in itself also renders them more physically vulnerable (Krug *et al.*, 2002). In extreme cases, rape and sexual violence result in the death of the victim; they may be killed by their assailant/s, be subsequently killed by family members or members of the community (honour killing); they may die from the physical injuries incurred, or commit suicide. Genital and non-genital injuries are common and may include mutilation and disfigurement. Women may experience impairment or loss of reproductive functioning and find themselves permanently devalued as marriage partners (Krug et al., 2002).

The risk of developing a sexually transmitted infection following rape is between 4% and 56%, depending on the local prevalence of such infections (Wilken and Welch, 2003). For women who are trafficked into sex work, the risk is even higher. The risk of HIV infection following rape is generally considered to be low, though this depends on the local prevalence of HIV. The risk increases with physical trauma. Rates of pregnancy following rape are around 5% for adult women of child-bearing age (Holmes et al., 1996), although this assumes a single 'one-off' sexual assault, rather than repeated rape, conducted with the explicit aim of destroying the enemy through impregnating their women.

Mental health problems in survivors of sexual assaults are common and include depression and suicide, post-traumatic stress disorder (PTSD), generalized and phobic anxiety, alcohol and substance misuse, as well as sexual dysfunction and poor physical health (Steketee and Foa, 1977; Waigandt et al., 1990; Resnick et al., 1997; Krug et al., 2002; Kilpatrick and Acierno, 2003; Schnurr and Green, 2004; Gilbert et al., 2008). Mental health problems following rape tend to be long term and are unlikely to resolve spontaneously, without access to specialist mental health care (Resnick et al., 1997).

Treatment and interventions

The UNHCR has set out the principles of identifying and responding to the needs of refugees and asylum seekers who have been sexually victimized (UNHCR, 1995). The key challenge in this population is to increase their willingness to disclose experiences of sexual violence. Establishing the safety of any refugee or asylum seeker is a pre-requisite to offering support and assistance, as they will not disclose their experiences or engage in treatment if they feel unsafe or fear reprisals. Sensitive, confidential interviewing methods are necessary to encourage individuals to report sexual victimization, without this further jeopardizing their sense of safety. The need for an interviewer of the same gender must be considered, as well as an interpreter, who is not a family member or known to the woman (Wilson et al., 2007).

Services for victims of sexual violence should be culturally competent and based on a range of good practices that have been found effective in victims of child sexual abuse, domestic violence, sexual assault, torture, and in asylum seekers, refugees, and migrants (Wilson *et al.*, 2007). These include strategies for crisis intervention, confidentiality, security, shelter, social and legal support, forensic assessment, medical treatment, counselling, psychotherapy, couple therapy, and family interventions (Agger, 1994; Zimmerman *et al.*, 2003). Treatments and interventions need to address the physical, psychological, and social consequences of sexual violence, as well as the multiple traumas and losses that often accompany such experiences. Services that are integrated and coordinated, i.e. which combine access to physical and psychological health care, social and legal advice, are most likely to be effective (Campbell and Ahrens, 1998, Wilson *et al.*, 2007). In the UK, Sexual Assault Referral Centres (SARCs) have been set up to provide holistic care for women who have been sexually assaulted, regardless of whether they have reported to the police, or whether legal action is being pursued (Lovett *et al.*, 2004). Alternatively, referral to specialist centres in the UK such as the Medical Foundation for the care of Victims of Torture (www.torturecare.org.uk), which has considerable expertise in treating individuals who have experienced sexual as well as other forms of violence, could be considered. Where there is no identifiable 'medical problem' requiring a healthcare intervention, facilitating contact with and support from refugee and community groups may be the most effective in promoting social support and acceptance.

Special issues and groups in context

Human trafficking

The Office of the United Nations High Commissioner for Human Rights (2000) has defined human trafficking as the 'recruitment, transportation or harbouring of persons by means of threat or use of force or other forms of coercion, of abduction, of fraud or deceptions for the purpose of exploitation'. The trafficking of women and girls is one of the world's fastest growing crimes and a gross violation of human rights (Office of the United Nations High Commissioner on Human Rights, 2001). The United States (US) government estimates that 600,000 to 800,000 people worldwide are trafficked into forced labour and prostitution each year (US State Department, 2004: 6). This report also estimates that '80 per cent of the victims trafficked across international borders are female and 70 per cent of those females are trafficked for sexual exploitation' (US State Department, 2004: 23).

Globally, women and children are trafficked for various purposes, including sexual servitude, domestic labour, sweatshop and agricultural labour, marriage (as 'mail-order brides'), begging, and in the case of children, for illegal adoption (Fergus, 2005). Trafficked boys and child soldiers in conflict-prone regions are also vulnerable to exploitation for labour and sex. Although men are commonly identified as traffickers and exploiters, women acting as recruiters, brothel-owners, and 'clients' of commercial sexual exploitation are more common than is sometimes realized (US State Department, 2008). Trafficked people represent diverse cultures. Some leave developing countries for more prosperous destinations, seeking to improve their lives through low-skilled jobs. Women, eager for a better future, are susceptible to promises of jobs abroad as *au pairs*, housekeepers, waitresses, or models—which fail to materialize and instead result in forced prostitution. Some families give children to relatives or friends, who promise education and opportunity but then sell the children into exploitative situations for money (US State Department, 2008). But poverty alone does not explain modern-day trafficking, which is driven by fraudulent recruiters, employers, and corrupt officials who seek to reap unlawful profits from others' desperation. Recent estimates of the profits from this illegal global trade are as high as $217.8 billion a year (International Labour Organization, 2005).

Trafficking can result in a series of further abuses, including debt-bondage, forced labour, slavery-like conditions, rape, torture, imprisonment, and even murder (Fergus, 2005). An epidemiological study conducted across Europe surveyed women who had been recently released from trafficking (Zimmerman *et al.*, 2003; 2008). The women belonged to 14 different countries (mostly non-EU states). More than half (53%) were trafficked to EU member states, 38% to other European States, and 8% to non-European States. 60% reported being either physically or sexually abused before being trafficked. Almost all women (95%) reported experiencing physical or sexual violence while in the trafficking situation, with 71% experiencing both. Over half (57%) of the women reported suffering between 12 and 23 concurrent physical symptoms upon entering care, with 63% reporting memory problems. More than 8 in 10 women reported headaches on entering care, and nearly 7 in 10 still reported headaches after more than 3 months in care. Over 60% reported sexual and reproductive health symptoms, including pelvic pain, vaginal discharge, and gynaecological infections. Upon entering care, over half (56%) of the women reported symptoms levels suggestive of PTSD. This symptom level compares with those found among survivors of war trauma and in torture victims. PTSD symptoms declined considerably on receiving care, with only 6% demonstrating such symptoms after 90+ days. Trafficked women's depression, anxiety, and hostility levels were extremely high: within the top tenth percentile of population norms for adult females. Ninety five per cent reported feeling depressed upon entry into post-trafficking care services, with 38% reporting suicidal thoughts. Depression appeared to be the most persistent symptom, showing very little reduction even after 90+ days in care. Seventeen per cent of the women reported daily alcohol consumption and 14% reported illegal drug use during the trafficking experience.

A victim centred approach to trafficking needs to address the three 'R's: rescue, rehabilitation, and reintegration, and to encourage learning and sharing of best practice in these areas (US State Department, 2008). It also needs to recognize the practical implications of consequences like cognitive problems, which may affect victims' credibility with authorities, and their capacity to co-operate in criminal investigations and make sound decisions regarding their safety. This is especially true for the first ninety days in care, given the severity of symptoms during this period. It should also be noted that trafficking survivors are a diverse group, differing in age, culture, nationality, personality, childhood experiences, marital status, and levels of education. As a framework for care, it has been suggested that service provision for trafficking survivors be divided into three stages (Zimmerman *et al.*, 2003):

1 The crisis intervention stage where the focus is on providing emergency and basic support services (including emergency medical treatment);

2 The adjustment stage where women begin to experience relative stability and adapt to their new circumstances. Here, medical treatment for a variety of symptoms become relevant; and

3 A longer-term symptom management stage. Here, some women continue to reorient themselves and look to the future, while others become increasingly distressed as they reflect upon their experiences and face stress-filled decisions and events.

Torture

Torture is practised in over 100 countries today and sexualized violence or sexual assault may be used as a form of torture. A recent study of 63 female asylum seekers in Sweden found that 76% reported rape (anal and vaginal) (Edston and Olsson, 2007). Most of them had suffered additional forms of persecution, including beatings and restrictions on their movements and activities. Female victims of torture were more likely than male victims to report sexual assault or gender based violence. The specific acts described include being held naked, being taunted and sexually humiliated, assaults on genitals, including electric shocks, withholding of sanitary protection (e.g. Asgary *et al.*, 2006; Edston and Olsson, 2007). Torture involving sexual assault and gender based violence is particularly degrading and humiliating for the victim (Lindner, 2001). The recent Abu Ghraib Baghdad prison scandal revealed the use of sexual degradation and humiliation in dealing with war captives as a form of abuse, eliciting worldwide disapproval (McCarthy, 2004).

Epidemiological research in war survivors, many of whom are also refugees, indicates that stressors such as threats of rape, genital fondling and molestation, witnessing the torture of others, and being stripped naked are profoundly humiliating and are as distressing as physical torture that involves actual physical pain. These experiences are recognized as representing a profound violation of dignity and basic human rights (Giacaman *et al.*, 2007).

Physical pain, in itself, is not the most important determinant of traumatic stress in survivors (Basoglu *et al.*, 2007). A case-control study of 55 tortured and 55 non-tortured ex-political prisoners of both sexes in Turkey found that post torture psychological problems, including anxiety, depression, and PTSD were related more to self reported distress during the torture, than to the severity and extent of the torture experience (Basoglu and Paker, 1995). More recent research in 279 survivors of war trauma from former Yugoslavia showed that physical torture (and rape) did not contribute to long-term psychological outcomes over and above the effects of non-physical stressors like those listed earlier (Basoglu *et al.*, 2007). Perceived distress and lack of control over stressors, rather than mere exposure to them, was associated with a greater likelihood of PTSD and depression. Feelings of shame and humiliation appear to contribute independently to the development of PTSD (Andrews *et al.*, 2000) and increased general health complaints in victims of torture (Hartling and Luchetta, 1999; Giacaman *et al.*, 2007) and crime (Andrews *et al.*, 2000). Basoglu *et al.* (2007) hypothesize that humiliating treatment and attacks on personal integrity, cultural values, morals, or religious beliefs may induce feelings of helplessness in the individual through not being able to act on anger and hostility generated by such aversive treatment. Further, they conclude that aggressive interrogation techniques or detention procedures involving deprivation of basic needs, exposure to aversive environmental conditions, forced nudity, threats, humiliating treatment, and other psychological manipulations conducive to anxiety, fear, and helplessness in the detainee are not substantially different from physical torture in terms of the extent of mental suffering they cause, the underlying mechanisms of traumatic stress, and their long-term traumatic effects. Thus, psychological manipulations, ill treatment, and torture during interrogation share the same psychological mechanism in exerting their traumatic impact. All three types of acts are geared towards creating anxiety, fear, and uncertainty in the detainee while at the same time conferring a profound sense of helplessness and loss of control. Such manipulations designed to remove control from the detainee can have a severe traumatic impact, even when they do not involve physical torture.

When survivors arrive as asylum seekers and refugees in destination countries, services that seek to screen, assess, and manage mental health problems need to be sensitive to these issues. They need to be especially aware that sexually degrading and humiliating treatment can potentially lead to adverse mental health outcomes of a similar type and severity as rape and other forms of sexual assault.

Female genital mutilation

Female genital mutilation (FGM) refers to 'all procedures involving partial or total removal of the external female genitalia or other injury to the female genital organs whether for cultural, religious or other non-therapeutic reasons' (WHO, 2000). This may then interfere with the natural functions of girls' and women's bodies.

It is classified into four major types (WHO, 2008).

Type I: Partial or total removal of the clitoris and/or the prepuce (clitoridectomy);

Type II: Partial or total removal of the clitoris and the labia minora, with or without excision of the labia majora (excision);

Type III: Narrowing of the vaginal orifice with creation of a covering seal by cutting and appositioning the labia minora and/or the labia majora, with or without excision of the clitoris (infibulation);

Type IV: All other harmful procedures to the female genitalia for non-medical purposes, e.g. pricking, piercing, incising, scraping, and cauterization.

The procedure has no health benefits, causes severe pain, and has several adverse health consequences, both immediate and long-term. It can be regarded and may be experienced as a violent act against the sexual integrity of women and is therefore a form of gender based violence. Women who are subjected to FGM may eventually need reconstructive surgery to allow for sexual intercourse and childbirth, or for the normal passage of menstrual flow (WHO, 2000). FGM is mostly carried out on young girls sometime between infancy and age 15, although it is occasionally carried out on adult women (UNICEF, 2005a). An estimated 100–140 million girls and women worldwide are currently living with the consequences of the first three types of FGM (WHO, 2000). In Africa, about 3 million girls are at risk for FGM every year (Yoder *et al.*, 2004). The practice is most common in the western, eastern, and north-eastern regions of Africa and has been documented in some countries in Asia and the Middle East. It is also common among immigrant communities from these regions in Europe and North America (WHO, 2008).

FGM is recognized internationally as a violation of the human rights of girls and women. The United Nations has supported the right of member states to grant refugee status to women who fear being mutilated if they are returned to their country of origin (UNHCR, 1996). Though fear of FGM as a basis for asylum is a developing area of UK law, the UK Immigration Appellate Authority Asylum Gender Guidelines (2000), the UK Borders Agency (2006) and the House of Lords (in Fornah, 2006) have supported the UNHCR view.

The practice is usually carried out by traditional circumcisers, who often play other key roles in such communities, for instance as birth attendants. However, FGM is increasingly being performed by medically trained personnel (OHCR, 2008). In societies in which it is practised, FGM is a manifestation of gender inequality rooted in sociocultural, economic, and political structures. It is supported by both men and women and anyone departing from the norm may face condemnation, harassment, and ostracism. Drivers include a desire for a sense of community membership, cultural identity and coming of age, marriage, and beliefs that the practice makes the genitalia more 'beautiful' and enhances the man's sexual pleasure. The practice may also be upheld by beliefs associated with religion (Budiharsana, 2004; Gruenbaum, 2006; Abdi, 2007; Johnson, 2007). Even though the practice can be found among Christians, Jews, and Muslims, none of their holy texts prescribes female genital mutilation and the practice pre-dates both Christianity and Islam (WHO, 2008). As such, FGM is a social convention governed by rewards and punishments, which are a powerful force for continuing the practice. Thus, it is difficult for families to abandon the practice without support from the wider community. Analysis of international health data shows a close link between women's ability to exercise control over their lives and their belief that female genital mutilation should be ended (UNICEF, 2005b).

Adverse health consequences include severe haemorrhage and shock, tetanus, infection and sepsis, urinary retention and problems with defecation, recurrent urinary tract infections, cysts, abscesses and genital ulcers, chronic pain, decreased sexual enjoyment and infertility, an increased susceptibility to HIV and other sexually transmitted diseases, complications in childbirth, and newborn deaths (OHCR, 2008). Mental Health sequelae can include a fear of sexual intercourse, PTSD, anxiety, depression, and memory loss (Whitehorn, 2002; Behrendt and Moritz, 2005; Lockhat, 2006). Behrendt and Moritz (2005), on conducting a case-control study on a sample of 47 Senegalese women in Dakar, found that 30.4% of circumcised women met criteria for PTSD. A further 47.9% met criteria for other anxiety disorders or an affective disorder. Only one of the uncircumcised women had a psychiatric diagnosis. All but one circumcised participant remembered the day of her circumcision as extremely traumatizing. Another case-control study from an Egyptian sample revealed that rates of somatization, anxiety, and phobias were significantly higher in the FGM group, as were rates of dyspareunia, loss of libido, and failure of orgasm (Elnashar and Abdelhady, 2007). These findings are concordant with those from other studies and indicate that the cultural significance of the practice is not protective against psychological complications (Behrendt and Moritz, 2005; Lockhat, 2006; Nour *et al.*, 2006; Elnashar and Abdelhady, 2007).

Mental health service providers must be trained to identify problems resulting from female genital mutilation and to treat them. This may be particularly difficult in communities where the practice is strongly associated with cultural identities and is 'normalized' as a consequence. This obstacle can be surmounted by culturally competent approaches that are alert to the needs of victims, while simultaneously sensitive to the powerful social imperatives that influence the practice.

Male victims of sexual violence

Of the thousands of men who seek refuge and asylum abroad, many are survivors of sexual violence and torture (Lunde *et al.*, 1980, 1981; Agger, 1988; Norredam *et al.*, 2005).

Male sexual trauma can be characterized according to the methods used (Lunde and Ortmann, 1990; Peel, 2002) as follows:

1 Direct genital trauma, which includes hitting, kicking, or applying electric shocks to genitals and/or anus, insertion of objects into urethral meatus and/or anus, and cigarette burns to penis;

2 Non-consensual sexual acts: pawing, anal rape, forced masturbation, and forced fellatio; and

3 Mental assaults: forced nakedness, sexual humiliation, and threats.

The actual prevalence of sexual trauma among male refugees and asylum seekers is uncertain. However, it has been estimated that 5000 to 8000 men were raped in the former Yugoslavia and that thousands of men and boys were raped during the Iraqi invasion of Kuwait (James, 2001). Sexual violence against men mostly takes place during detention and imprisonment and is perpetrated by guards, interrogators, or other prisoners. Agger (1989), reviewing the literature on sexual torture, found that 52% of male political prisoners who sought help after torture had been sexually abused. In a study of male political prisoners in El Salvador, Agger (1988) found that 76% had experienced at least one form of sexual torture. Peel *et al.* (2000) studied 607 men from 45 countries, finding that 25% had been sexually assaulted.

Of these, 21% had been raped, 47% had sustained assaults to the genitals, 27% had sustained electric shocks to the genitals, and a further 21% had had an object inserted in the anus or urethral meatus. In a different study, Peel *et al.* (2000) investigated sexual trauma among male Tamil refugees who had been imprisoned, and found a prevalence of 21%. However, it is likely that these figures are underestimates because of the taboo and stigmatization to discussing male sexual trauma inherent in most cultures.

Such experiences have high physical and mental health costs, leading to long-term adverse outcomes. Physical outcomes may include chronic genital pain (including erectile pain), Peyronie's disease, lower urinary tract symptoms, and erectile dysfunction (Norredam, 2005). Survivors may also be exposed to HIV and other sexually transmitted diseases. Mental Health sequelae can include PTSD and Major Depressive Disorder (Turner, 2000).

Service providers have to be alert to the particular difficulties in screening for sexual trauma in male survivors. A substantial body of evidence indicates that men who have been victims of sexual assault have particular difficulty in disclosure and accessing services (Kaufman *et al.*, 1980; Mezey and King, 2000). For instance, a study of British male victims of sexual assaults in general showed that 79% of raped men sought no help for a mean period of 16 years after the assault (King and Woollett, 1997). This has been attributed to a variety of causes, including fear of stigmatization and the shame of a perceived loss of masculinity. Sex role socialization may contribute to the reservations such men have in acknowledging and expressing feelings of distress and vulnerability. This may have to do with such feelings being equated with weakness and inadequacy, both contrary to traditional social paradigms of 'maleness'. In the same way that men are assumed to be not vulnerable to sexual assault, they may also be expected 'to be a man' when subject to such assault, i.e. cope effectively in the face of adversity. Thus, being a male rape victim and expressing distress about it appear to contravene two central tenets of masculinity (Mezey and King, 2000). These cultural taboos and barriers to disclosure make sensitive screening for such trauma among refugee and asylum seeker populations particularly important.

Conclusions

The persistence of regional conflicts and political instability has led to a situation where increasing numbers of people are forced to leave strife-torn countries and seek asylum and refuge abroad (Castles *et al.*, 2003). This has intersected with globalization, the fall in transaction and travel costs, and the ties of the Commonwealth, leading to substantial numbers of refugees and asylum seekers arriving in the UK, legally or otherwise (Glover *et al.*, 2001). However, people fleeing conflict and oppression to seek asylum increasingly face restrictive immigration policies (Crisp, 2003).

Thus, refugees and asylum seekers who have experienced significant loss and trauma in the past, simultaneously face a number of legal and social challenges in the present and the future. The evidence indicates that many refugees and asylum seekers have been subjected to some form of sexualized violence, including sexual torture, trafficking and rape, forced marriage, and female genital mutilation. These experiences cause significant trauma to the victims and lead to adverse health and social outcomes. Refugees and asylum seekers are often faced with the difficult task of negotiating Home Office interviews, having to re-live traumatic and distressing events, with few supports in a strange environment and culture. Under-reporting and partial reporting of experiences of sexual violence are major issues in this context. Sensitive, confidential interviewing by interviewers of the same gender may encourage individuals to report sexual victimization, without this further jeopardizing their sense of safety or their asylum status. Coordinated and integrated services, which are culturally sensitive and which provide medical and psychological health care, social and legal care, and advice and support, are most likely to be acceptable and effective.

References

Abdi, M.S. (2007). *A Religious Oriented Approach to Addressing FGM/C among the Somali Community of Wajir.* Nairobi: Population Council.

Agger, I. (1988). Psychological Aspects of Torture: Psychological Aspects of Torture with Special Emphasis on Sexual Torture: Sequels and Treatment Perspectives. Paper presented to the WHO Advisory Group on the Health Situation of Refugees and Victims of Organized Violence (Gothenburg).

Agger, I. (1989). Sexual torture of political prisoners: an overview. *Journal of Traumatic Stress* 2(3): 305–318.

Agger, I. (1994). *The Blue Room: Trauma and Testimony among Refugee Women.* London: Zed Books.

Andrews, B., Brewin, C., Rose, S., and Kirk, M. (2000). Predicting PTSD symptoms in victims of violent crime: the role of shame, anger and childhood abuse. *Journal of Abnormal Psychology* 109: 69–73.

Andrews, G., Corry, J., Slade, T., Issakidis, C., and Swanston, H. (2004). *Child Sexual Abuse. Comparative Quantification of Health Risks.* Geneva: WHO.

Asgary, R., Retalios, E., Smith, C., and Paccione, G. (2006). Evaluating asylum seekers/torture survivors in urban primary care: A collaborative approach at the Bronx Human Rights Clinic. *Health and Human Rights* 9(2): 164–179.

Basoglu, M. and Paker, M. (1995). Severity of trauma as predictor of long-term psychological status in survivors of torture. *Journal of Anxiety Disorders* 9: 339–350.

Basoglu, M., Livanou, M., and Crnobaric, C. (2007). Torture versus other cruel, inhuman and degrading treatment: Is the distinction real or apparent? *Archives of General Psychiatry* **64**: 277–285.

Beevor, A. (2003). *Berlin: The Downfall, 1945*. Penguin: London.

Behrendt, A. and Moritz, S. (2005). Posttraumatic stress disorder and memory problems after female genital mutilation. *American Journal of Psychiatry* **162**: 1000–1002.

Bogner, D., Herlihy, J., and Brewin, C.R. (2007). Impact of sexual violence on disclosure during Home Office interviews. *British Journal of Psychiatry* **191**: 75–81.

Budiharsana, M. (2004). Female Circumcision in Indonesia: Extent, Implications and Possible Interventions to Uphold Women's Health Rights. Jakarta: Population Council.

Campbell, R. and Ahrens, C.E. (1998). Innovative community services for rape victims: an application of multiple case study methodology. *American Journal of Community Psychology* **26**(4): 537–571.

Castles, S., Crawley, H., and Loughna, S. (2003). States of Conflict: Causes and Patterns of Forced Migration to the EU and Policy Responses. London: Institute of Public Policy Research.

Cenada, S. and Palmer, C. (2006). Lip Service or Implementation? Home Office Gender Guidance and Women Asylum Seekers. London: Asylum Aid.

Crisp, J. (2003). Refugees and the global politics of asylum. In S. Spencer (Ed.), *The Politics of Migration*, pp. 75–87, London: Blackwell Publishing.

Edston, E. and Olsson, C. (2007). Female victims of torture. *Journal of Forensic and Legal Medicine* **1416**: 368–373.

Elnashar, R.A. and Abdelhady, R. (2007). The impact of female genital cutting on health of newly married women. *International Journal of Gynecology and Obstetrics* **97**: 238–244.

Fergus, L. (2005). Trafficking in women for sexual exploitation. Briefing no. 5. Australian Centre for the Study of Sexual Assault. Australian Institute of Family Studies.

Fornah (FC) *versus* Secretary of State for the Home Department. (2006). Session 2005–2006, UKHL 46. House of Lords.

Giacaman, R., Abu-Rmeileh, N.M.E., Husseini, A., Saab, H., and Boyce, W. (2007). Humiliation: the invisible trauma of war for Palestinian youth. *Public Health* 121, 563–571.

Gilbert, R., Widom, C.S., Browne, K., Fergusson, D., Webb, E., and Janson, S. (2008). Burden and consequences of child maltreatment in high income countries. *Lancet* **373**(9657): 68–81.

Glover, S., Scott, C., Loizillon, A., *et al.* (2001). Migration: An Economic and Social Analysis. RDS occasional paper no. 67. London: Home Office.

Gruenbaum, E. (2006). Sexuality issues in the movement to abolish female genital cutting in Sudan. *Medical Anthropology Quarterly* **20**: 121.

Hartling L.M. and Luchetta, T. (1999). Humiliation: assessing the impact of derision, degradation, and debasement. *Journal of Primary Prevention* **19**: 259–278.

Henttonen, M., Watts, C., Roberts, B., Kaducu, F., and Borchert, M. (2008). Health services for survivors of gender-based violence in Northern Uganda: a qualitative study. *Reproductive Health Matters* **16**(31): 122–131.

Holmes, M., Resnick, H.A., Kirkpatrick, D.G., and Best, C.L. (1996). Rape-related pregnancy: estimates and descriptive characteristics from a national sample of women. *American Journal of Obstetrics and Gynecology* **175**(2): 320–325.

Home Office. (2003). Sexual Offences Act. London: Home Office.

Home Office. (2004). Asylum Policy Instruction 'Gender Issues in the asylum claim'. London: Home Office. http://www.ind.homeoffice.gov.uk/documents/ asylumpolicyinstructions/apis/genderissueintheasylum.pdf?view=Binary

Home Office and Scottish Executive. (2007). UK Action Plan on Tackling Human Trafficking. London: TSO. www.homeoffice.gov.uk/documents/human-traffick-action-plan

International Labour Organisation. (2005). A Global Alliance against Forced Labour. Available online at http://www.ilo.org/declaration/Follow-up/Globalreports/lang--en/ index.htm, accessed 18 January 2009.

James, J. (2001). Silent conflict – helping the survivor of sexual violence. *Emergency Nurse* 9: 15–18.

Jewkes, R., Sen, P., and Garcia-Moreno, C. (2002). Sexual violence. In E.G. Krug, L.L. Dahlberg, J.A. Mercy, A.B. Zwi, and R. Lozano, (Eds.), *World Report on Violence and Health,* p. 149, Geneva, Switzerland: World Health Organization.

Johnson, M. (2007). Making mandinga or making Muslims? Debating female circumcision, ethnicity, and Islam in Guinea-Bissau and Portugal. In Y. Hernlund and B. Shell-Duncan, (Eds.), *Transcultural Bodies: Female Genital Cutting in Global Context,* pp. 202–223, New Brunswick, NJ: Rutgers University Press.

Kaufman, A., Divasto, P., Jackson, R., Voorhees, D., and Christy, J. (1980). Male rape victims: non institutionalized assault. *American Journal of Psychiatry* 137: 221–223.

Kelly, L., Lovett, J., and Regan, L. (2005). A gap or a chasm? Attrition in Reported Rape Cases. Child and Women Abuse Studies Unit. Home Office Research Study 293. London: Home Office.

Kilpatrick, D.G. and Acierno, R.E. (2003). Mental health needs of crime victims: epidemiology and outcomes. *Journal of Traumatic Stress* 16 (2): 119–132.

King, M. and Woollett, E. (1997). Sexually assaulted males: 115 consulting a counselling service. *Archives of Sexual Behaviour* 26: 579–588.

Krug, E.G., Dahlberg, L.L., Mercy, J.A., Zwi, A.B., and Lozano, R. (Eds). (2002). *World Report on Violence and Health.* Geneva, Switzerland: World Health Organization.

Lindner, E.G. (2001). Humiliation and the human condition: mapping a minefield. *Human Rights Review* 2: 46–63.

Lockhat, H. (2006). *Female Genital Mutilation: Treating the Tears.* London: Middlesex University Press.

Lovett, J., Regan, L., and Kelly, L. (2004). *Sexual Assault Referral Centres: Developing Good Practice and Maximising Potentials.* London, UK: Home Office Research Study 285.

Lunde, I., Rasmussen, O.V., Lindholm, J., and Wagner, G. (1980). Gonadal and sexual functions in tortured Greek men. *Danish Medical Bulletin* 27(5): 243–245.

Lunde, I., Rasmussen, O.V., Wagner, G., and Lindholm, J. (1981). Sexual and pituitary–testicular function in torture victims. *Archives of Sexual Behaviour* 10(1): 25–32.

Lunde, I. and Ortmann, J. (1990). Prevalence and sequelae of sexual torture. *Lancet* 336: 289–291.

McCarthy, A.C. (2004). Torture: thinking about the unthinkable. *Commentary* 118: 17–25.

Mezey, G.C. and King, M. (1989). The effects of sexual assault on men – a survey of 22 subjects. *Psychological Medicine* 19: 205–209.

Mezey, G. (1994) Rape in war. *Journal of Forensic Psychiatry,* 5 (3) 583–597.

Mezey, G.C. and King, M.B. (2000). *Male Victims of Sexual Assault* (2nd Edn). Oxford: Oxford University Press.

Myhill, A. and Allen, J. (2002). Rape and Sexual Assault of Women: The Extent and Nature of the Problem. Findings from the British Crime Survey. Home Office Research Study 237. London: Home Office.

Norredam, M., Crosby, S., Munarriz, R., Piwowarczyk, L., and Grodin, M. (2005). Urologic complications of sexual trauma among male survivors of torture. *Urology* 65: 28–32.

Nour, N.M., Michels, K.B., and Bryant, A.E. (2006). Defibulation to treat female genital cutting: effect on symptoms and sexual function. *Obstetrics and Gynecology* 108: 55–60.

Office of the United Nations High Commissioner for Human Rights. (2000). Protocol to Prevent, Suppress and Punish Trafficking in Persons, Especially Women and Children, Supplementing the United Nations Convention Against Transnational Organized Crime. GA Res. 55/25, Annex 2, UN GAOR 55th Sess., Supp. No. 49, at 60, UN Doc A/45/49/Vol. 1. Available at: http://www.ohchr.org/english/law/protocoltraffic.htm accessed January 26, 2009.

Office of the United Nations High Commissioner for Human Rights. (2001). Traffic in Women and Girls. Commission on Human Rights 57th Sess., E/CN.4/RES/48.

OHCR, UNAIDS, UNDP, UNECA, UNESCO, UNFPA, UNHCR, UNICEF, UNIFEM, WHO (2008). Eliminating Female Genital Mutilation: An Interagency Statement. Geneva: World Health Organization.

Peel, M., Mahtani, A., Hinshelwood, G. and Forrest. D. (2000). The sexual abuse of men in detention in Sri Lanka. *Lancet* 355: 2069–2070.

Peel, M. (2002). Male sexual abuse in detention. In M. Peel and V. Iacopino, (Eds.), *The Medical Documentation of Torture*. London: Greenwich Medical Media.

Resnick, H.S., Acierno, R.E., and Kilpatrick, D.G. (1997). Health impact of interpersonal violence. Section II: Medical and mental health outcomes. *Behavioral Medicine* 23(2): 65–78.

Schnurr, P. and Green, B. (Eds.). (2004). *Trauma and Health: Physical Health Consequences of Exposure to Extreme Stress*. Washington, DC: American Psychological Association.

Senn, T., Carey, M., Vanable, P., Coury-Doniger, P., and Urban, M. (2007). Characteristics of sexual abuse in childhood and adolescence influence sexual risk behaviour in adulthood. *Archives of Sexual Behaviour* 36: 637—645.

Shanks, L. and Schull, M.J. (2000). Rape in war: the humanitarian response. *Canadian Medical Association Journal* 163 (9): 1152–1156.

Steketee, G. and Foa, E.B. (1977). Rape victims: post traumatic responses and their treatment. *Journal of Anxiety Disorders* (1): 69–86.

Turner, S. (2000). Surviving sexual assault and torture. In G. Mezey and M. King (Eds.), *Male Victims of Sexual Assault*, pp. 97–112, Oxford: OUP.

United Kingdom Borders Agency (2006). Asylum Policy Instructions: Gender Issues in the Asylum Claim October 2006. At: www.ukba.homeoffice.gov.uk/sitecontent/documents/policyandlaw/asylumpolicyinstructions, accessed 21 January 2009.

United Kingdom: Asylum and Immigration Tribunal/Immigration Appellate Authority, Immigration Appellate Authority (UK) (2000). Asylum Gender Guidelines, 1 November 2000. Online. UNHCR Refworld. At: http://www.unhcr.org/refworld/docid/3ae6b3414.html, accessed 21 January 2009.

US State Department (2004). 'Trafficking in persons report', United States State Department, http://www.state.gov/g/tip/rls/tiprpt/2004/, accessed 20 January 2005.

US State Department (2008). Trafficking in Persons Report. U.S. Department of State Publication 11407. Office of the Undersecretary for Democracy and Global Affairs and Bureau of Public Affairs.

UNICEF (2005a). Female Genital Mutilation/Female Genital Cutting: A Statistical Report. New York: UNICEF.

UNICEF (2005b). *Changing a Harmful Social Convention: Female Genital Mutilation/ Cutting.* Innocenti Digest. Florence: UNICEF.

UNHCR (1995). Sexual Violence Against Refugees: Guidelines on Prevention and Response. Geneva: UNHCR.

UNHCR (1996). 'FGM', draft, 21 Feb. 1996, General Legal Advice. Division of International Protection. Geneva, Switzerland: UNHCR.

Waigandt, A., Wallace, D.L., Phelps, L., and Miller, D.A. (1990). The Impact of Sexual Assault on Physical Health Status. *Journal of Traumatic Stress* 3(1): 93–101.

Wakabi, W. (2008). Sexual violence increasing in Democratic Republic of Congo. *Lancet* 371(9606): 15–16.

Walby, S. and Allen, J. (2004). Domestic Violence, Sexual Assault and Stalking: Findings from the British Crime Survey. Home Office Research, Development & Statistics Directorate, London.

Ward, J. and Vann, B. (2002). Gender-based violence in refugee settings. *The Lancet.* Supplement 360: s13–14.

Whitehorn, J. (2002). Female genital mutilation: cultural and psychological implications. *Sexual Relationships and Therapy* 17: 161–170.

WHO (2000). *Female Genital Mutilation.* Fact Sheet No 241, June 2000. Geneva: World Health Organization. At: http://www.who.int/mediacentre/factsheets/fs241/en/a.

Wilson, R., Sanders, M., and Dumper, H. (2007). Sexual Health, Asylum Seekers and Refugees. A Handbook for People Working with Refugees and Asylum Seekers in England. London: FPA.

Wilken, J. and Welch, J. (2003). Management of People Who Have Been Raped. *British Medical Journal* 326: 458–459.

Yoder, P.S., Abderrahim, N., and Zhuzhuni, A. (2004). Female Genital Cutting in the Demographic and Health Surveys: A Critical and Comparative Analysis. Calverton: Macro International Inc.

Zimmerman, C., Yun, K., Shvab, I., *et al.* (2003). The Health Risks and Consequences of Trafficking in Women and Adolescents. Findings from a European Study. London: London School of Hygiene & Tropical Medicine (LSHTM).

Zimmerman, C., Hossain, M., Yun, K., *et al.* (2008). The health of trafficked women: a survey of women entering post-trafficking services in Europe. *American Journal of Public Health* 98(1): 55–59.

Chapter 18

Paternalism or autonomy? Ethics, ideology, and science in refugee mental health interventions

Derrick Silove and Susan Rees

The first refugee mental health services in the modern era were initiated over 30 years ago (Kinzie *et al.*, 1980; Somnier and Genefke, 1986; Mollica *et al.*, 1987), with many other agencies subsequently being established in refugee resettlement countries around the world. It is striking that in this pioneering phase, human rights and medical concerns converged in giving impetus to this movement, with physicians' groups in organizations such as Amnesty International playing a key role in identifying the need for rehabilitation programmes for refugees, particularly survivors of torture. In subsequent times, however, the human rights and medical domains increasingly have been represented as opposing philosophical forces, a tension that has given rise to important ethical dilemmas as the field has evolved. These tensions can be located within the broader context of health ethics, particularly in relation to the concepts of *primum non-nocere* (first, do no harm), beneficence, paternalism, and autonomy (Gillon, 1985; Smith, 2005). As we will indicate, although retaining their generic meanings, terms such as autonomy and paternalism have special meanings and applications in the refugee field. This chapter considers how ambiguities relating to these ethical concepts have influenced debate and practice in the refugee mental health field, across areas of service development, treatment, and research. A focus on clinical ethics, well addressed by Kinzie and colleagues (1980), falls outside the scope of the chapter.

Protection, paternalism, and autonomy: special meanings in the field of refugee mental health

The tension between autonomy and paternalism is one of the core ethical challenges confronted by all fields of health practice (Thomasma, 1983; Quill and

Brody, 1996; Farr Curlin *et al.*, 2007). Autonomy refers to the rights and capacity of persons (referred to as patients) to make their own decisions about their health and well-being, whereas paternalism implies that physicians or other health professionals have a privileged position in directing the course of treatment. Generally, the two principles are regarded as being in opposition, with the enlightened approach favouring the promotion of autonomy over what is seen as an antiquated custom of medical paternalism. In the present chapter, we illustrate that in the refugee field, as in other areas of medicine, notions of autonomy and paternalism require a more nuanced analysis. The complexity of the refugee experience, including exposure to state persecution, displacement, flight, and ongoing social and psychological challenges related to resettlement, create a complex set of needs (Rees and Pease, 2007). In that context, policy, service, and practice may at various times include elements of what we refer to as a benign form of paternalism while at the same time giving central focus to the ultimate aim of promoting autonomy.

The political dilemma facing refugees

The emergence of the nation state as the unit of political organization in the modern world has made the status of citizenship an unavoidable reality for all people around the globe. By implication, citizens are engaged in a social contract with the state, one that should confer reciprocal benefits and duties. In more enlightened nations, the state has a responsibility to protect the rights of all citizens and to treat them with beneficence and care (an ideal rarely fully realized in practice). In turn, the citizen is required to abide by the laws and customs of the state. In the positive sense, the state therefore has a paternalistic or protective function, broadly analogous to that of a parent who is entrusted with the safety and well-being of the child. For refugees, the state of origin has abrogated this role: instead of upholding the principle of beneficence, it has acted with malevolence, exploiting its power in a manner that has led to the persecution, torture, and abuse of its citizens. In this instance, international law allows for the persecuted person to reject the authority of the state and to seek protection from another nation, with dedicated international agencies, particularly the United Nations High Commissioner for Refugees (UNHCR), being established to facilitate the process.

In reality, many refugees encounter grave difficulties in securing the protection they seek. Commonly, they are confined in refugee camps where their citizenship status remains uncertain for many years. Others live as stateless persons in countries bordering the conflict or as asylum seekers awaiting the outcomes of their refugee applications. In all these instances, the key experience is one of insecurity and anxiety about whether the state in which they currently reside, or any other, will provide them with the durable protection afforded regular citizens.

In addition, many of the settings in which displaced persons find themselves (in refugee camps, as undocumented 'illegals', as asylum seekers) are characterized by conditions of restriction, confinement, and socio-economic deprivation. Freedom of movement may be curtailed, refugees may not have the right to work or to participate in education, and they may be denied reunion or contact with family members (Silove *et al.*, 1997). Hence, refugees often face conditions of life in which they are not afforded either adequate protection or the right to exercise their autonomy. In that context, autonomy and paternalism cannot be construed as entirely polar opposites—the refugee is denied the benefits of state protection (a form of benevolent paternalism) and also suffers from a curtailment of basic freedoms.

Both elements appear to be directly relevant to the mental health of refugees. For example, amongst asylum seekers, the persistence of psychological distress is directly related to the length of time they are obliged to wait before obtaining protection visas as well as to the deprivations and restrictions they experience in their everyday lives (Silove *et al.*, 1997; Rees, 2003; 2004). Even refugees who achieve permanent residency may experience a residue of insecurity for years prior to re-establishing a durable sense of trust in the adopted country and its institutions (Rees and Pease, 2007). Hence, in the refugee context, elements of autonomy and benign paternalism may both have a place in designing effective interventions depending on the specific array of needs evident at any one time for each group.

Yet in spite of these complexities, practitioners in the field have appeared at times to adopt an extreme position in relation to their interpretation of the principles of autonomy and paternalism. To illustrate this division, we present a somewhat graphic characterization of the polar opposite positions, noting that in reality, most practitioners are located on a continuum of perspectives ranging between the two extremes. The paternalistic characterization usually is applied to 'clinicians', often medical personnel or clinical psychologists who are typified as advocating top-down treatments and who give priority to methods derived from the health sciences. These personnel tend to apply psychiatric diagnoses such as post-traumatic stress disorder (PTSD) and depression (often being accused of reifying these categories) and tend to advocate treatments such as cognitive behavioural therapy (CBT), and/or psychotropic medications, reflecting a faith in expert-based cures for what are depicted as being essentially medical conditions[1]. In the autonomy camp are those,

---

[1] The authors note that this bioreductionist approach to medicine and mental illness has been largely superseded in theory, and to varying degrees in practice, since the conception

usually but not exclusively non-medical personnel, whose primary focus is on the social domain. They draw on diverse theoretical sources including the principles of human rights, community development, and cultural diversity to argue for programmes that empower refugees to regain control over their own lives. Commonly, these advocates are critical of what is referred to as the paternalistic medical model, promoting instead a multidimensional and community development approach to intervention, including solution focused group work, problem solving, intensive case support including referral to social agencies for assistance with health, housing, language acquisition, and employment, and advocacy to promote social, cultural, and human rights. This perspective is commonly associated with scepticism about the value of what are seen as 'technical' psychological or medical interventions, particularly CBT (see hereunder), with a more client-centred or group counselling approach being favoured. Research focusing specifically on post-traumatic stress disorder (PTSD) is often viewed with some suspicion, being regarded as intrusive and potentially damaging, particularly insofar as it risks retraumatizing refugees by eliciting painful memories of the past. Added to this, the experiences of refugees are considered too complex and multifaceted to make scientific inquiry of psychiatric type relevant, particularly when the research draws on positivistic/quantitative methods, an approach which is seen to be reductionistic.

The design of specialist rehabilitation services for refugees

Given this background, it is understandable that early formulations of service approaches for the rehabilitation of refugees highlighted the importance of adopting a multi-dimensional, psychosocial approach (Silove *et al.*, 1991), one that included a focus on empowerment, human rights, cultural issues, resettlement, and community development. The approach was posited as differentiating mental health work in the refugee field from the more confined medical model approach that was applied in the routine clinical practice applied in generic psychiatric clinics. Some services went to elaborate lengths to design their physical environments in a manner that was 'non-clinical', in recognition that torture often occurred in settings that mimicked hospital or other institutional settings, in some instances perpetrated or overseen by medical personnel. In keeping with this concern, counsellors would be proactive in accompanying refugees to the dentist or to hospitals, especially if they required invasive procedures. In emphasizing the risks associated with a

---

of the biopsychosocial model (Engel, 1980). Hence this characterization of the 'strict' medical model rarely matches the reality in practice.

clinical setting, this perspective served to further encourage a wariness of all aspects of the traditional medical model.

Not all services adopted this non-medical 'psychosocial' model. Some pioneering refugee services were based in hospital settings, led by psychiatrists. To our knowledge, there are no data indicating whether refugees were more or less likely to attend services in either type of setting. In addition, there is a deficit of data with which to compare the efficacy of each model in reducing trauma symptoms, or in improving the refugees' capacity to settle and operate more autonomously in the new country.

We note, however, that some elements of the non-medical approach may in fact have proved to be paternalistic, for example, when workers have been active in accompanying patients to attend other services. Refugees often have extensive health needs, making attendance at clinics and hospitals an important aspect of their early resettlement experiences. Whereas it may be the case that some refugees require personalized support to attend medical services in the early phase, the continuation of such a model is neither feasible nor desirable with respect to promoting autonomy in the longer term. Instead, cognitive behavioural techniques such as systematic desensitization may actually achieve the aim of autonomous functioning in this area more rapidly and effectively, by facilitating the refugee's capacity to overcome phobic-avoidant tendencies and attend these services independently.

Nevertheless, the focus on protecting refugees from exposure to trauma cues was understandable in the early development of psychosocial services: refugees were being seen in the initial phase of resettlement when their levels of distress and insecurity were at a height, and service providers were in the pioneering phase of practice without access to an established set of procedures, or to the benefits of knowledge accrued through service evaluation research.

Post-conflict countries

A parallel ideological divide is evident between advocates of mental health clinics and psychosocial programmes in the field of international aid for countries exposed to conflict and displacement (van Ommeren *et al.*, 2005). As a consequence, there has been great difficulty in developing a unified policy in psychosocial and mental health in this area, with ideologically based notions rather than a sound evidence base driving the design and implementation of programmes. The overall effect, itself of great ethical concern, has been a reduced lobbying power for advocates of mental health interventions for refugee and conflict-affected populations in the developing world.

A recent WHO publication focusing on mental health care programmes in acute emergencies reflected on this conflict between advocates of the so-called trauma model, broadly aligned with the medical model, and those promoting psychosocial programmes (van Ommeren *et al.*, 2005). The division between these perspectives was regarded as a major obstacle for programme planners who found it difficult to arbitrate between what appeared to be the irreconcilable claims of protagonists for competing approaches. The risk is that the consequent uncertainties will continue to discourage funders and policy makers from giving priority to the psychological needs of refugees and other conflict-affected populations, thereby compounding the longstanding stigma and history of neglect associated with mental health issues in the developing world. Hence the stakes from an ethical and human rights perspective are very high. One evident consequence of the ideological divisions within the field was that the early version of the Sphere Project's minimum standards for disaster response did not cover mental health at all (van Ommeren *et al.*, 2005). This deficiency has been addressed partially in the recently adopted IASC guidelines (Humanitarian Charter and Minimum Standards in Disaster Response, 2004) although even that extensive document does not confront some of the key issues in a forthright manner.

What constitutes psychosocial and mental health programmes in these settings is itself an area of contention. Psychosocial programmes commonly focus on vulnerable groups such as widows, ex-child soldiers, veterans, and single mothers, amongst others, with the emphasis being on collective activities that aim to empower each disadvantaged group. The rationale underlying this model is that within each society, there is a reservoir of resiliency supported by traditional coping mechanisms, which, if mobilized, allow members to adapt effectively over time. It is argued that interventions should aim to facilitate the process of natural recovery by supporting local initiatives without imposing approaches derived from other contexts. Viewed from this perspective, the establishment of mental health clinics represents a top-down model in which expatriate 'experts' import Western treatments for conditions such as PTSD that some have argued have little salience in other cultures (Bracken *et al*,1995; Summerfield, 2001). Hence, according to this pervasive conceptual polarization, the psychosocial model promotes autonomy whereas the clinic-based method replicates in microcosm a culture of authoritarianism and paternalism.

There are, however, many difficulties with any attempt to defend such a clear-cut dichotomization. PTSD is only one of the several mental disorders needing attention in refugee and post-conflict populations. There is increasing recognition that untreated mental illness amongst conflict-effected and refugee population represents a source of substantial disability and social disruption, not just for the affected person but also for the family and wider social network (Silove *et al.*, 2000; 2008). Periods of prolonged conflict compound problems of socio-economic underdevelopment, resulting in the undermining of mental health services (if they exist at all). It is not uncommon for families to resort to restraining psychotic members, for example, by tying them to trees. Although not well documented, anecdotal evidence suggests that in the midst of conflict, the severely mentally ill are at risk of abandonment, exploitation, and abuse. A common outcome is that persons with psychosis are found concentrated in gaols. Hence a focus on the severely mentally ill should be a high ethical and human rights priority in the aftermath of humanitarian emergencies. Failure to provide the mentally ill with care reduces any opportunity for that subgroup to regain the capacity to exercise even a rudimentary level of autonomy. There is also some empirical evidence that a group with trauma-related disorders continue to experience ongoing disability in the post-conflict phase often without access to treatment (Silove *et al.*, 2008).

Whereas most psychosocial programmes take active steps to promote traditional practices and indigenous leadership, it seems inevitable that the very existence of these initiatives, like any western involvement, will contribute to the overall acceleration of social change that is typical of the post-conflict environment. Aid agencies bring with them their own philosophies, approaches to management, and ways of working that can never be entirely value-neutral. It is moreover impossible to avoid the power imbalance created by the presence of expatriate personnel who have had the advantages of advanced levels of education and greater access to resources.

It is equally inaccurate to depict clinical services as been invariably culturally insensitive. In settings of best practice, such services have demonstrated the feasibility of integrating cultural understandings of distress and traditional healing approaches into comprehensive models of care. Emphasis is given to training indigenous mental health workers to implement both Western and traditional approaches to managing traumatic stress and other mental health problems. In addition, priority is given to promoting local leadership and community participation in directing and shaping the development and management of mental health services.

Psychotherapeutic approaches and science

There also is an evident divergence in approaches to treatment between the refugee field and the general area of clinical traumatology. Research with survivors of civilian trauma (accidents, rape, occupational injury) has produced evidence supporting the effectiveness of specific forms of cognitive behavioural therapy in which exposure to memories of the trauma commonly plays a central role. Recent guidelines for the treatment of PTSD have concluded that trauma-focused CBT is the therapy of choice for this condition (Australian Centre for the Treatment of Post-traumatic Mental Health, 2007). Questions remain however as to the applicability of this method, that systematically exposes the person to the trauma memories, to refugee survivors of trauma. Whether or not refugees, and in particular, torture survivors benefit from CBT, particularly, an approach that systematically exposes the person to trauma memories, is a topic that continues to attract heated debate. Four key objections have been raised about the use of trauma-focused, brief CBT in these settings, namely, (1) that psychotherapy in general is alien to non-Western cultures; (2) more specifically, that CBT is overly directive (and hence paternalistic); (3) that systematic exposure to memories of traumas such as torture and rape can be retraumatizing; and (4) that brief interventions of this kind do not address the complex and long-term nature of the psychosocial problems facing refugees. Some years ago, the first author of this chapter commented on the paradox of offering CBT to survivors of trauma: first, the person was exposed to the initial trauma event; then they experience distressing and repeated replays of the experience in the form of flashbacks and nightmares; and finally, trauma-focused therapists guide them through a systematic process of repeating the memories in imagination during the course of treatment (Silove, 1992).

The widespread resistance to CBT in the refugee field can be traced back to philosophical and ideological controversies that prevailed in Psychology in the 1960s and 1970s. Strong objections were raised about the growing use of behavioural therapy, which was seen as a form of psychological control akin to social engineering, an identification that was intensified by the controversial claims of advocates such as B.F. Skinner. With that history, and even though the approach has evolved over time, it is not surprising that CBT has been regarded with suspicion by practitioners in the refugee field, where social, human rights, and political factors are relevant in considering the optimal approach to interventions. Again, at the one pole in the discourse are those who are characterized (or stereotyped) as clinicians who advocate CBT methods; at the other are those who depict themselves as defending the human rights of torture survivors, and who tend to criticize the simplistic assumptions of CBT.

This conflict has been given extensive publicity in a prolonged and spirited exchange published in the prestigious British Medical Journal. A leading researcher in the field wrote a commentary asserting that after 30 years, treatment services for refugees were still not applying evidence-based treatments (namely CBT) for survivors of torture, in spite of research showing that the commonly applied multi-modal psychosocial interventions did not work (Başoğlu, 2006).

In response, experienced clinicians (Jaranson *et al.*, 2007) argued that brief treatments such as CBT do not address the enormity of the impact of torture, a form of abuse that 'destroys the fundamental sense of trust in other human beings, raises deeply disturbing existential questions, and results in despair' that cannot be compared with the consequences of other traumas. As others have done, these commentators argue for recognition of a complex form of PTSD response amongst survivors of torture, requiring longer-term and more comprehensive interventions.

A key issue highlighted in the ensuing debate is the paucity of scientific evidence attesting to the efficacy of any treatments in the refugee field. There is an evident imperative therefore to develop a sound scientific foundation for practice in the field so that conjecture and controversy are replaced by evidence. In the field, however, conventional science is often identified with the medical model and hence with paternalism, an ethos of anti-science that has inhibited research into interventions in the field (Leaning, 2001). It is noteworthy that the slender evidence that exists offers tentative support for a role for CBT interventions in treating severe traumatic stress reactions, with practitioners demonstrating the feasibility of modifying the approach to match each context and cultural setting (Otto and Hinton, 2007; Neuner *et al.*, 2004). In contrast, longitudinal studies have shown minimal improvements amongst refugees attending comprehensive rehabilitation programmes using multidimensional interventions, even in centres with extensive experience in the field (Carlsson *et al.*, 2005). A more recent study, however, has shown modest gains for a broad-based multidimensional intervention for torture survivors in Nepal (Tol *et al.*, 2009). What is most striking in considering the body of evidence as a whole, however, is how few resources have been committed to undertaking studies that subject competing therapeutic models to a critical test.

Conclusions

This chapter has focused on some key ethical issues underpinning approaches to interventions for refugees and torture survivors. We have attempted to illustrate the complexities of applying general medical ethical principles to the field, particularly the risk in assuming that ethical concepts such as autonomy and paternalism are polar opposites. Instead, we have attempted to demonstrate that there is a complex balance of these influences in designing and applying interventions. We suggest therefore that ideologically driven approaches need to be replaced by models that are tested by a systematic process of ongoing evaluation and critical analysis. A process of international consensus-building is needed to develop a standard set of assessment procedures to allow comparison of research findings across treatment agencies.

In spite of a conviction by some that the risks of research in refugee populations outweigh the benefits, it remains clear that systematic investigations can be undertaken in an ethical manner (see also Leaning, 2001), and in a way that yields immediate as well as potentially longer-term gains to enhance recovery. Most services have waiting lists so that a wait-list control design is possible and justifiable in designing intervention studies. Alternatively, given the current state of knowledge, it is clearly defensible to conduct randomized controlled trials comparing CBT-based treatments with the standard multimodal interventions used routinely in services.

Those who argue *a priori* that refugees should not be subjected to research are at risk of themselves acting paternalistically. There is no reason to believe that refugees lack an interest and commitment to advancing the scientific understanding of interventions that may assist them or others in similar predicaments in the future. Furthermore, to deny refugees treatments that may work, for example CBT in selective cases, may also constitute an act of paternalism. Refugees should at least be given the right to make informed choices about the interventions they may receive, particularly if there are competing claims about the efficiency of different approaches. It may be that unless a subgroup of refugees disabled by severe PTSD or depressive symptoms are offered specific therapies (such as CBT and/or medication), they will not be able to participate effectively in the new society irrespective of the opportunities offered them by comprehensive psychosocial programmes. For example, it is possible that high levels of PTSD and depressive symptoms impair the refugee's ability to learn the native language of the resettlement country, a major impediment to integration and effective functioning and a source of further frustration and stress.

In conclusion, we note that ideology and fervour are vital elements driving the establishment of a new field. As the field matures, however, any intervention-based endeavour in the health or social science arena is obliged to subject its practices to critical test, a process that requires a sober, and objective perspective. That point has arrived for the refugee mental health field. Instead of regarding science and ethics as potentially opposing forces, we should see the two as allies in the endeavour of achieving the greatest benefit for our patients—establishing interventions that work.

References

Australian Centre for Posttraumatic Mental Health (2007). Australian Guidelines for the Treatment of Adults with Acute Stress Disorder and Posttraumatic Stress Disorder: Practitioner Guide. Australian Centre for Posttraumatic Mental Health.

Basoglu, M. (2006). Rehabilitation of traumatised refugees and survivors of torture. *British Medical Journal* **333**: 1230–1231.

Bracken, P.J., Giller, J.E., and Summerfield, D. (1995). Psychological responses to war and atrocity: the limitations of current concepts. *Social Science and Medicine* **40**: 1073–1082.

Carlsson, J.M., Mortensen, E.L., and Kastrup, M. (2005). A follow-up study of mental health and health-related quality of life in tortured refugees in multidisciplinary treatment. *Journal of Nervous and Mental Disorders* **193**: 651–657.

Farr Curlin, R., Lawrence, M., and Chin, J.L. (2007). Religion, conscience, and controversial clinical practices. *New England Journal of Medicine* **356**: 593–600.

Gillon, R. (1985). (Primum non-nocere) and the principle or non-maleficence. *BioMed Journal* (Clininical Research Edition) **291**: 130–131.

Humanitarian Charter and Minimum Standards in Disaster Response (2004). Geneva: Sphere Project. Available from: http://www.sphereproject.org/handbook/index.htm

Jaranson, M. (2007). Standard therapy for all torture survivors?: A reply to Metin Basoglu. 30 January 2007. Accessed from BMJ.com/cg/eletters. (July 3 2009).

Kinzie, J.D., Tran, K.A., Breckenridge, A., and Bloom, J.D. (1980). An Indochinese refugee psychiatric clinic: culturally accepted treatment approaches. *American Journal of Psychiatry* **137**: 1429–1432.

Leaning J. (2001). Ethics of research in refugee populations, *The Lancet* **357**: 1432–1433.

Mollica, R.F., Wyshak, G., and Lavelle, J. (1987). The psychosocial impact of war trauma and torture on Southeast Asian Refugees. *American Journal of Psychiatry* **144**: 1567–1572.

Neuner, F., Schauer, M., Klaschik, C., Karunakara, U., and Elbert, T. (2004). A comparison of narrative exposure therapy, supportive counseling, and psychoeducation for treating posttraumatic stress disorder in an African refugee settlement. *Journal of Consulting and Clinical Psychology* **72**: 579–587.

Otto, M.W. and Hinton, D. (2007). Treatment of pharmacotherapy–refractory posttraumatic stress disorder among Cambodian refugees: A pilot study of combination treatment with cognitive–behaviour therapy vs sertraline alone. *Behaviour Research and Therapy* **41**: 1271–1276.

Quill, T. and Brody, H. (1996). Physician recommendations and patient autonomy: Finding a balance between physician power and patient choice. *Annals of Internal Medicine* **125**: 763–769.

Rees, S. (2003). Refuge or retrauma? The impact of prolonged asylum seeker status on the well being of East Timorese women asylum seekers residing in the Australian community. *Australasian Psychiatry*. Supplement **11**: S96–S101.

Rees, S. (2004). East Timorese asylum seekers in Australia – extrapolating a case for resettlement. *Australian Social Work* **57**: 259–272.

Rees, S. and Pease, B. (2007). Domestic violence in refugee families in Australia: Rethinking settlement policy and practice. *International Journal of Immigrant and Refugee Studies* **5**: 1–19.

Silove, D., Tarn, R., Bowles, R., and Reid, J. (1991). Psychosocial needs of torture survivors. *Australian and New Zealand Journal of Psychiatry* **25**: 481–490.

Silove, D. (1992). Psychotherapy and trauma. Current Opinion in Psychiatry **5**: 370–374.

Silove, D., Sinnerbrink, I., Field, A., Manicavasagar, V., and Steel, Z. (1997). Anxiety, depression and PTSD in asylum seekers: Associations with pre-migration trauma and post-migration stressors. *British Journal of Psychiatry* **170**: 351–357.

Silove, D., Ekblad, S., and Mollica, R. (2000). The rights of the severely mentally ill in post-conflict countries. *Lancet* **255**: 1548–1549.

Silove, D., Bateman, C.R., Brooks, R.T., *et al.* (2008). Estimating clinically relevant mental disorders in a rural and an urban setting in postconflict Timor Leste. *Archives of General Psychiatry* **65**: 1205–1212.

Smith, C.M. (2005). Origin and uses of Primum Non Nocere – above all, do no harm! *Journal of Clinical Pharmacology* **45**: 371–377.

Somnier, F.E. and Genefke, I.G. (1986). Psychotherapy for victims of torture. *The British Journal of Psychiatry* **149**: 323–329.

Summerfield, D. (2001). The invention of post-traumatic stress disorder and the social usefulness of a psychiatric category. *BioMed Journal* **322**: 95–98.

Tol, W.A., Komproe, I.H., Jordans, M.J.D., Thapa, S.B., Sharma, B., and De Jong, J.T.V.M. (2009). Brief multi-disciplinary treatment for torture survivors in Nepal: A naturalistic comparative study. *International Journal of Social Psychiatry* **55**: 39–56.

Thomasma, D. (1983). Beyond medical paternalism and patient autonomy: a model of physician conscience for the physician–patient relationship. *Annals of Internal Medicine* **98**: 243–248.

Van Ommeren, M., Saxena, S., and Saraceno, B. (2005). Aid after disasters. *BioMed Journal* **330**: 1160–1161.

Chapter 19

Impact on clinicians

Sean Cross and Jim Crabb

Introduction

The United Nations High Commission for Refugees (UNHCR) states that there are over 30 million people of concern to them (UNHCR, 2007). Most are located in Asia and Africa, with many living in large camps as a result of a number of problems that may have forced people from their homes. The numbers seeking asylum in Western nations increased significantly after the end of the Cold War and into the 21st century. It has been noted that refugees and asylum seekers bring with them a series of health challenges (Burnett and Peel, 2001b). As a result the impact upon clinicians working with them can be significant. Some of these challenges are universal and independent of where clinicians may work with refugees—others are specific to certain settings. It would be foolish to state that exactly the same impacts occur regardless of whether a clinician is working in a North London clinic or in a border camp in Sudan; however, this chapter will try to focus on the general themes that have emerged in the literature.

To simplify the fluid and complex relationship between refugee client and clinician in an attempt to analyse the effect that this may have on a mental health worker, we will look at the possible impacts at three different levels: 1) Those aspects or characteristics intrinsic to both the refugee and the clinician as individuals; 2) Aspects specific to the refugee or asylum seeker experience, which may impact on the clinician; and 3) Those aspects specific to the therapeutic relationship between clinician and client. These are false boundaries with significant overlap but enable a series of challenges to be laid out in a reasonably logical fashion.

It is important to note in the introduction that the legal classification of individuals in this area of work is complex. As recorded earlier, the UNHCR divides the numbers of those of concern into refugees, asylum seekers, and internally displaced persons. For ease of writing during this chapter the term 'refugee' is used without necessarily implying the exact legal meaning associated with it, with the more specific terms saved for those times where it is specifically relevant to the point being made.

Finally by way of introduction, a danger inherent in this exercise is to problematize all potential impacts. It is clear that many of the issues that will be raised can be seen as difficulties, but it is also hoped that some of the impacts will be viewed as positive, as is certainly the case with our own clinical experiences.

Aspects intrinsic to the refugee and clinician that may impact

Refugees are by definition those who have fled, for a variety of reasons, due to a 'well founded fear of being persecuted' (UN, 1951). Such flight usually involves travelling significant distances, often crossing cultures and state boundaries. It is not uncommon for some clinicians to be members of the same cultural heritage as those seeking help, but on the whole, certainly within the West, this is not usually the case. Therefore, at a fundamental level in most cases the issue of difference arises requiring cultural competency in assessment and management.

To be culturally competent, all clinicians need to be aware of their own cultural inheritance and potential prejudices. Leaving aside for the time being the issue of language and interpreter use, it is recognized that it is remarkably easier to gain or impart information with someone who is similar to oneself in a whole range of different ways—see Table 19.1. A variety of verbal and non-verbal communication mechanisms can be used within a context of shared cultural knowledge. Difficulties invariably arise as differences grow—whether these are related to language, religious values, or broader cultural factors—and this will most certainly impact on the clinician. However, communicating across these differences is an essential skill for any clinician working with refugees to learn.

The extent of any impact will vary and familiarity with multicultural settings may reduce many of these aspects. However, for those whose work normally caters to a less diverse population, the impact may be greater. In the UK for example, from the year 2000 a policy of 'dispersal' of new asylum seekers to towns and cities across the country and away from London and the southeast of England occurred. It was even recognized by the Home Office

Table 19.1 Summarizing some of the many ways in which difference may occur

Age	Gender	Class
Ethnicity	Religion	Language
Sexual orientation	Nationality	Political persuasion

(UK Ministry of Internal Affairs), that such a policy had an impact on local services and clinicians normally unaccustomed to working with such groups (Johnson, 2001).

Any of the differences mentioned in Table 19.1 earlier may result in a lack of shared knowledge. Into that vacuum assumptions may arise, from which prejudice may spring. Building cultural competence and shared knowledge requires one to have an awareness of relevant issues, which even if somewhat alien, are accepted as valid. 'Culturally aware' assessment and management processes have been described at great length (Fontes, 2008). Table 19.2 summarizes many of the issues that arise in cross-cultural interactions. These can be viewed as generic for dealing with any kind of cultural difference but a refugee population can present particularly pertinent difficulties. At a basic level, for example, the epidemiology of refugee populations within the West reveals a disproportionate skew towards youth and male gender—in the UK in 2007 more than 75% of asylum seekers were under 35 years old and 70% of these were male (Home Office, 2007). This almost certainly occurs because of the hardships associated with the refugee flight, but brings a range of potential impacts not

Table 19.2 Summarizing important ideas in a culturally aware process

Be aware of oneself	Be aware of other	Be aware of circumstance
Beliefs about how certain problems *should* present according to one's own cultural norms	Variations in presentation of the same problem, e.g. different idioms of distress	The wider socio-political context within which you are working
How one's own cultural norms affect the formulation process	The variety of symptom cluster profiles that may occur, e.g. different emphases on the somatic	Acceptance of the reality of institutionalized prejudice processes
Any general assumptions and prejudices held by one's own culture about others	The basic norms and values of other cultures without assuming they are automatically held	Understand that acculturation can result in hybrid responses becoming common
The way one has previously accepted or challenged these assumptions and prejudices	Avoidance of both negative and positive assumptions of others	Multiculturalism may mean different groups access and use the same service differently
Knowledge of the assumptions and prejudices made by other cultures about one's own	Assessment of the impact of assumptions or prejudices directed at your culture	
One's own non-verbal communication methods	Other kinds of non-verbal communication methods	

least because this group may be perceived as being more threatening. However, a deeper impact than basic demography is politics. The political context behind the seeking of refugee status tends to result in much greater importance being attached to such matters than would normally occur within a clinician–client relationship. Knowledge of the socio-political situation in many troubled parts of the world can be an invaluable tool in enabling a fuller dialogue.

Beyond these basics is the importance of accurate interpretation of possible psychopathology such as an understanding of variations of idioms of distress across cultures. In addition, attitudes to medicine, psychiatry, and healing as well as expectations of what may be offered therapeutically all bring potential impacts on the clinician. Some of these aspects will be taken up further later in this chapter but acknowledgement of them is an important starting point.

Aspects of the 'refugee experience' that may impact on the clinician

There are two important aspects of the refugee experience that this section will focus on with regard to possible impacts upon the clinician: 1) the consequences of the realities of the refugee's current social existence and 2) the repercussions of any original trauma.

The realities of the refugee experience, even when relative safety is reached, can be enormously focused on loss. Not only possible loss of family or friends, but also loss of contacts, security, job, money, status, and many others—fleeing is seldom planned in an organized fashion. Some of the differences noted earlier in Table 19.1 can be warped in a way that the clinician may not be used to experiencing. For example, it is not unusual for highly educated, successful, politically aware, and engaged individuals to present to clinicians in significant poverty. It has been commented upon that enforced poverty is very common and a consequence of some Western government policies (Refugee Council, 2002). When these are unexpected, the impact on the clinician may be marked and unless recognized and managed appropriately, can lead to difficulties in the therapeutic relationship, which will be further dealt with in the next section.

The impact of trauma

Trauma of one form or another is prevalent within the refugee experience. Direct targeted torture or more generic but traumatic violence experiences are common. These stories in turn are recounted to the clinician and their impacts can be significant. It is common for many mental health professionals to regularly hear unpleasant stories. However, the refugee population is a cohort in whom such tales tend to be much more prevalent and with whom it is common to experience little in the way of cathartic accounts of justice. The potential effect on the clinician has been recognized for some time. All are variations on themes of traumatization, one step removed from the direct experience in a 'secondary' way. A number of different models are described in the literature. These vary in the extent to which they draw on counter-transference psychodynamic theory, but whatever the theoretical framework underlying the models, they all form an important justification for adequate support and supervision structures being in place for clinicians.

General 'burnout' is described in clinicians working with those who have experienced trauma (van der Ploeg *et al.*, 1990; Pross, 2006). Symptoms include apathy, feelings of hopelessness, rapid exhaustion, disillusionment, melancholy, forgetfulness, and irritability. The clinician may also have an alienated, impersonal, and cynical attitude towards their clients together with a tendency to blame themselves coupled with a sense of failure. Sometimes the clinician will develop similar physical symptoms to the client who may evoke intense feelings such as rage directed towards those responsible for the suffering. The clinician may also experience helplessness in the face of overwhelming amounts of work to be done, which can, in turn, lead to negative feelings about the client. In the phenomenon of burnout, cynicism and hopelessness can replace faith in the clinician's capacity to heal (Wilson, 2004). Perhaps as a result of burnout, trauma therapists have been found to be more cynical about the inherent goodness in people than their colleagues working in mainstream services (Smith *et al.*, 2007).

In a compassion fatigue model, clinicians have been described as developing trauma symptoms with confusion and isolation from peers and family supports (Figley, 2002). This is thought to occur as a direct reaction of exposure to the client's traumatic material and so develops independently regardless of the therapist's experience or personality. A specific reaction pattern has also been described where the clinician will experience shock, anxiety, feelings of being overwhelmed, and somatic complaints in response to the client's traumatic material (Smith *et al.*, 2007).

Vicarious traumatization has been defined as the transformation of the helper's inner experience as a result of empathic engagement with the trauma of another, specifically when the clinician's own cognitions concerning safety, trust, and control are overwhelmed by exposure to the traumatic material (McCann and Pearlman, 1990). This can result in significant problems developing for the clinician. An 'infection' model hypothesizes that in vicarious traumatization the clinician becomes flooded with memories, nightmares, fear, and distrust. In this situation, the mental state of the clinician is characterized by depression and cynicism.

In reality there is usually little distinction between secondary traumatization, burnout, compassion fatigue, or vicarious traumatization. It has been argued that the categories are perhaps of little use in everyday clinical practice except to highlight the inherent dangers of exposure (Salston and Figley, 2003).

A further useful way of classifying the potential consequences to the clinician is in terms of time. The effects of trauma work at the time of interview, immediately afterwards, and in the long term should be noted, as each may result in different impacts for which the clinician should prepare (Veer, 1998).

Secondary re-traumatization is of particular concern for any clinician who themselves may have in the past experienced trauma. In the management of refugees, this is not uncommon—many charities and voluntary organizations may themselves have clinicians who were previously refugees. 'Wounded healers' is a Jungian term, often used in trauma work that describes clinicians who have experienced their own significant personal trauma. Whilst this may put them at an advantage in being able to empathize with their clients, concern has been expressed that day-to-day work with trauma may impair the clinician's ability to process their own experiences. It has also been noted that traumatic reactions can be induced in clinicians by material other than trauma. On balance however, although many dangers may be inherent from the descriptions given earlier, it has also been recorded that when properly managed, long-term trauma therapy has not been found to negatively influence experienced therapists on self-reported measures (Smith *et al.*, 2007).

Given these concerns guidance has been suggested on how to avoid many of these situations by taking preventive measures as summarized in Table 19.3 (Pross, 2006).

Aspects of the clinician–client relationship that may impact on the clinician

When working with refugees the therapeutic relationship between the client and therapist is central to engaging the individual in treatment, easing suffering, and helping them establish their life in a new country. The therapeutic relationship will often evolve more than in a 'typical' case as the refugee adapts to new processes of treatment and to the cultural mores of their new host country. For many therapeutic relationships, a basic difference will be evident immediately due to the use of interpreters. As with all interpreter use, the impact on the clinician may be marked (Farooq and Fear, 2003). Additionally, powerful expectations and assumptions will influence the emerging therapeutic relationship. These include how the refugee views treatment, how the refugee views the individual managing the treatment, and how the health professional views the progress of the client.

Table 19.3 Summarizing putative factors for prevention of 'Burnout' (Pross, 2006)

- Clinician self-care – avoiding overwork, having regular time for hobbies, leisure, family, and friends
- Solid professional training in diagnosis and (psycho)therapy
- Therapeutic self-awareness
- Regular examination by colleagues
- External supervision
- Limiting caseload
- Continuing professional education and learning new concepts in trauma
- Opportunities for research and training sabbaticals
- Keeping a balance between empathy and a proper professional distance to clients
- Protecting caregivers against being misled by clients with fictitious PTSD
- Having an institutional setting in which the roles of therapists and evaluators are separate
- Social recognition for caregivers
- Forming alliances with mainstream medical and academic institutions
- Overcoming the financial and legal outsider status of centres that work with refugees
- Integration of centres that work with refugees into the general healthcare system.

This material was first published in TORTURE Journal, volume 16 no. 1.

Expectations the client may have about treatment

The foundation of a strong therapeutic alliance in Western health care has been thought to consist of three components: warmth, empathy, and positive regard (Rogers, 1951). It is important to bear in mind that this cornerstone of the therapeutic process together with the concept of a collaborative relationship is based on Western, liberal tradition. The assumption that the client is a consumer who is able to make choices about their health care within a shared collaborative relationship between client and therapist may be unfamiliar in some cultures. Clients from a different background may expect the 'expert' to hand down instructions, commands, or actual physical assistance in a hierarchical fashion without their being an active participant in this process. There may of course be other reasons a refugee is reluctant to embrace warmth, empathy, positive regard, and a collaborative approach. When an individual has been in fear for their life or is threatened with deportation, it can be completely reasonable for them to mistrust a clinician who may be considered an agent of a hostile state. Confusion over differing instruments of the new host state—such as healthcare and immigration/security agencies—can be common, in particular over the level of any communication between them. Similarly experiences of trauma will lead to fear and distrust in the client who may also not disclose the extent of their difficulties due to fear of consequences

(Pernice and Brook, 1994). In these instances, it is important for clinicians to appreciate the fact that the therapeutic relationship, particularly in the early stages of treatment, may be more emotionally distant then they are used to. It is important for the clinician to meet the needs of their client and balance their approach accordingly. Adopting a collaborative approach in the first instance may confuse, alienate, or distance the refugee from the treatment process, whereas taking an over directive approach may re-enact the refugees' previous experience of trauma from which they have fled.

A refugee may have little or no experience of the treatment being offered to them and in which it is assumed they will participate. This is particularly true when psychological interventions are employed. Most traditional psychotherapies used in a Western setting are based on the assumption that vocalizing distress and past events is inherently healing. This may not be the case in certain cultures where experiences may remain unspeakable. It is all too easy for the therapist to unwittingly breech etiquette which may prevent further disclosure and in extreme cases the relationship may break down altogether (Pernice and Brook, 1994). In these situations it may be best to focus on the 'here and now' helping the individual to function as fully as they can in their new surroundings. In some circumstances, largely non-verbal techniques such as Eye Movement Desensitisation and Reprocessing (EMDR) may be appropriate particularly if processing of traumatic memories is an issue. Other aspects of psychological therapy can also be problematic. Boundaries for sessions (e.g. keeping therapy to 1 hour) may be seen as authoritarian and negative in the light of the refugee's experiences. Holding on to emotions from one meeting to the next can also be an intolerable and alien concept for the client. It has been suggested that therapists should explain the meaning of boundaries such as time keeping to the individual and arrive at an arrangement that is agreeable to all parties (D'Ardenne and Mahtani, 1999). It can also be difficult for the clinician and client to gauge their progress throughout therapy. For example, in some cultures respect towards authority can be communicated through politeness, positive affirmative answers to questions, and a desire to communicate that the individual is doing well. This will result in mixed messages being given to the therapist and a confusing clinical picture.

In instances were medication is employed there can be differing expectations between client and clinician. Refugees from certain parts of the world may expect psychotropic medication to provide relief after a short course in the same way a physical treatment would do. In certain cultures psychological distress can be managed by traditional healers. Medication given during these consultations can produce instant violent reactions (e.g. rash or vomiting) that may be interpreted by the user as demonstrating its strength or power against their illness. Individuals from these cultures can be distrustful and disappointed when given a Western medicine with minimal side effects that they may see as weak. This in turn can undermine their confidence in the clinician.

Expectations the client may have about the clinician

Refugees typically have multiple physical, psychological, and social problems (Burnett and Peel, 2001a; McColl *et al.*, 2008). They tend to exist outside mainstream healthcare and social services systems and therefore there can be a tendency for a single clinician (often working for a voluntary agency) to assume multiple roles that would ordinarily be taken on by a multi-disciplinary team. This can have important safety implications if a clinician is risk managing a complex situation or performing a role they are not trained for. A single clinician performing many roles can also have a marked impact on the relationship dynamic. A lack of role clarity has been linked to the emotional burden experienced by the therapist whereas a direct relationship has been demonstrated between the amount of psychosocial problems a client has and the amount of emotional stress found in the therapist (Smith *et al.*, 2007). A refugee also may have unrealistic expectations about the power and influence that a single health professional may be able to exert over their social situation such as involvement in processing an asylum application. Unaddressed, these assumptions can erode the therapeutic relationship.

The relationship dynamic is complicated by the fact that clinicians who put in extra effort can often be seen as more genuine by refugees. Although this can often strengthen the therapeutic alliance, it can alternatively hinder an individual regaining a sense of control and empowerment needed to recover from their experiences (Linden and Grut, 2002).

Expectations the clinician may have about the client

Much has been written using psychodynamic models in refugee work and provides a useful and familiar framework for many Western trained clinicians. Problems related to counter transference have been reported, often as a result of the blurring of roles and boundaries described earlier. Empathic enmeshment is a description of what occurs when the clinician does not have enough inner distance from the client. Descriptions of this suggest it leads to confusion, lack of progress, helplessness, and anger. In the opposite position of empathic repression, which can occur after a period of over involvement, too much internal distance and too little empathy leads to disappointment, helplessness, and guilt (Wilson, 2004). In both positions it may be tempting for the clinician to abandon the case, ignoring basic human suffering and distress which are explained away as being 'normal' for a different culture and therefore unchangeable or outside the remit of health professionals.

It has also been suggested that certain traits in the personality of the clinician can become pathological in the therapeutic relationship. A desire for power and control on behalf of the helper may compensate for their own feelings of inadequacy and helplessness outside of work (particularly in the case of 'wounded healers' described earlier). In these situations this drive may initially be displayed through frantic activity on behalf of the client and the passionate championing of their case. In its most pathological expression a situation may develop where the clinician becomes an omnipotent force with the refugee client reduced to little more then a helpless child. There may also exist narcissistic traits in the clinician who wishes to receive adoration from society and grateful clients. Finally, it has been suggested that a therapist may also unconsciously explore their own dark fantasies through seeking out trauma work (Hawkins and Shohet, 2000). The presence of any of these traits in a clinician would not automatically prevent the individual working with refugees; however, they reinforce the importance of adopting the approaches outlined in Table 19.3—particularly those of therapeutic self-awareness, regular self-examination, and external supervision.

Conclusions

As has been described, the impact on a clinician working with refugees can be significant. Awareness of these issues is an essential first step when considering the help that is provided to this group who are often in desperate need. Such provision may then be given in a way that is appropriate and hopefully healing in its outcome without an adverse impact on the clinician themselves.

References

Burnett, A. and Peel, M. (2001a). Asylum seekers and refugees in Britain. The health of survivors of torture and organised violence. *British Medical Journal* **322**: 606–609.

Burnett, A. and Peel, M. (2001b). Health needs of asylum seekers and refugees. *British Medical Journal* **322**: 544–547.

D'ardenne, P. and Mahtani, A. (1999). *Transcultural Counselling in Action,* London: Sage.

Farooq, S. and Fear, C. (2003). Working through interpreters. *Advances In Psychiatric Treatment* **9**: 104–109.

Figley, C.R. (2002). *Treating Compassion Fatigue,* New York, NY; London: Brunner-Routledge.

Fontes, L.A. (2008). *Interviewing Clients Across Cultures: A Practitioner's Guide,* New York; London: Guilford.

Hawkins, P. and Shohet, R. (2000). *Supervision in the Helping Professions: An Individual, Group and Organizational Approach.* Buckingham: Open University.

Home Office (2007). Home Office Statistical Bulletin: Asylum Statistics United Kingdom 2007; http://www.homeoffice.gov.uk/rds/pdfs08/hosb1108.pdf

Johnson, M. (2001). Asylum Seekers in Dispersal – Healthcare Issues. *Home Office On Line Report 13/03* http://www.homeoffice.gov.uk/rds/pdfs2/rdsolr1303.pdf Crown Copyright.

Linden, S. and Grut, J. (2002) *The Healing Fields: Working with Psychotherapy and Nature to Rebuild Shattered Lives.* London: Frances Lincoln.

McCann, L. and Pearlman, L.A. (1990). Vicarious traumatization: a framework for understanding the psychological effects of working with victims. *Journal Of Traumatic Stress* **3**: 131–149.

McColl, H., McKenzie, K., and Bhui, K. (2008). Mental healthcare of asylum-seekers and refugees. *Advances in Psychiatric Treatment* **14**: 452–459.

Pernice, R. and Brook, J. (1994). Relationship of Migrant Status (Refugee or Immigrant) to Mental Health. *International Journal of Social Psychiatry* **40**: 177–188.

Pross, C. (2006). Burnout, vicarious traumatization and its prevention. *Torture* **16**: 1–9.

Refugee Council (2002). Poverty and Asylum in the UK –http://www.refugeecouncil.org.uk/policy/position/2002/poverty.htm

Rogers, C.R. (1951[2003]). *Client-Centred Therapy: Its Current Practice, Implications and Therapy.* London: Constable.

Salston, M. and Figley, C.R. (2003). Secondary traumatic stress effects of working with survivors of criminal victimization. *Journal of Trauma Stress* **16**: 167–174.

Smith, A.J.M., Kleijn, W.M., Trijsburg, R.W., and Hutschemaekers, G.J.M. (2007). How therapists cope with clients' traumatic experiences. *Torture* **17**: 203–215.

UN (1951). Convention Relating to the Status of Refugees.

UNHCR (2007). *Statistical Yearbook 2006: Trends in Displacement, Protection and Solutions* http://www.unhcr.org/statistics.html UNHCR.

Van Der Ploeg, H.M., Van Leeuwen, J.J., and Kwee, M.G. (1990). Burnout among Dutch psychotherapists. *Psychological Reports* **67**: 107–112.

Veer, G.V.D. (1998). *Counselling and Therapy with Refugees and Victims of Trauma: Psychological Problems of Victims of War, Torture, and Repression.* New York: John Wiley.

Wilson, J.P. (2004). Empathy, trauma transmission and countertransference in posttraumatic psychotherapy. In J.P. Wilson and B. Drosdek, (Eds.), *Broken Spirits: The Treatment of Traumatized Asylum Seekers, Refugees, War and Torture Victims.* Brunner-Routledge.

Chapter 20

Mental health service provision for asylum seekers and refugees

Kamaldeep Bhui, Nasir Warfa, and
Salaad Mohamud

Introduction

International migration is a fact of modern life. International trade enhanced by the development of communication technologies and easier travel, on one hand, and political instability and poverty in many parts of the world, on the other, have changed the dynamics of migration in the past few decades. There are many reasons for people to migrate. Migration experts mainly categorize them into push and pull factors. People have always left their homes to settle in other lands, either because of 'pull' factors that encourage migration or 'push' factors that encourage or compel them to involuntarily leave their homeland. The extent of globalization is now testament to how much easier migration has become, and how much one part of the world relies on another for humanitarian aid and asylum at times of crisis. Today there are varieties of migrant groups other than economic migrants: asylum seekers, undocumented migrants, and other vulnerable people such as unaccompanied children and trafficked persons.

Contemporary migration is complex and challenges migration policies and theories of migration. Migration also challenges social and immigration policies based on simplistic theoretical frameworks (Watters, 2001). As people move between countries, they connect individual and environmental health factors between one country and another (Davidson *et al.*, 2004). This type of mobility has an effect that goes beyond the physical displacement of persons or populations. People travel with their culture, religion, and traditions. They also travel with their health beliefs and micro-communities that may recreate in the shape of pre-migration social networks, contexts, and experiences. Furthermore, migrants may carry genetic material between different socio-economic and environmental contexts, potentiating new gene environment interactions, with possible adverse consequences for their health and well-being.

In addition, new migrants, like the mainstream population, would require access to public services. Thus, new migrants place demands on health services and public health policy. Their situation would also raise questions about social and employment policy that can harness the skills that migrants bring.

Refugees and asylum seekers: challenges to mental health services

Refugees and asylum seekers bring challenges for services that are common to all migrants, including different cultural beliefs and language needs. However, there are challenges unique to asylum seekers and refugees as a consequence of exposure to war, conflict, persecution, and escape from their country of origin (Warfa and Bhui, 2003, Craig *et al.*, 2006). Once in the host nation, asylum determination of whether a person is a refugee is most often left to certain government agencies within the host country. This could sometimes lead to unfair decisions in some countries with a very restrictive official immigration policy. The long period of time it takes to recognize refugees and asylum seekers in the host countries tends, in many instances, to aggravate both physical and mental health difficulties (Van Ommeren *et al.*, 2001; Laban *et al.*, 2005). The immigration procedure relating to granting refugee status may last for a few months to a few years. This long waiting period places great strains on asylum seekers who during this time are forced to reside in special refugee centres as in many parts of Europe; or they are dispersed to areas where they might face discrimination and attack from local residents. Hallas *et al.* (2007) who studied asylum seekers in designated centres in Denmark found an association between the period of stay and referrals for mental disorders. They reported that referrals for psychiatric disorders increased with the length of stay (0 to 1600 days) in the asylum centres. Asylum seekers and refugees also face extra challenges due to asylum and refugee policy or health policy that structures the delivery of health care in special ways for asylum seekers and refugees. In the chapter on Psychiatric Diagnoses and Assessment Issues for Refugees and Asylum Seekers, we explained how discriminatory immigration policies towards asylum seekers and refugees have caused considerable psychological problems among this group.

In other words, political processes to manage migrants, asylum seekers, and refugees pose specific challenges to health services. Thus, these policies and processes are important as they can convey unwelcoming and perhaps discriminatory attitudes as well as undermine efforts to provide comprehensive health care and social safety. Although this chapter does not address the prevalence of mental disorders amongst immigrants, it is relevant that factors

Table 20.1 Summary of the unique challenges faced by refugee groups and service providers

Common challenges faced by refugee groups	Unique Challenges in Service Provision (UCSP)
• Isolation	• Dealing with torture and consequential mental disorders
• Language barriers	
• Experiences of discrimination	• Providing services within restrictive asylum law
• Loss of social status	
• High rates of unemployment	• Providing care to mobile populations
• Socio-economic deprivation	• Providing services to patients with complex life experiences
• Acculturation difficulties	• Providing services to patients to multiplicity of need and co-morbidity issues
• Bereavements and separations	
• Past experiences of traumatic life events	• Providing services to patients with diverse cultural and religious backgrounds
• Post-migration social problems	• Providing services to patients with language barriers
• Poor access to healthcare services	
• Frequent residential mobility	

influencing service delivery are likely to influence the nature and extent of disorders and their prevalence. Watters (2001) and Silove *et al.* (2000) made links between discriminatory immigration policies in the West and the higher levels of mental health problems found among refugees and asylum seekers.

To begin with, mental health care is often organized on a geographical basis, by local government or health provider boundaries. For populations that are residentially unstable, this places special strain on services and also makes them more likely to drop out of treatment programmes. Traditionally, residential mobility might have involved endogenous people in search of better employment, housing, or education. The organization of services across geographical boundaries may be necessary for the most vulnerable, and those moving between areas may end up not receiving care packages. Residential mobility is not necessarily related to improvements in accommodation or movement to a less deprived area as we found in our work with Somali refugees in South and East London where we retrospectively mapped deprivation indices of residential venues over a five year period for Somali immigrants.

Residential moves involving significant distances also impact on children as these require a change of schools. School transitions have been described as a stressful process in that young children and adolescents must adjust quickly to unfamiliar surrounding, new friends, and teachers as well as the demands and expectations placed on them relating to their academic performance.

Number of studies show that entering a new school is linked with academic and behavioural problems, increasing anxiety over meeting school expectations, and problems gaining acceptance among peers (Crockett et al., 1989). Some stressors such as parental divorce, low family socio-economic and family dysfunction have also been found to impact adversely on both geographical relocation and deviant outcomes (Astone and McLanahan, 1994; Eckenrode et al., 1995). In the UK, however, longitudinal studies on the relationship of geographical mobility and mental ill-health are scarce. One of the few surveys carried out (Lamont, et al., 2000) reported that greater geographical mobility by the schizophrenic patients could be an important factor for the high demands of psychiatric bed use and the difficulties in keeping contact with patients in London. Frequent change of residential address was also associated with patients from more deprived inner London areas than patients from outer areas. In Birmingham, Vostanis et al. (1998) suggested that homeless families and their children's access to primary and secondary health care may be disrupted because of frequent change of address. He also found that mental health problems remained higher in re-housed mothers and their children.

Also crucial is the issue of access to healthcare services. The legal status of migrants in receiving societies often determines access to health and social services. For example, a migrant who is granted permanent residence enjoys the same access to services as the citizens of the host society, but this is not usually the case for labour migrants or irregular migrants. In the UK, asylum seekers are eligible for National Health Service (NHS) treatment only if they have made an application to remain in the country or have been detained by the immigration authorities (Department of Health, 2004). Those who have not made an application for asylum or have had an application refused are not eligible for NHS treatment. The exceptions to this rule are emergency care, treatment of sexually transmitted infections (excluding HIV), and other conditions that threaten public health. Yet, paradoxically, despite these protections against spend on asylum seekers, admission to hospital on a treatment order under mental health legislation (i.e. the disorder is known and treatment is required) mandates the cost of social and mental health care be met. How this affects decision making in applying the mental health act has not been investigated.

The role of language, religion, geographical mobility, immigration status, shared history, and proximity to host country and familiarity with service systems can influence whether services are used, or whether prescriptions and preventive health recommendations are taken up (Powell, et al., 2004). However, uptake is made more difficult if challenges we noted earlier all interact with each other. For example, pre-migration experiences of refugees vary considerably, but many have either witnessed or directly experienced trauma prior to escape from their native countries. Refugees might have also lived long-term in refugee camps in the developing world and traumatic stressors may relate to refugee camp life.

Assessment and intervention

Assessments and treatment by the use of an interpreter is complex, especially when assessing the mental state, personality, and conscious and unconscious affects and drives. How much more difficult is this made when the individual is so traumatized that they feel unsafe speaking to anyone about their past, unsafe because of internal eruptions of emotions and perceived external threats to safety (Warfa, 2006); in speaking to professionals, strangers may represent 'authority figures' that in their homeland were oppressive. Detention processes themselves may be experienced as forms of imprisonment, oppression, and as unduly restrictive, perhaps adding to risks of mental health problems (Silove et al., 2000). Furthermore, restrictions on welfare benefits and employment rights (for example in the UK) can place asylum seekers and refugees in a predicament and at the bottom of the social ladder in a society. The British Refugee Council has documented the impact of restrictions on welfare benefits and employment rights on the mental well-being of asylum seekers (http://www.refugeecouncil.org.uk/). They may never recover the social status they once held in their home country, or achieve in accord with their educational and occupational histories. It is unclear whether this is due to the impact of conflict and the asylum process on their personality and resilience, or whether it is due to the early conditions they experienced in the host country.

Nevertheless, refugees who have successfully immigrated to the Western world may continue to have psychological distress and difficulties adapting and adjusting years later. For example, many Southeast Asian patients, other than those with schizophrenia and bipolar disorders, who continued to seek mental health care years after entry into the US, have not made successful adjustments when they compared themselves with their neighbours (Chung and Bemak, 1996). Like many other refugees, these refugees learnt little English, had difficulties finding proper jobs, and were entirely dependent on government housing and welfare handout that was increasingly getting complicated. Worst of all, they were in despair that their children, once their hope for the future, were dropping out of school, and became disrespectful to them. However, as Lavik et al. (1996) pointed out, relationships between living conditions in exile and mental ill-health do not automatically arise from simple cause-and-effect relationships. Living conditions may influence mental health, and mental health problem may create more adjustment difficulties in the host country. A good example is the Guatemalan refugees described by Sabin *et al.* (2003). After twenty years in exile, it was difficult for these refugees to have hope for the future or believe that there was anything they could do to improve their lives. Consequently, many of these refugees experienced profound demoralization that calls for a social solution at least as important as a medical one (Chodoff, 2002).

The following three case studies exemplify specific and unique dilemmas in the provision of mental health services to refugees and asylum seekers.

___

Case study one: assessment challenges

Ms A: a 28-year-old married woman, a refugee from East Europe, with two children aged 5 and 1, is referred to a psychotherapy department for dynamic therapy. She has received counselling in primary care, and this is reported to show significant progress in processing material about loss of family and homeland. She arrives for a psychotherapy assessment with her 1-year-old child, and appears profoundly depressed and suicidal. Yet, the assessment can not be undertaken with sensitivity and depth due to her attending to her child, as she does not wish to disclose or cry in front of her child. A health visitor is engaged to look after the child for future assessments, and it transpires her husband also agrees to offer child care, but he defaults frequently. She finally receives three assessments on her own, and she refuses to use an interpreter. She does not understand what therapy is about, but needs all sort of social help. She reports nightmares about loss and about being subjected to violence, remains very depressed and appears not to be able to link past with present in trial interpretations. She receives CBT and is not able to attend the sessions or make use of the therapy, indeed child-care breaks down and she separates from her partner.

___

As a clinical practitioner, what is your response to her treatment need? Is psychotherapy helpful? Will she benefit and should the therapist make other social interventions, for example, manage childcare; should her insistence to not have an interpreter be respected?

___

Case study two

Mr AA is a 28-year-old single man of Somali origin; he has refugee status, and lives in a local authority housing project, but his placements break down and he ends up homeless again, having to seek help from an emergency hostel. He comes to the attention of a local homeless team, who notice he has paranoid symptoms, some disinhibition, self neglect, and poverty, and he chews khat and takes alcohol on a daily basis. He is often seen outside his property on the street, and assessed by the team who think he may have schizophrenia, or a personality disorder, and elements of PTSD. His khat chewing makes him more disorganized in behaviour, but when he chews less khat he is much more able to have a conversation and does not appear so ill. He has not shown irritability, but lives in destitution and cannot establish a stable property that he can manage. Should he be sectioned to be treated for schizophrenia and assessed off khat and alcohol, or should he be offered a depot and admitted for that alone? The local authority want him admitted and treated but the homeless team does not think he meets criteria for admission or forced treatment under the mental health act, especially as when he stops chewing Khat he seems socially needy but not mentally ill.

How is this case different from the first one? Are the issues similar or different? Do you think both cases present specific challenges to services? What are these unique challenges?

Case study three

Our third case study involves a 35-year-old man (Mr SB), who is single, and appears to have schizophrenia. He was first diagnosed following an admission under the mental health act, and he then is placed on depot medication while being resettled in the community. He is unable to manage his own affairs and ends up being in temporary accommodation. He takes about a year to gradually enter a college course, and then to begin planning for a more permanent place of residence. He is also gradually switched to oral medications, which are monitored by staff at his hostel. He chews khat but this has not been a substantial problem, at least it is not excessive and is not obviously related to psychotic symptoms. He has few relatives, two sisters, in the same city. They have not met with him for many years. He makes contact with them as he begins to recover and consider more permanent settlement. However, they feel he is not ill, and that he is living in very impoverished environment, and that this environment is responsible for his loss of interest in his appearance and in working. He has not been able to get employment in the UK, but had begun work as a teacher in Somalia. He is not married, and his two sisters say this explains his 'depression'. They think that the problems he faces are to do with living in the UK and suggest he go home and seek a marital partner, as this they feel is the source of his difficulties. An elaborate plan is negotiated over many weeks; this includes providing sufficient oral medication for a month, and instructions to any receiving doctor or hospital about his diagnosis and about concerns about descending into homelessness. He is reluctant to use a depot again. He travels and does not return within the year. On return some 18 months later, the team is made aware through other Somali patients that he has returned. In the course of searching him out, they discover him sleeping under a bridge, homeless again and not having taken medication for a long time. He has some symptoms of paranoia, is suspicious of the team, and his previous care-coordinator, and there are complaints of remembering events that culminated in the loss of his brother in Somalia during the war. The two sisters are nowhere to be found, and appear to no longer be in contact with him. He is resettled, placed on depot, stabilized, and returns to college to undertake further courses in computing. A year later, his sisters make contact with the team as they are trying to find him. They visit him, again at the temporary place of residence, a supported hostel. They wish him to travel to Somalia again and say he is now married and his wife is awaiting his return.

The cases set out earlier challenge beyond the refugee experience. These are sometimes to do with being part of a transnational community. Travel between a familiar homeland and new place of residence may be frequent and challenges continuity of care. The absence of comprehensive services in the country of origin also makes it difficult to plan for continuous care, but also risks institutionalization in systems of care that may not lead to optimal recovery. Family relations are also not always explicit and stigma and fear about mental illness may lead to significant avoidance of mental health services and disengagement not due to the patient's preferences but family preferences. Alternative explanatory models of illness may give rise to quite distinct expectations of treatment and fears about treatment. These cases also show the challenges mental health services face in the care of asylum seekers and refugees, and when providing services to people from divergent cultural groups, but also special feature for people who are seeking asylum and refugee status. The issues include:

- ◆ Assessment precision
- ◆ Diagnostic challenges
- ◆ Co-morbidity
- ◆ The need for multiple interventions
- ◆ Social network, capital, and support lacking
- ◆ Risks often not manageable in the community as no support or observation system
- ◆ Uncertain residential instability and legal status: entitlements to treatments are challenged
- ◆ Psychologically protective (defensive) moves and requests that obscure mental state (for example, I don't wish to use an interpreter; or non-uptake of psychological interventions but take up of social and legal interventions)
- ◆ Questions about the effectiveness of models of treatment
- ◆ It becomes common, in the face of these problems to conclude that the asylum seekers and refugees are 'untreatable', or have 'unmet need', and their needs are not met by the clinical interventions or the resources available. In such circumstances, it is unclear for clinicians and managers what they should do, what their obligations are, and what additional resources can be commanded to deliver care.

Pathway interventions and one-stop shops

Although the case histories outline dilemmas presenting to specialist services, mental disorders can emerge at many points in the journey to refugee status.

Services may need to operate at multiple levels, at multiple locations, and with multiple health and social interventions from departure in the home country to arrival in the UK. Managed programmers of asylum (for example, US or Australia) appear to provide clarity about expectations, but may be selecting the most able and least ill. The provision of a clear time limited package of care to encourage rapid integration and employment may be important to obviate the damage done by uncertainty and forced unemployment.

Policy makers, politicians, and specialist services might tackle trauma exposure by tackling the cause of conflict through political process and liaison with services and training the workforce in the countries of origin; in-transit difficulties will be difficult to address as the escape journeys are often risky, precarious, and uncertain and perhaps through illegal means. The way asylum seekers are then processed on seeking asylum may undermine and challenge their chances of acculturation and adaptation to become citizens in their new homeland. Family separation, social network fragmentation, unemployment, education and training opportunities, and residential mobility all undermine the ability of asylum seekers and refugees to become embedded in an economy of health and social care and to optimize their health and social functioning. These factors operate as risk factors for mental distress, complicate mental disorder, are a consequence of social and asylum processes, and limit the ability to use help and services and interventions.

Moreover, there are still varying degrees of inequality when it comes to the access migrants and refugees have to the health system in the West—the human dignity of migrants seeking health care is still being violated, and migrants are discriminated against on account of their origins, their way of life, and their convictions (Domenig, 2004). People of refugee background often come from countries with vastly different health systems. Access to care for some refugees is therefore hindered by a lack of familiarity with available services (Portes et al., 1992). Many refugee patients might not be fully informed, if at all, about upcoming treatment, such as operations or other invasive medical interventions. Often they do not understand the diagnosis that they were given and therefore are unable to deduce any subsequent therapeutic or other consequences. It is known that pathways to care differ across ethnic groups but there are few studies of pathways to care for asylum seekers and refugees, with varying concerns about over representation in hospital settings; in a study of London's inpatient units we did not confirm this showing asylum seekers and refugees were under represented (Bhui et al., 2006). Some data suggest a higher risk of serious self-harm among young refugees, who are admitted to hospital (Hodes et al., 2008).

Encouraging psycho-social interventions

Poverty and lack of employment clearly can compound poor social status with limited power in society. Educational level and occupational background will obviously influence post-migration adjustment. However, if the migration is forced or unplanned, the chances are that individuals with higher qualifications may not find suitable jobs and resort to doing menial jobs (Stewart and Nicholas, 2002), which may lower their self-esteem and lead to isolation. In an interesting study, Zilber and Lerner (1996) found that, among immigrants to Israel who had arrived the year before, levels of emotional stress were correlated with individual factors including their professions and past history of distress. In general, unemployment has been considered a risk factor for mental ill health in refugees. A higher level of education was associated with a lower level of mental health (Bhui *et al.*, 2003; Papadopoulos *et al.*, 2004). With time this advantage may be lost as their frustration grows because they are unable to reach a corresponding position in the host society. It is worth mentioning here that some of these educated men and women had been leaders in their home countries and had high self-esteem and recognition. In exile, they may not be able to maintain that level of self-esteem and recognition. For these refugees, referring them to employment and voluntary services may improve their psychological recovery and better uptake of health services.

In terms of family separation and social support, unlike many economic migrants, who can dream about and plan their departure, refugees often flee their homelands in a hurry, leaving part or sometimes all of their loved ones behind. Once in the host country, refugees' separation problem is rarely rapidly resolved (Warfa *et al.*, 2006). Instead, people claiming leave to remain face legal hurdles that may take years to be sorted out. As a consequence, those coming alone and waiting for their families to join them may experience distress and suffer from lack of emotional support. They may feel guilty, powerless, and depressed about a separation over which they have little or no control (Warfa, 2006). For refugees, the question of what an extended separation means to the various members of the family and what their different expectations are is the one they ask themselves frequently. In a study of South East Asian refugees Beiser and Hyman (1997) found that separation from spouses had higher psychological impact than separation from parents and sibling. Marital status appeared to be an important factor such that married refugees whose spouses were with them in Canada had lower levels of depression than single, divorced, or widowed adults (Beiser *et al.*, 1993).

In conclusion, the issues demonstrate that many determinants of migrant mental health present a challenge to decision makers and service providers who need to plan and provide effective and accessible health services for communities with diverse languages, cultural backgrounds, migration circumstances, and socio-economic status. For mental health services, co-morbid problems are a challenge but then cultural barriers to delivery of treatments are also problematic. Interventions that are routinely provided may not be provided with sufficient time for assessment, or for adaptation of interventions for unique cultural contexts. Indeed guidelines and protocols, the hallmarks of good clinical practice, may be too restrictive and undermine the possibility of creative and more effective adaptation of interventions. One-stop shops are proposed, but fundamental service re-configurations and adaptations are needed, including of specific interventions, if the future effectiveness of care practices and services are to be optimized.

References

Astone, N.M. and McLanahan, S.S. (1994). Family structure, residential mobility and school drop-out: A research note. *Demography* **31**(4): 575–584.

Beiser, M., Johnson, P.J., and Turner, R.J. (1993). Unemployment, underemployment and depressive affect among Southeast Asian refugees. *Psychological Medicine* **23**(3): 731–743.

Beiser, M. and Hyman, I. (1997). Refugees' time perspective and mental health. *American Journal of Psychiatry* **154**(7): 996–1002.

Bhui, K., Abdi, A., Abdi, M., *et al.* (2003). Traumatic events, migration characteristics and psychiatric symptoms among Somali refugees. *Social Psychiatry and Psychiatric Epidemiology* **38**: 35–43.

Bhui, K., Craig, T., Mohamud, S., *et al.* (2006). Mental disorders among Somali refugees: developing culturally appropriate measures and assessing sociocultural risk factors. *Social Psychiatry and Psychiatric Epidemiology* **41**(5): 400–408.

Chodoff, P. (2002). The medicalization of the human condition. *Psychiatric Services* **53**(5): 627–628.

Chung, R.C. and Bemak, F. (1996). The effects of welfare status on psychological distress among Southeast Asian refugees. *Journal of Nervous & Mental Diseases* **184**: 346–353.

Craig, T., Jajua, P., and Warfa, N. (2006). Mental healthcare needs of refugees. *Psychiatry Journal. The Medicine Publishing Company Ltd.* **5**(11): 405–408.

Crockett, L.J., Peterson, A.C., Graber, J.A., Schulenberg, J.E., and Ebata, A. (1989). School transitions and adjustment during early adolescence. *Journal of Early Adolescence* **9**(3): 181–210.

Davidson, N., Skull, S., Burgner, D., *et al.* (2004). An issue of access: Delivering equitable health care for newly arrived refugee children in Australia. *Journal of Paediatrics and Child Health* **40**: 569–575.

Department of Health. (2004). Proposals to Exclude Overseas Visitors from Eligibility to Free NHS Primary Medical Services: A Consultation. London: DoH. www.dh.gov.uk/assetRoot/04/08/22/67/04082267.pdf, accessed 26 November 2004.

Domenig, D. (2004). Transcultural change: a challenge for the public health system. *Applied Nursing Research* **17**(3): 213–216.

Eckenrode, J., Rowe, E., Laird, M., and Brathwaite, J. (1995). Mobility as a mediator of the effects of child maltreatment on academic performance. *Child Development* **66**: 1130–1142.

Hallas, P., Hansen, A.R., Stæhr, M.A., Munk-Andersen, E., and Jorgensen, H.L. (2007). Length of stay in asylum centres and mental health in asylum seekers: a retrospective study from Denmark. *BMC Public Health*. http://www.biomedcentral.com

Kinzie, J., Sack, W., Angell, R., Clark, G., and Ben, R. (1989). A three year follow-up of Cambodian young people traumatised as children. *Journal of the American Academy of Child and Adolescent Psychiatry* **28**: 501–504.

Laban, C.J., Gernaat, H.B., Komproe, I.H., van der Tweel, I., and De Jong, J.T. (2005). Postmigration Living Problems and Common Psychiatric Disorders in Iraqi Asylum Seekers in the Netherlands. *Journal of Nervous and Mental Disease* **193**(12): 825–832.

Lamont, A., Ukoumunne, O.C., Tyrer, P., Thornicroft, G., Patel, R. and Slaughter, J. (2000). The geographical mobility of severely mentally ill residents in London. *Social Psychiatry and Psychiatric Epidemiology* **35**(4): 164–169.

Lavik, N.J., Hauff, E., Skrondal, A., and Solberg, O. (1996). Mental disorder among refugees and the impact of persecution and exile: some findings from an out-patient population. *British Journal of Psychiatry* **169**(6): 726–732.

Papadopoulos, I., Lees, S., Lay, M., and Gebrehiwot, A. (2004). Ethiopian refugees in the UK: Migration, adaptation and settlement experiences and their relevance to health. *Ethnicity and Health* **9**(1): 55–73.

Portes, A., Kyle, D., and Eaton, W.W. (1992). Mental illness and help-seeking behaviors among Mariel Cuban and Haitian refugees in south Florida. *Journal of Health and Social Behavior* **23**(4): 282–298.

Powell, R.A., Leye, E., Jayakody, A., Mwangi-P., F.N., and Morison, L. (2004). Female genital mutilation, asylum seekers and refugees: the need for an integrated European Union agenda. *Health Policy* **70**: 151–162.

Sabin, M., Cardozo, B.L., Nackerud, L., Kaiser, R., and Varese, L. (2003). Factors associated with poor mental health among Guatemalan refugees living in Mexico 20 years after civil conflict. *Journal of American Medical Association* **290**: 635–642.

Silove, D., Steel, Z., and Watters, C. (2000). Policies of Deterrence and the Mental Health of Asylum Seekers. *Journal of American Medical Association* **284**: 604–611.

Stewart, E. and Nicholas, S. (2002). Refugee doctors in the United Kingdom. *British Medical Journal* **325**(7373): S166.

Van Ommeren, M., de Jong, J.T., Sharma, B., Komproe, I., Thapa, S., and Cardena, E. (2001). Psychiatric disorders among tortured Bhutanese refugees in Nepal. *Archives of General Psychiatry* **58**(5): 475–482.

Vostanis, P., Grattan, E., and Cumella, S. (1998). Mental health problems of homeless children and families: longitudinal study. *British Medical Journal* **316**(7135): 899–902.

Warfa, N. and Bhui, K. (2003). Refugees and Mental Healthcare. Psychiatry, Special topics, **2**(6): 26.

Warfa, N., Bhui, K., Craig, T., *et al.* (2006). Post-migration geographical mobility, mental health and health service utilisation among Somali refugees in the UK: a qualitative study. *Health Place* **12**(4): 503–515.

Watters, C. (2001). Emerging paradigms in the mental health care of refugees. *Social Science and Medicine* **52**: 1709–1718.

Zilber, N. and Lerner, Y. (1996). Psychological distress among recent immigrants from the former Soviet Union to Israel, I. Correlates of level of distress. *Psychological medicine* **26**: 493–501.

Chapter 21

Conclusions: what next?

Dinesh Bhugra, Tom Craig, and
Kamaldeep Bhui

No two refugees' or asylum seekers' experiences are likely to be similar; they
are not homogenous as a group either. The challenges for policymakers and
clinicians are similar but differ, as in clinical settings ethical issues may be
more significant than policy imperatives. Policies may control the process and
the number of immigrants but the misery and clinical experience of refugees
and asylum seekers in the consulting room raise a different set of issues.

The purpose of this book has been to highlight clinical issues related to refugees and asylum seekers. These issues are almost universal but additional information and factors may play a role in ensuring that individuals get the best and
most appropriate treatment they need. In any assessment, both proximal and
distal factors need to be explored. Proximal factors include familial, housing,
and employment issues, which will vary according to the ethnicity, migration
status, and trauma related to the experience of becoming a refugee or an asylum
seeker. Distal factors including broader issues related to culture, social factors,
and cultural adjustment may be explored. Good clinical practice demands that
all these factors are explored in every patient seen in a clinical setting. For refugees and asylum seekers, additional proximal and distal factors such as loss of
family, friends, possible social support, and cultural bereavement and culture
shock will need to be explored in detail to get a fuller picture. Furthermore,
issues related to other migrants, acculturation, changes in family structures
with varying levels of acculturation in the family and the group as a whole need
to be taken into account while making a management plan. Ethnic differences
in pharmacodynamics and pharmacokinetics and in metabolism, with religious rites and rituals associated with problems related to acceptance of Western
medicine need to be borne in mind while looking at therapeutic adherence.

Clinicians, as members of society, do have a role in working with policy
makers and other stakeholders to ensure that refugees and asylum seekers get
the best treatment available. The tension between politicians and clinicians,
especially related to refugees and asylum seekers, may never be over, but a
creative tension can most certainly lead to positive solutions. As policymakers

and clinicians both may not get rid of political conflicts although one can aspire to an ideal world where refugees and asylum seekers, when seeking help, shelter, and our support, receive them unconditionally. It is imperative that the physical and the emotional needs are dealt with so that they become more productive members of society and contribute to the new society.

Many refugees and asylum seekers will be traumatized, either by the events they faced in the pre-migration phase or after the migration process, which can be unsettling. It is important that clinicians do not medicalize the normal human emotions and reactions, and that they deal with these in an appropriate social and cultural context. A sense of relief of having arrived at a 'safe' place may be short-lived and may become tinged with anxiety and worry, especially if the legal status after migration is not clear and takes a long time to be resolved.

There is no doubt that children or unaccompanied adolescents will have their problems, especially when they are at an extremely vulnerable developmental and emotional stage. Women and older individuals will have a different set of problems which would need to be resolved. As with their other patients, clinicians are not in a position to offer everything to everyone, but they should have a repository of knowledge and information, which can be used to ensure that early and appropriate help is available.

Clinicians cannot be experts in every culture, but practical input from the local community can allow them to access information. Innovative strategies, such as using a culture broker who can educate both the team and the community, may enable developments of cost-effective services.

In this volume the focus has been on the mental health of refugees' and asylum seekers' mental health and also on specific topics related to certain issues and therapeutic interventions. We also looked at global policy in this context, at pre-migration and post-migration and also following the process itself, which is a significant life event, though further detailed follow-ups are necessary to understand both pathology and coping strategies.

Changes in family structure and social support do create problems in settling down. It is likely that migrant refugee groups may wish to stay together but that in itself may create ghettos and increase racial views and stigmas. On the other hand, placing vulnerable individuals in isolated communities far away from others who have similar experiences may make them feel further alienated. When vulnerable unaccompanied adolescents are challenged on their age and may be repatriated, it raises further challenges for clinicians. Different countries have varying levels and types of assistance available to refugees and asylum seekers. Such assistance is not only financial and material, but also emotional; and various cultures will provide emotional assistance in different ways, which may be seen as rejecting, alienating, patronizing, or supportive. In the adjustment and acculturation process, some of these factors may need to be explored. Thus the interaction between the individual and their own culture and both the group and individual interaction with the new culture becomes a complex one. These interactions are further complicated by legal aspects and resources needed and made available.

Pre-migration factors are often identifiable but there may not be any time or opportunity necessarily to prepare for the process, and it is the post-migration period, which becomes of interest both to clinicians and to researchers. Traumatic events related to migration may further complicate matters; additionally, physical infections or organic factors may also play a role in the adjustment to the new culture and also in the pathology and help seeking. Interventions—whether psychological, psychotherapeutic, or pharmacological—must be tailored to the needs of the patients presenting and they must be culturally appropriate and accessible. There need to be clinical diagnoses, but often it will be difficult to pigeonhole people and it is essential that patient needs take precedence in totality in making any therapeutic plans. Refugees and asylum seekers may not have been directly affected by the trauma but may have experienced it indirectly, which does not make it any less stressful.

Not only does there need to be a global rethink of policy on refugees and asylum seekers, but research networks across countries and cultures should start to bring together human experience and understanding of trauma and resilience along with coping strategies. Rather than simply focusing on rates of disorders and categories, an understanding of overlap of categories and idioms of distress will enable clinicians to provide emotionally accessible services. In an ideal world, there would be no refugees or asylum seekers, but that is highly unlikely. What the profession can offer is its duty of compassion, understanding, and keeping patient's interests paramount above all.

Index